Cancer Control

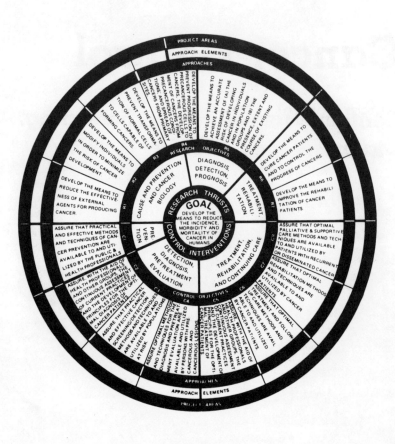

Cancer Control

Contemporary Views on Screening, Diagnosis, and Therapy

including a colloquy
on the Delaney Clause

Edited by
Irving I. Kessler, M.D., Dr.P.H.
Professor and Chairman
Department of Epidemiology
 and Preventive Medicine
University of Maryland School of Medicine
Baltimore

University Park Press
Baltimore

UNIVERSITY PARK PRESS
International Publishers in Science, Medicine, and Education
233 East Redwood Street
Baltimore, Maryland 21202

Copyright © 1980 by University Park Press.

Typeset by American Graphic Arts Corporation.

Manufactured in the United States of America by
The Maple Press Company.

Library of Congress Cataloging in Publication Data
Main entry under title:

Cancer control.

    Bibliography: p.
    Includes index.
    1. Cancer—Prevention. 2. Medical screening. 3. Cancer—Preven-
tion—Social aspects—United States. I. Kessler, Irving I.   II. Title: Delaney
Clause.
RC268.C34   616.9'94   79-23830
ISBN 0-8391-1539-3

Contents

Contributors vii
Foreword ix
Preface xi

Part I Critiques of Cancer Control
  1 The Scope of Cancer Control
     Irving I. Kessler 3
  2 Prospects for Cancer Control through Diagnosis and
     Screening
     Nathaniel I. Berlin 57
  3 Possibilities and Limitations in Screening for Cancer
     William Pomerance 67

Part II Theoretical Considerations
  4 Decision Making in Cancer Screening by Risk Factor
     Analysis
     Anita K. Bahn, Prakash L. Grover, and
     Daniel G. Miller 79
  5 Signal Detection Theory in the Early Diagnosis of
     Cancer
     Lee B. Lusted 105

Part III Diagnostic and Therapeutic Problems
  6 Immunodiagnosis of Cancer in Man
     Ronald B. Herberman 121
  7 The Epidemiologic Significance of Cytologic and
     Histologic Data
     Leopold G. Koss 143
  8 The Implications of Chemotherapy for Cancer
     Control
     C. Gordon Zubrod 155

Part IV Advances in the Detection of Breast and Other Cancers
  9 Breast Fluid Analysis in Breast Cancer Detection
     Nicholas L. Petrakis 165
 10 Considerations in Breast Cancer Screening
     Sam Shapiro 183

11 Cancers of the Lung, Pancreas, and Brain: Problems
    and Progress in Early Detection
    Charles Ralph Buncher 193

Part V   The Delaney Clause: A Colloquy
12 Evolution of the Delaney Clause
    Gilbert S. Goldhammer.......................................209
13 A Healthy Law for Consumers
    Anita Johnson 215
14 The Delaney Clause and Food Safety
    Robert W. Harkins 223
15 Whither the Delaney Clause?
    Irving I. Kessler...243

Index 271

Contributors

Anita K. Bahn, M.D., Sc.D.
Professor of Research Medicine
(Epidemiology)
University of Pennsylvania School of
Medicine
Philadelphia, Pennsylvania 19104

Nathaniel I. Berlin, M.D.
Director, Cancer Center
Northwestern University
Chicago, Illinois 60611

Charles Ralph Buncher, Sc.D.
Director, Division of Epidemiology
and Biostatistics
University of Cincinnati Medical
Center
Cincinnati, Ohio 45267

Gilbert S. Goldhammer, Consultant
Intergovernmental Relations and
Human Resources Subcommittee
House of Representatives
Washington, D.C. 20515

Prakash L. Grover, Ph.D., M.P.H.
Epidemiologist
Fox Chase Cancer Center
Philadelphia, Pennsylvania 19111

Robert W. Harkins, Ph.D.
Director, Research and Development
Johnson & Johnson Development
Corporation
New Brunswick, New Jersey 08903

Ronald B. Herberman, M.D.
Chief, Laboratory of Immunodiagnosis
National Cancer Institute
Bethesda, Maryland 20205

Anita Johnson, Staff Attorney
Environmental Defense Fund
Washington, D.C. 20036

Irving I. Kessler, M.D., Dr.P.H.
Professor and Chairman
Department of Epidemiology and
Preventive Medicine
University of Maryland School of
Medicine
Baltimore, Maryland 21201

Leopold G. Koss, M.D.
Professor and Chairman
Department of Pathology
Albert Einstein College of Medicine at
Montefiore Hospital and Medical
Center
Bronx, New York 10467

Lee B. Lusted, M.D.
Clinical Professor
Departments of Radiology and
Academic Affairs
Scripps Clinic and Research
Foundation
La Jolla, California 92037

Daniel G. Miller, M.D.
President and Medical Director
Preventive Medicine Institute–Strang
Clinic
New York, New York 10016

Nicholas L. Petrakis, M.D.
Professor and Chairman
Department of Epidemiology and
    International Health
University of California
San Francisco, California 94143

William Pomerance, M.D.*
Chief, Diagnosis Branch
Division of Cancer Biology and
    Diagnosis
National Cancer Institute
Bethesda, Maryland 20205

—————————
*Deceased.

Sam Shapiro, Director
Health Services Research and
    Development Center and,
Professor, Health Services Adminis-
    tration
School of Hygiene and Public Health
The Johns Hopkins University
Baltimore, Maryland 21205

C. Gordon Zubrod, M.D.
Director, Comprehensive Cancer
    Center for the State of Florida
University of Miami School of
    Medicine
Miami, Florida 33152

Foreword

It has become increasingly evident in recent years that prevention and early detection offer the most promising long range solutions to the control of mortality and morbidity from cancer. Furthermore, because cancer is second only to cardiovascular disease as a cause of death in the elderly, any success in the prolongation of life through aging research will probably require more effective methods to prevent, reverse, and treat cancer.

Environmental factors of various kinds are important in the etiology of many human cancers. Carcinogens in the work place are implicated, as well as exposures to a wide variety of physical and chemical agents in the general environment. It is important to note that these substances do not necessarily act alone but that interactions between them and other factors as well are probably essential. Thus, the pathogenesis of cancer is affected by many influences including nutrition, hormone levels, immunologic status, and the interaction of chemicals with infectious agents. An important current example is the enhancement of the risk of pleural mesotheliomas by the interaction of asbestos exposure with cigarette smoking.

In order to reach their activated state, virtually all chemical agents in the environment must be metabolized by the host. In the tissues, activation reactions compete with inactivation reactions, the attributable carcinogenic risk probably representing a balance between the two.

Although much more needs to be learned about the metabolism of known chemical carcinogens in human tissues, there is at least a 100-fold variation between individuals in their metabolism of many important chemicals. This may explain the large differences in cancer risks among various population groups and individual people. It may soon become possible to develop tests that are predictive of cancer risk in individuals and to undertake preventive measures as appropriate.

Chemoprevention, a relatively new concept in cancer control, has been attracting considerable interest lately. This concept implies dietary, pharmacologic, or other interventions that may decrease the risk of a given level of carcinogen exposure or even reverse preneoplastic lesions. Interventions are already possible in experimental animals that modify both initiation and progression of certain neoplasms. The probability of reversing the cancer phenotype is suggested by the results of recent animal experiments. They represent exciting research areas for the future.

Since the work of Berenblum it has become apparent that the development of cancer in many sites is a multistage process involving the conversion of initiated cells into one or more neoplastic populations, with invasive cancer being the end result.

Among the events occurring after initiation are promotion and progression. Much is known about promotion, especially in the skin, where environmental or dietary tumor-inducing agents in animals, and possibly humans, act as promoters or initiators. More needs to be learned about progression, namely, the process whereby in situ lesions ultimately invade and metastasize. This appears to be important in organs where preneoplastic lesions and carcinomas in situ tend to be numerous and bilateral, for example, in the breast or lungs.

In this volume, Dr. Kessler and his contributors review many of the promising arenas of cancer control and their implications for the future, especially in the prediction of human cancer risk. At present, such predictions are usually based on animal tests that are expensive, relatively insensitive, and pose difficulties in extrapolation of results to man. Ultimately, the achievement of cancer control will require a fuller understanding of the molecular mechanisms so that more sensitive, accurate, and rapid tests for cancer, directly applicable to man, can be developed.

Benjamin F. Trump, M.D.
Professor and Chairman
Department of Pathology
Director, Maryland Cancer Program
University of Maryland

Preface

This is a time of unprecedented public interest and governmental investment in cancer. Deaths from this disease are approaching 400,000 per annum, and the economic costs exceed tens of billions of dollars. Related research expenditures from public and private sources each year far surpass one billion dollars. The figures would have to be multiplied to reflect the impact of cancer around the world.

It may, therefore, be appropriate to step back from the hospital bed, the laboratory bench, and the political arena and attempt to assess the extent to which the scourge of neoplastic diseases is being or promises to be controlled. *Control* is broadly defined here and includes any preventive, diagnostic, or therapeutic modality that may reduce the mortality or morbidity attributable to cancer.

The volume begins with a discourse on the magnitude of the cancer problem and a general assessment of the many approaches to cancer control, their current status and future prospects. Two chapters address the potential and the limitations of controlling cancer through diagnostic means.

In an era of inflationary pressures and competitive demands on the tax dollar for consumer services, the allocation of fiscal and human resources to cancer control efforts—if these are to succeed—must be based upon planning that is both fiscally and scientifically sound. In this context, two theoretically based approaches to decision making in cancer screening are presented: one in relation to a multiphasic screening program, the other in terms of signal detection theory as applied to cancer control.

Two important diagnostic modalities, one new and the other quite old, are discussed. Cancer immunodiagnosis, still in its infancy, promises a noninvasive, sensitive, and specific tool that is still largely unrealized. By way of contrast, cytologic screening has already accomplished a great deal, although it is *per se* clearly inadequate to the task and, ironically, is being challenged of late, perhaps because controlled evaluative trials on such techniques as the Pap test have never been undertaken.

As exemplified by the impressive advances in the treatment of leukemia and breast cancer, the role of drugs—often in combination—has become increasingly important. The implications of chemotherapy for cancer control in the future are weighed by the eminent director of a comprehensive cancer center.

Several years ago mammography was recommended as an effective tool in the early detection of breast cancer and then largely withdrawn on the basis of presumed radiologic hazards. The risks and benefits of breast cancer screening are considered, and a promising new approach, involving analysis of routinely collected breast fluids, is described. Problems relating to three prevalent and notably unpreventable cancers, those of the lung, brain, and pancreas, are reviewed, with special emphasis on newly developed and noninvasive diagnostic techniques.

The volume concludes with a colloquy on the Delaney Clause, encompassing contributions by representatives of Congress, consumer groups, the food industry, and academia. While all agree that the public should not knowingly be exposed to human carcinogens, widely differing views are offered on the means for achieving this end. The inadequate state of our knowledge about cancer and its antecedents is, of course, largely responsible for the regulatory dilemma.

The contributors to this volume participated in a series of invited seminars at The Johns Hopkins University, organized during my tenure there as Professor of Epidemiology. The text chapters represent the distillation of their thinking on the several topics. In this process, all of us benefited from vigorous discussions that followed each presentation.

I am extremely grateful to the authors for their contributions and forbearance during the production of this volume. Thanks are also due to Mrs. Hildred Griffeth for the typing of the manuscript.

Irving I. Kessler, M.D.

Cancer Control

Part I
Critiques of Cancer Control

1
The Scope of Cancer Control

Irving I. Kessler

Organized efforts to control cancer in the United States may be said to have begun with the establishment of the American Society for the Control of Cancer in 1913. The slogan adopted, "Early Cancer Can Be Cured," was not intended to reflect the state of the art but rather to encourage the application of existing knowledge and techniques to the prevention, early detection, and treatment of cancer.

These efforts began to bear fruit during the ensuing two decades when the legislatures of several large states—notably Massachusetts and New York—appropriated funds for the development of statewide cancer control programs. These encompassed specialized tumor clinics, tumor registries, and diagnostic pathology services aimed at improving the quality of cancer care and the dissemination of knowledge to the general public.

The federal statute that established the National Cancer Institute in 1937 specifically mandated activities related to cancer control. These were strongly supported by the American Cancer Society, which was incorporated as the successor to the American Society for the Control of Cancer in 1944. Shortly thereafter the tempo of cancer control activities increased substantially, thanks not only to the federal government but to the increasing involvement of state and voluntary agencies as well.

By the early 1950s, the "Seven Danger Signals of Cancer" were being widely advertised and annual or periodic physical examinations were recommended as a mainstay of the control effort by many health professionals. The slogan "Every Doctor's Office A Cancer Detection Center" reflected an overly simplistic view of cancer control that was rather quickly and quietly dismissed. In its stead came a number of full-time cancer detection centers, including the famous Strang Clinic in New York.

At about this time, the value of Papanicolaou's method for exfoliative cytologic screening for cervical cancer was demonstrated and came to be

3

regarded as an essential component of most cancer control programs. The Federal Cancer Control Program was based in the Bureau of State Services of the U.S. Public Health Service between 1957 and 1970. Related activities were carried on by the Regional Medical Program, which was terminated in 1976. Most importantly, a Division of Cancer Control and Rehabilitation was designated as one of the five major divisions of the National Cancer Institute in 1974, after having been established under the Office of the Director 2 years earlier. Still more recently, philosophical and jurisdictional problems have led to yet another proposal for the reorganization of the Federal Cancer Control Program, the structure of which is not yet apparent.

The magnitude of the cancer problem, with particular emphasis upon the situation in the United States, is considered in the following section. This is followed by a discussion of cancer control techniques based largely upon the strategies recommended by the National Cancer Program Plan. Special attention is paid to those neoplasms that appear to be most amenable to control at this time or that have appeared so. Some controversies related to cancer control are broached, and, finally, some conclusions are drawn.

MAGNITUDE OF THE CANCER PROBLEM

A baby born in the United States today has in excess of one chance in four of developing cancer during his or her lifetime (Figure 1); of the total, approximately one-half will die of the disease. Risks decline in older age because of the increasing competitive mortality from coronary, cerebrovascular, and other diseases during this epoch of life. In general, whites incur greater lifetime cancer risks than nonwhites except for men above age 64, among whom there is an excess probability of lung cancer and prostate malignancies in nonwhites. At any given point in time, some three million persons are alive with cancer in the United States (Table 1).

The magnitude of the cancer problem is also apparent from its ranking as a cause of mortality (Figure 2). Among males and females of all ages, cancer accounts for more deaths than any other cause except heart disease (Table 2). It is the leading cause of death among women of ages 25–64 years and the second most prevalent killer of all other females except those at the two extremes of age. Cancer is the second leading cause of death among males 5–14 and 45 years of age and over. It is no less than fourth in rank among the leading causes of death for all other categories of persons classified by age group, sex, and race.

The risk of cancer varies considerably by sex and topographic site. Among males, lung cancer predominates and is followed by cancers of the colon/rectum, prostate, urinary bladder, and stomach. Among women, breast cancer is the most frequent neoplasm, followed by those of the

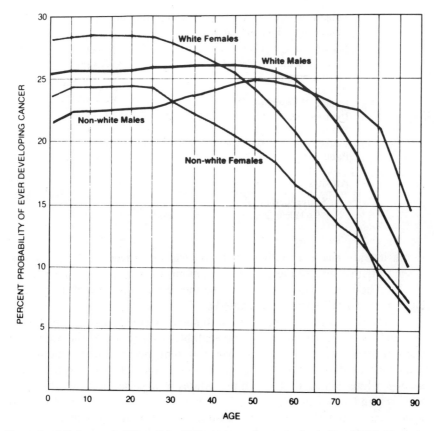

Figure 1.   Lifetime probability of developing cancer of any site (excluding skin) by age, sex, and race in the United States, 1969. Source: Levin et al., 1974.

colon/rectum, uterus, lung, and ovary. These rankings are quite similar, whether incidence or mortality rates are considered.

One indication of the degree to which cancers are or are not being controlled is the trend in their incidence over time. Lung cancer has shown a most dramatic increase among all race/sex groups (Table 3). Conversely, the most pronounced secular decline in incidence has been recorded for stomach cancer. Malignancies of the pancreas and female breast have also increased substantially in both whites and blacks. Esophageal cancer has remained constant or perhaps declined slightly among whites while increasing threefold among blacks of each sex. Colon cancer incidence is apparently increasing much more rapidly among blacks of each sex than whites, while rectum cancer has begun to decline in all groups except black males, among

Table 1.   Persons alive in 1971 with history of
cancer, in the United States

Breast	677,000
Colon/Rectum	495,000
Total uterus	387,000
Prostate	201,000
Lung and bronchus	85,000
Lymphomas	45,000
Stomach	39,000
Leukemias	37,000
Pancreas	5,000
Esophagus	4,000
All sites[a]	2,922,000

Source: Levin et al., 1974.

[a] Excluding skin and carcinoma in situ.

whom its rate has essentially stabilized. Ovarian cancer incidence has also leveled off in white women, while continuing to increase at a slow rate in blacks. The time trends observed in the incidence data parallel those calculated from mortality statistics (Table 4).

That cancers are caused, at least to some extent, by environmental factors and therefore are potentially preventable is suggested by the wide variations in the risk of cancer among different occupational groups. For example, standardized mortality ratios (i.e., risks of death from cancer) among white males in the United States range between 59 (for farm laborers and foremen) and 123 (for other laborers) (Table 5). Ratios for buccal cavity and pharynx cancers also involve a twofold gradation between farmers and other laborers. The range for esophageal cancer risk among white males is in excess of fivefold, while equivalent variations in cancer mortality risks are apparent among white females and among nonwhites of both sexes.

More direct evidence on the role of occupational factors in human cancer has been derived from studies on a variety of specific agents (Table 6). Many substances, ranging from arsenic to coal tar derivatives and x-rays, are associated with increased risks of skin and lung cancer. Aniline dyes have long been implicated as bladder carcinogens, while the leukemogenic potential of benzol and related agents is under active investigation. Such occupational carcinogens should obviously be taken into consideration whenever cancer control programs are being planned or evaluated.

International variations in cancer mortality are also of consequence in cancer control. There are many reasons for these variations, which often persist even after the appropriate adjustments for differences in age distributions have been made. These include variations among countries in degrees of access to medical diagnosis and treatment, differences in death certification practices of local physicians, policies regarding autopsies and autopsy rates, as well as geographic differences in the prevalence of environment carcinogens. Because none of these factors remain constant over time, differences in cancer mortality rates between—as well as within—countries are to be expected.

Secular trends in the age-adjusted cancer mortality rates of a number of developed countries are presented in Table 7. In general, the rates in males of the various countries increased by up to 20% or so during the decade between 1956–1957 and 1966–1967. The only exceptions are Switzerland, Finland, and Norway where the rates either fell or remained constant. In rather marked contrast to these trends are those recorded among the female populations in the same countries. Overall, the mortality rates declined by a few percentage points, most notably in Switzerland and Finland where declines in cancer risks were also observed among males. A notable exception is Portugal, where an 11% increase in rates was experienced by females to parallel the 22% increase among males. Changes of such magnitude and rapidity are usually attributable to secular improvements in certification of causes of

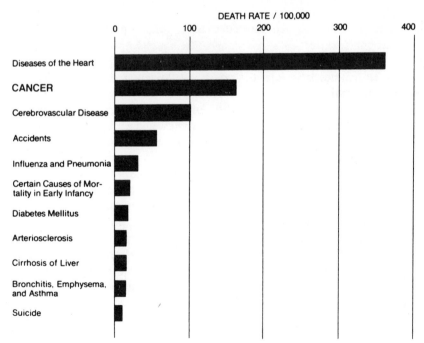

Figure 2.   Death rates for the 11 leading causes of death in the United States. Source: Levin et al., 1974.

Table 2.   Mortality figures for five leading causes of death, by age group and sex in the

All ages		1–4 years		5–14 years		15–24 years	
Male	Female	Male	Female	Male	Female	Male	Female
Heart diseases 417,918	Heart diseases 317,624	Accidents 2,564	Accidents 1,736	Accidents 5,695	Accidents 2,508	Accidents 19,396	Accidents 4,940
Cancer 180,157	Cancer 150,573	Congenital malformations 694	Congenital malformations 637	Cancer 1,389	Cancer 1,040	Homicide 3,333	Cancer 1,114
Cerebrovascular disease 93,456	Cerebrovacular disease 113,710	Pneumonia influenza 601	Cancer 449	Congenital malformations 481	Congenital malformations 420	Suicide 2,378	Homicide 824
Accidents 79,756	Accidents 34,882	Cancer 578	Pneumonia Influenza 442	Pneumonia Influenza 327	Pneumonia Influenza 324	Cancer 1,817	Suicide 750
Pneumonia Influenza 35,148	Pneumonia Influenza 27,591	Meningitis 141	Homicide 128	Homicide 215	Heart diseases 162	Heart diseases 642	Heart diseases 412

death and other artifacts, rather than to substantial improvements in therapy or cancer control efforts.

A substantial preponderance of cancer mortality among males as compared with females is apparent in nearly all the countries listed in Table 7. In fact, the male/female ratio in cancer mortality is not only high but appears to be increasing as well. In several of the countries, males are seen to incur risks of cancer mortality between 50% and 80% higher than those of their female compatriots. While, to some extent, such trends may be attributed to the decline of uterine cancer as a cause of death among women, the phenomenon remains largely unexplained.

An important measure of the effectiveness of a cancer control program can be the variation over time in the proportion of patients whose tumors are detected while still localized or limited to the primary site. In a stable population, this proportion should obviously rise if more and more of the population at risk is benefiting from early cancer detection. The percent of patients in the United States who underwent surgical resection within 4 months of cancer diagnosis has increased substantially over the past 3 decades (Table 8). The significance of this is twofold. First, the trend may reflect increasingly successful efforts at early diagnosis and treatment. Second, because surgical resection makes possible a greater accuracy in the classification of the clinical stages of cancer, observed secular trends in the

United States in 1970 (all races combined)

25–44 years		45–64 years		65+ years	
Male	Female	Male	Female	Male	Female
Accidents 18,865	Cancer 9,902	Heart diseases 128,955	Cancer 55,444	Heart diseases 274,181	Heart diseases 264,236
Heart diseases 13,445	Accidents 5,114	Cancer 65,556	Heart diseases 47,663	Cancer 102,769	Cerebro-vascular disease 96,738
Cancer 7,939	Heart diseases 4,793	Accidents 17,528	Cerebro-vascular disease 14,028	Cerebro-vascular disease 73,313	Cancer 82,511
Suicide 5,866	Suicide 2,506	Cerebro-vascular disease 17,165	Accidents 6,636	Pneumonia Influenza 21,434	Pneumonia Influenza 18,778
Homicide 4,907	Cerebro-vascular disease 2,446	Cirrhosis 11,908	Cirrhosis 6,158	Asthma[a] 16,756	Arterio-sclerosis 17,336

Source: Levin et al., 1974.

[a] Including bronchitis, emphysema, and asthma.

percentage of patients with localized tumors may reflect changes in thera-peutic modalities rather than in early detection per se.

In fact, increases in the proportions of localized neoplasms have been observed for only a few cancer sites including breast, prostate, bladder, corpus uteri, and melanoma of the skin. With respect to the most prevalent cancers, namely, colon, lung, and female breast, only slight increases in pro-portions of patients with localized disease have been recorded in recent decades. There was a paradoxical *decrease* in the proportion of localized cases of pancreas cancer diagnosed between the 1940s and the late 1960s. This may be attributable to the more frequent and accurate detection in recent years of metastatic neoplasms of this organ.

Another statistic potentially useful for evaluating the effectiveness of cancer control programs is the time trend in survival rates among patients with a given malignancy. If such rates are increasing, this would imply either earlier detection or more effective treatment. In fact, survival rates have improved for a number of cancers including the leukemias, Hodgkin's disease, multiple myeloma, melonoma, and cancers of the prostate, urinary bladder, larynx, and thyroid cancer (Table 9). Most of the improvements were registered during the 1940s and the 1950s, largely because of advances in treatment and in the effectiveness of oncologic surgery. Since that time, survival rates have leveled off or are improving much more slowly. Pancreas

Table 3.   Time trends in cancer incidence rates by site and race and sex: three surveys conducted by NCI in 1937, 1947, and 1969

Site	Race and sex	1937	1947	1969
Esophagus	White male	7.8	8.3	6.0
	White female	1.6	1.9	1.6
	Black male	6.0	9.7	19.5
	Black female	1.4	2.2	4.2
Stomach	White male	44.0	34.1	14.0
	White female	26.1	18.3	6.1
	Black male	38.3	39.6	20.5
	Black female	22.2	22.8	10.0
Colon	White male	22.4	26.2	33.1
	White female	24.0	27.8	27.6
	Black male	13.2	13.9	26.4
	Black female	11.8	16.2	37.1
Rectum	White male	19.0	22.1	17.3
	White female	12.2	15.2	10.7
	Black male	8.0	12.7	13.1
	Black female	8.4	13.6	9.9
Pancreas	White male	7.0	9.3	11.3
	White female	4.9	5.5	6.7
	Black male	5.0	11.6	15.0
	Black female	3.4	6.4	14.5
Lung	White male	13.7	29.5	68.9
	White female	4.0	6.5	13.5
	Black male	8.4	25.4	84.7
	Black female	3.4	5.8	18.2
Breast	White female	66.2	72.6	75.2
	Black female	49.4	53.9	67.8
Uterus (total)	White female	59.9	56.3	35.3
	Black female	108.8	95.6	49.0
Ovary	White female	12.7	14.7	13.3
	Black female	5.5	9.9	11.4
Prostate	White male	29.8	34.8	42.7
	Black male	30.7	49.9	77.6
Bladder	White male	15.3	18.6	22.5
	White female	7.4	8.0	5.9
	Black male	5.6	7.0	15.3
	Black female	5.5	7.9	4.5

Source: Levin et al., 1974.

cancer continues to earn its reputation as a universally fatal and short-term malignancy. Overall, the trends in relative survival rates offer little evidence that cancer control programs in the United States are becoming more effective.

THE NATIONAL CANCER PROGRAM PLAN

In his State of the Union Speech and Health Message of 1971, former President Nixon called for a coordinated national effort against cancer, with special emphasis on research and control. The Congress provided substantial funds for the development of a National Cancer Program Plan, which was to be accomplished through joint efforts of the National Cancer Institute, the National Advisory Cancer Council, and some 250 laboratory-based and clinical scientists from the academic community. The Plan, which evolved from a series of 42 meetings in late 1971 and early 1972, is comprised of two major elements: an Overall Strategic Plan and a more detailed Operational Plan. Each of these, in turn, is made up of research components designed to acquire new information about the cancer process and control components aimed at reducing mortality and morbidity from cancer by applying existing knowledge more effectively (Table 10).

The research and control components of the National Cancer Program Plan are directed at three so-called "target areas" oriented about the natural history of malignant neoplasms. Thus, one target area relates to pathogenesis or cause, from the research perspective, and to prevention, from the cancer control aspect. Once a neoplasm has been initiated, primary prevention is no longer possible, but prognosis may be markedly improved through early detection and treatment. At the other extreme, when dealing with an invasive and perhaps metastatic lesion, research and control objectives must necessarily encompass improvements in methods for late treatment and rehabilitation.

A number of general objectives were proposed in the National Cancer Program Plan for each of the three target areas. With respect to cancer cause or prevention, four objectives were suggested: 1) reducing the effectiveness of environmental carcinogens, 2) increasing the resistance of human subjects to the carcinogenic process, 3) preventing the malignant transformation of normal cells, and 4) preventing the progression of premalignant conditions and metastases. The latter objective pertains, in fact, to two target areas, that is, those aimed both at prevention and detection.

Also directed at cancer detection and prognosis are the objectives of identifying individuals in a population who are at substantial risk of developing particular cancers, and, with respect to those whose cancers have already been initiated, of detecting the lesions as early as possible, and cor-

Table 4. Time trends in age-adjusted cancer death rates

Whites		Nonwhites	
Males	Females	Males	Females
Increasing Trends			
Pancreas	Pancreas	Buccal cavity and pharynx	Buccal cavity and pharynx
Larynx	Bronchus and lung	Esophagus	Esophagus
Bronchus and lung	Ovary	Intestines	Intestines
All urinary organs	Kidney	Pancreas	Pancreas
Kidney	Brain and other parts of nervous system	Larynx	Bronchus and lung
Brain and other parts of nervous system	Hodgkin's disease	Bronchus and lung	Breast
Hodgkin's disease	Leukemia and aleukemia	Prostate	Ovary
Leukemia and aleukemia		All urinary organs	All urinary organs
		Kidney	Kidney
		Bladder and other urinary organs	Bladder and other urinary organs
		Brain and other parts of nervous system	Brain and other parts of nervous system
		Hodgkin's disease	Leukemia and aleukemia
		Leukemia and aleukemia	

Decreasing Trends

Buccal cavity and pharynx	Esophagus	Thyroid gland	Stomach
Tongue	Stomach	Bone	Cervix uteri
Stomach	Larynx		Bone
Bone	Cervix uteri		
	Bladder and other urinary organs		
	Thyroid gland		
	Bone		

Stable Trends

Esophagus	Buccal cavity and pharynx		Tongue
Bladder and other urinary organs	Tongue		Larynx
Thyroid gland	Breast		Thyroid gland

Irregular Trends

Intestines	Intestines	Tongue	Rectum
Rectum	Rectum	Stomach	Hodgkin's disease
Breast	All urinary organs	Rectum	
Prostate		Breast	
Male genital organs except prostate		Male genital organs except prostate	

Source: Lilienfeld, Levin, and Kessler, 1972.

Table 5. Standardized mortality ratios for all sites of cancer combined and for cancer of selected sites by broad occupational group, white male population of United States ages 20–64, 1950

Broad occupational group	All sites	Buccal cavity and pharynx	Esopha- gus	Stomach	Large intestine	Rectum	Lung and bronchus	Bladder	Skin	Leukemia and aleukemia
All persons ages 20–64	100	100	100	100	100	100	100	100	100	100
Professional, technical, and kindred workers	91	83	68	64	124	111	82	97	93	114
Farmers and farm managers	81	62	35	91	81	64	55	73	133	127
Managers, officials and proprietors, except farm	95	83	64	74	110	94	95	85	105	111
Clerical and kindred workers	92	100	77	69	118	103	94	115	93	93
Salesworkers	102	93	70	75	114	113	103	111	137	106
Craftsmen, foremen, and kindred workers	111	107	117	108	104	118	132	125	132	105
Operative and kindred workers	101	105	122	102	105	111	110	99	128	92
Service workers, except private household	109	141	149	102	106	119	125	123	N.A.	91
Laborers, including farm laborers and foremen	105	133	166	116	95	94	103	96	213	96
Farm laborers and foremen	59	64	85	79	53	32	53	76	N.A.	72
Laborers, except farm and mine	123	161	182	130	108	113	123	104	172	106

Source: Bailar, King, and Mason, 1964.

N.A. = Not available.

Table 6. Carcinogenic agents that may be associated with various occupations

Agent	Sites of cancer	Areas where noted
Specific agents		
Arsenic	Skin, lung	United States, Great Britain, Germany, France, Argentina, Taiwan, African countries
Coal tar, pitch	Skin, lung	United States, Great Britain
Petroleum	Skin, lung	United States, France, Great Britain, Austria
Shale oils	Skin	United States, Great Britain
Lignite tar and paraffin	Skin	Great Britain, France
Creosote oils	Skin	United States, Great Britain
Anthracene oils	Skin	Great Britain
Soot carbon black	Skin	United States, Great Britain
Mustard gas	Lung	Japan
Cutting (mineral) oils	Skin, respiratory, and upper alimentary tract	Great Britain, Australia
Products of coal carbonization	Lung, bladder	Great Britain, United States, Japan
Sunlight	Skin	United States, Argentina, Australia, France, et al.
Chromates	Lung	United States, Great Britain, Germany, Canada
Asbestos	Lung, pleura, peritoneum, GI tract	United States, Great Britain, Germany, Canada, South Africa, Holland, Australia, USSR, Italy, et al.
Aromatic amines, dyes, rubber	Bladder, possibly biliary tract salivary glands	United States, Germany, Great Britain, Switzerland, et al.
X-rays and radium	Skin, lung, leukemia	United States, et al.
Nickel	Lung, nasal cavity and sinus	Great Britain, Norway, Canada
Benzol	Leukemia	United States, et al.
Isopropyl oil	Lung, larynx, nasal sinus	United States
Radioactive chemicals	Bones, nasal sinus	United States
Chemicals (various)	Lymphoma, pancreas	United States
Nonspecific (Occupations):		
Wood furniture working	Nasal cavity, sinuses	Great Britain, United States
Leather working	Nasal cavity, sinuses, bladder	Great Britain, United States
Soft coal mining	Stomach	United States (1 report)

Source: Bailar, King, and Mason, 1964.

15

Table 7. Age-adjusted cancer mortality rates in various countries, by sex, 1956–1957 and 1966–1967, with male-female ratios and percent change

Country	Male			Female			Male/female ratio	
	1956–1957	1966–1967	Percent change	1956–1957	1966–1967	Percent change	1956–1957	1966–1967
Australia	130.9	143.2	+9	100.4	96.8	−4	1.30	1.48
Austria	187.6	192.7	+3	136.9	130.3	−5	1.37	1.48
Belgium	153.2	182.9	+19	122.9	120.3	−2	1.25	1.52
Canada	133.9	146.8	+10	114.4	109.0	−5	1.17	1.35
Chile	147.0	149.8	+2	138.4	137.1	−1	1.06	1.09
Denmark	152.6	158.2	+4	141.6	132.6	−6	1.08	1.19
England and Wales	170.9	182.5	+7	113.4	114.9	+1	1.51	1.59
Finland	186.7	183.1	−2	116.2	102.8	−12	1.61	1.78
France	155.1	174.1	+12	105.9	100.3	−5	1.46	1.74
Germany, Federal Republic	160.0	174.1	+9	128.7	126.5	−2	1.24	1.38
Ireland	131.4	142.9	+9	110.6	115.1	+4	1.19	1.24
Israel	116.0	121.5	+5	116.7	114.5	−2	0.99	1.06
Italy	130.6	152.0	+16	99.7	99.3	0	1.31	1.53
Japan	127.6	141.3	+11	94.0	94.9	+1	1.36	1.49
Netherlands	148.5	175.5	+18	122.2	120.7	−1	1.22	1.45
New Zealand	137.4	146.2	+6	107.5	109.5	+2	1.28	1.34
Northern Ireland	149.4	151.3	+1	114.5	107.0	−7	1.30	1.41
Norway	124.9	124.7	0	106.5	100.1	−6	1.17	1.25
Portugal	93.1	113.6	+22	75.9	84.4	+11	1.23	1.35
Scotland	183.2	202.8	+11	127.8	124.6	−3	1.43	1.63
Sweden	119.9	126.1	+5	109.2	104.5	−4	1.10	1.21
Switzerland	182.5	164.4	−10	127.6	107.6	−16	1.43	1.53
South Africa	158.0	171.0	+8	117.2	113.4	−3	1.35	1.51
United States, white	139.6	146.8	+5	111.1	104.6	−6	1.26	1.40
United States, nonwhite	151.1	178.5	+18	125.9	121.9	−3	1.20	1.46

Source: Segi and Kurihara, 1972.

16

Table 8. Time trends in percentage of cancer patients with localized disease at diagnosis and percentage treated surgically

Site	1940–1949			1950–1954			1955–1964			1965–1969		
	Number of cases	Percent local	Percent surgical	Number of cases	Percent local	Percent surgical	Number of cases	Percent local	Percent surgical	Number of cases	Percent local	Percent surgical
Stomach	6,567	20	31	5,166	15	42	9,983	18	46	3,889	18	48
Colon	7,066	36	58	7,525	38	76	19,461	41	81	10,152	42	84
Rectum	6,154	37	55	5,604	42	72	11,515	45	76	5,512	46	78
Pancreas	1,989	19	20	2,046	13	21	5,374	14	8	2,888	11	10
Lung and bronchus	4,264	18	11	6,663	17	20	22,585	19	26	15,941	18	27
Female breast	12,696	38	81	11,886	41	84	25,698	45	88	14,911	47	90
Cervix uteri	6,988	44	12	5,963	52	23	10,557	52	22	4,888	47	22
Corpus uteri	3,632	62	55	3,486	69	69	7,614	74	75	4,400	78	79
Ovary	2,476	26	61	2,259	26	63	5,240	28	68	3,085	27	71
Prostate	4,845	46	60	5,212	51	59	13,790	57	61	7,384	63	64
Bladder	3,898	66	70	3,975	67	81	10,177	75	85	5,295	79	87
Melanoma of skin	754	54	73	924	56	83	2,862	68	91	1,996	73	93

Source: Levin et al., 1974.

Table 9.   Time trend in 3-year relative survival, by site

Site	1940–1949 No. cases	1940–1949 3-year survival (percent)	1950–1959 No. cases	1950–1959 3-year survival (percent)	1965–1969 No. cases	1965–1969 3-year survival (percent)
Stomach	7,390	12	9,987	15	3,889	15
Colon	7,488	36	16,153	49	10,152	50
Rectum	6,979	35	10,901	47	5,512	49
Pancreas	2,009	2	4,391	2	2,888	2
Larynx	1,462	47	3,259	60	2,725	67
Lung and bronchus	4,772	6	16,072	10	15,941	11
Female breast	12,184	63	22,105	71	14,911	72
Cervix uteri	7,075	53	10,280	64	4,888	63
Corpus uteri	3,509	66	6,529	74	4,400	76
Ovary	2,339	30	4,296	33	3,085	35
Prostate	6,008	49	11,647	59	7,384	66
Bladder	4,337	48	8,350	58	5,295	62
Melanoma of skin	749	49	1,982	63	1,996	74
Brain and cranial meninges	2,437	28	4,679	28	3,810	37
Thyroid	697	67	2,377	81	1,445	86
Hodgkin's disease	1,013	35	2,008	44	1,990	61
Multiple myeloma	391	10	1,328	13	1,116	27
Acute leukemia	922	4	2,837	14	2,432	30
Chronic leukemia	1,599	24	3,627	35	1,587	41

Source: Axtell, Cutler, and Meyers, 1972.

Table 10.   National Cancer Program Plan: Research components

Target areas	General objectives
I. CAUSE/PREVENTION/BIOLOGY	1. Reduce effectiveness of *external agents* in producing cancer
	2. *Modify individuals* in order to minimize their risk of developing cancer
	3. *Prevent transformation* of normal cells to cells capable of forming cancers
	4. *Prevent progression* of precancerous cells and conditions to cancer; prevent metastases
II. DETECTION/DIAGNOSIS/PROGNOSIS	5. *Assess the risk* of cancer in individuals and populations; establish the frequency and natural history of each type of cancer
III. TREATMENT/REHABILITATION	6. *Cure or control* the progress of cancer in man
	7. Improve the *rehabilitation* of cancer patients

Source: National Institutes of Health. 1974. National Cancer Program Operational Plan FY 1976–1980. U.S. Department of Health, Education, and Welfare, Publication No. 75-777, Washington, D.C.

rectly predicting their ultimate course. With respect to treatment and rehabilitation, that is, the third target area, the Plan's general objectives are to cure or control the progress of cancer as well as to maximize the rehabilitation of cancer patients.

For each of the three target areas, there are cancer control objectives (Table 11) parallel to the research objectives just described. These relate principally to increasing the accessibility and utilization of existing cancer control methods as well as new methods resulting from research stimulated by the National Cancer Program. This distinction between research and operational tools in the fight against cancer is a crucial one. An example is given in the next section of how a theoretically inferior cancer detection instrument can in fact be more effective than a theoretically superior one under conditions in which acceptance by or accessibility to the target population is sufficiently greater.

The seven research objectives developed for the National Cancer Program were elaborated upon, refined, and eventually broken down into a much larger number of relatively specific operational approaches (Table 12). The remainder of this chapter is largely oriented around these approaches, their strengths, weaknesses, and immediate relevance in cancer control.

Reducing the Effectiveness of External Agents

A crucial objective in cancer control is to render environmental carcinogens ineffective or less effective in their human hosts. A first step toward achiev-

Table 11. National Cancer Program Plan: Control components

Target areas	General objectives
I. PREVENTION	1. Means for *cancer prevention:* available, utilized
II. DETECTION/DIAGNOSIS/ PRETREATMENT EVALUATION	2. Means for *cancer screening and early detection:* available, utilized
	3. *Diagnostic practices:* continuously assessed and optimized
	4. Means for *diagnosis and pretreatment evaluation:* available, utilized
III. TREATMENT/REHABILITATION/ CONTINUING CARE	5. *Treatment practices:* continually assessed and optimized
	6. Means for *treatment and follow-up care:* available, utilized
	7. Means for *rehabilitation:* available, utilized
	8. Means for *palliation and supportive care:* available, utilized

Source: National Institutes of Health. 1974. National Cancer Program Operational Plan FY 1976–1980, U.S. Department of Health, Education, and Welfare, Publication No. 75-777, Washington, D.C.

Table 12.   National Cancer Program Plan: Approaches to research objectives

1. REDUCE EFFECTIVENESS OF EXTERNAL AGENTS

a. Identify environmental carcinogens
b. Assess the human relevance of a.
c. Identify human cancer viruses

d. Counteract the carcinogenicity
   of external agents
e. Elucidate determinants of differences
   in susceptibility to cancer

2. MODIFY INDIVIDUALS TO MINIMIZE RISK

a. Enhance effectiveness of immune
   responses
b. Modify metabolic pathways
c. Modify genetic constitution or gene
   expression

d. Eliminate precancerous lesions
e. Elucidate determinants of differences
   in susceptibility to cancer

3. PREVENT MALIGNANT TRANSFORMATION

a. Elucidate genetic and epigenetic factors

b. Elucidate immunologic mechanisms

c. Elucidate role of cell surfaces and
   membranes
d. Elucidate mechanisms of normal
   differentiation and dedifferentiation

4. PREVENT DEVELOPMENT OF CANCER FROM TRANSFORMED CELLS

a. Elucidate interactions of cells and host
b. Interfere with tumor initiation

c. Detect and eliminate cancer microfoci
d. Apply mathematical models to the
   process

5. ASSESS CANCER RISK IN INDIVIDUALS AND POPULATIONS

a. Develop predictors of high and low risk
b. Identify cancer-associated or
   precancerous states

c. Improve screening methods
d. Improve diagnostic methods
e. Elucidate determinants of differential
   rates of growth and dissemination

6. CURE OR CONTROL THE PROGRESS OF CANCER

a. Improve surgery, radiation, chemotherapy, and immunotherapy techniques
b. Modify cell control mechanisms to
   reverse malignant transformation

c. Enhance host resistance
d. Develop predictors of responses
   to treatment regimens

7. IMPROVE REHABILITATION OF CANCER PATIENTS

a. Improve restorative, supportive, and
   palliative techniques

b. Elucidate psychosocial aspects of cancer
   treatment

Source: National Institutes of Health. 1974. Digest of Scientific Recommendations for the National Cancer Program. U.S. Department of Health, Education, and Welfare, Publication No. 74-570, Washington, D.C.

ing this goal is the identification of the specific agents, whether chemical, radiologic, or microbiologic.

Clinical Studies   More often than not, human carcinogens have been detected through the astute observations of clinical practitioners, rather than by laboratory investigation or epidemiologic study.

For example, the carcinogenicity of aniline dyes to the human bladder was first suggested by a German surgeon on the basis of his observation of three bladder tumors among 45 workers employed in a fuchsine manufacturing plant (Rehn, 1895). His hypothesis, that urinary bladder cancer was the result of chronic irritation of the organ's mucous membrane by chemical compounds excreted in the urine over a period of many years, is still in vogue today. The relationship with synthetic dyes was further elucidated some years later by a Swiss physician who demonstrated that the incidence of bladder cancer was 33 times greater among dye workers than other men (Leuenberger, 1912). In more recent times, these insightful clinical observations have been confirmed by controlled epidemiologic studies.

Perhaps the most famous example of the clinical detection of an environmental carcinogen was the discovery by Percival Pott (1775) that chronic exposure to soot causes scrotal cancer among chimney sweeps. This observation was made long before the development of modern concepts of cancer pathogenesis. Almost exactly a century later, the information assembled by Pott was refined somewhat by Von Volkmann (1875), who observed three cases of skin cancer in various sites among individuals chronically exposed to tar or paraffin. That these substances are the agents responsible for chimney sweeps' cancer was later demonstrated clinically by Butlin (1892) and experimentally by Yamagiwa and Ichikawa (1918) in rabbits. The specific carcinogen responsible for these tumors, 3,4-benzpyrene, was eventually identified by a research scientist, Sir Ernest Kennaway and his colleagues (1924, 1930).

Centuries earlier, the Swiss physician Paracelsus described the *Mala Metallorum*, a fatal lung disease—actually cancer—that occurred among the Schneeberg miners of the Erzegebirge mountains between present-day Czechoslovakia and East Germany. In 1556, Agricola attributed the disease to the inhalation of coal dust. Uranium miners at nearby Joachimstal, the source of Madame Curie's radium, were observed to experience a marked increase in lung cancer mortality due to the inhalation of radioactive dusts (Rostoski, Saupe, and Schmorl, 1926). As was the case with the aniline dyes, our knowledge concerning the carcinogenic properties of radioisotopes evolved from astute clinical observations refined in the laboratory and subsequently confirmed by systematic epidemiologic investigation in human populations.

Other examples of the role of the clinician in identifying environmental carcinogens include the acquisition of knowledge on the role of x-rays in skin cancer (Von Frieben, 1902), radioactive luminous paint of watch dials in bone sarcoma (Martland and Humphries, 1929), and asbestos in pleural mesothelioma (Wagner, Sleggs, and Marchand, 1960).

Experimental Techniques   In addition to clinical studies, a wide variety of experimental techniques have been systematically employed in the search for environmental carcinogens. For many years, efforts have been made to correlate chemical structure with biologic (i.e., carcinogenic) activity. An example is the spectroscopic and other research undertaken to synthesize and test hydrocarbons that were chemical variations of dibenzanthracene, first identified as a carcinogen by Kennaway (1924). Benzene rings were added and subtracted, alkyl groups were substituted in different positions in the nucleus, hexagon rings were replaced by pentagon rings, C was substituted by N and by S, and so on (Hieger, 1949). Substantial progress has been made, but it is not yet possible to evaluate the potential carcinogenicity of substances in man on the basis of their chemical configurations alone.

The fact that chemical carcinogens interact with subcellular macromolecules offers another potential tool for cancer control. For example, the binding of 7,12-dimethylbenzanthracene to cellular DNA is closely linked to its carcinogenicity in the mouse. Similarly, β-propiolactone induces tumors in direct proportion to the extent of its binding to mouse skin DNA (Süss, Kinzel, and Scribner, 1973). Such findings are relevant not only to the detection of environmental carcinogens but also to the importance of host factors in susceptibility to specific cancers.

Other macromolecular indicators of carcinogenesis are presently undergoing active investigation. The most promising of these appear to be two antigens of the genital herpesvirus that are associated with active growth of uterine cervix cancer (Aurelian et al., 1973; Aurelian, Strnad, and Smith, 1977; Strnad and Aurelian, 1978). One of these, a virion envelope polypeptide of molecular weight 161,000, termed AG-4, is a structural protein antigen of the genital herpesvirus HSV-2. Normal women lack AG-4, as measured by the presence or absence of 19S immunoglobulin antibodies against it, except for a brief period following primary HSV-2 infection. Women with a variety of other cancers, including cervical adenocarcinoma, likewise fail to test positively for AG-4. On the other hand, more than 90% of subjects with untreated invasive squamous carcinoma of the cervix test positive. Between 3 and 6 weeks following surgery or radiotherapy, essentially all such women test negative. With clinical recurrence of the disease, more than 90% again test positive. Approximately two out of three women with documented carcinoma in situ and one woman in three with cervical dysplasia are also AG-4 positive. The test appears to be identifying those women whose intraepithelial or preneoplastic lesions are destined to progress.

These findings offer substantial confirmation of the etiologic role of HSV-2 in the pathogenesis of squamous carcinoma of the uterine cervix. The findings also suggest the possible use of AG-4 testing in screening women for the early detection of this neoplasm. The utility of AG-4 testing in determining prognosis and recurrence in patients previously treated for invasive cervical cancer is also promising.

AG-e, another herpesvirus-specific antigen, is present in exfoliated cervical anaplastic cells but not in normal cells. This antigen, composed of two structural proteins located in the virion envelope, induces a transient antigen-driven cell-mediated immune response. Women without cervical neoplasia are nonreactive. A variety of other possible macromolecular indicators of carcinogenesis, such as carcinoembryonic antigen (CEA) have not yet proved to be of substantial value in the identification or early detection of environmental carcinogens (Gold et al., 1973)

In Vitro Systems   Although human carcinogens to date have been largely identified on the basis of clinical observations, the public's increasing concern with cancer and the consequent proliferation of regulations dealing with its control have created the need for the rapid screening of substances for their potential cancer-provoking effects. Thus, an important goal in the National Cancer Program has been the development of cellular in vitro systems for demonstrating carcinogenicity.

Mutagenicity assays, such as the Salmonella/Ames test, are among the more popular short-term tests. These are based on the assumption that cancer is related to cellular DNA changes and that the detection of such changes should be predictive of a substance's potential carcinogenicity. Their rationale depends on the presumption of a substantial correlation between mutagenicity in the system and carcinogenicity in man.

Other in vitro systems have been designed to detect morphologic transformations in human cell systems by putative oncogenic viruses or chemicals, sister chromatid exchange, mitotic recombination in yeast, induction of plasminogen activator, or sex-linked recessive lethality in *Drosophila*, among others. Each of the short-term tests has its own limitations, both with respect to sensitivity and specificity as well as with respect to the range of chemical classes falling within its screening purview. Thus, for example, when the potential carcinogenicity of saccharin was evaluated by 10 short-term tests, three positive and seven negative results were obtained. This left the issue essentially unresolved (Office of Technology Assessment, 1977).

The most widely accepted and utilized test system for carcinogenicity is the long-term assay in animal models. Golberg (1975) finds it "difficult to foresee a future plan of study of toxicological potential that is not based in the first phase on the use of whole animals." Long-term assays may involve one or more species, generations of animals, routes of administration, doses, and a variety of other experimental conditions. The conditions are imposed by the need to extrapolate the results of the assay from animal to man.

Difficulties in Assessing the Relevance of Agents in Humans   Another important contemporary subject of research in carcinogenesis concerns the differences in the metabolic systems of various animal species that affect their responses to exogenous carcinogens. Since man in all likelihood does not metabolize saccharin, for example, it would seem presumptuous to extrapolate to homo sapiens the results of experiments with animal species capable of metabolizing this substance. An equally difficult problem stems from the lack of appropriate animal models for certain human cancers, such as those of the uterine cervix, prostate, and pancreas. Inferential problems associated with the use of animal models are discussed further in Chapter 15.

The effectiveness of external carcinogens might also be reduced by elucidating how carcinogenic influences are transmitted to future generations. Such influences may be genetic or otherwise vertically transmitted. Wilm's tumors, osteogenic sarcomas, retinoblastomas, leukemias, and other childhood neoplasms may involve such mechanisms and deserve further study. So, too, does the "oncogene," whose role in the transmission of breast and other cancers in adulthood remains unresolved. The problem of vaginal cancer arising in the offspring of women given diethylstilbestrol during pregnancy offers a classic example of the potential vertical transmission of carcinogens (Herbst et al., 1975).

A reduction in the effectiveness of external carcinogens could also result from the exploitation of improved techniques for quantifying potential chemical carcinogens, biologic agents, or ionizing radiations in the environment as well as in presumptively exposed individuals or groups. Urine, saliva, exhaled air, blood, biopsies, and necropsies can all testify to the body's loading of putative carcinogens in both general populations and selected subgroups at high risk. Regular environmental monitoring of air, water, and other media can provide useful information on levels of exposure to known carcinogens in geographically or occupationally defined populations.

The public's increasing concern with cancer and the subsequent proliferation of governmental regulations concerned with its control have created the need for the rapid screening of substances for their potential cancer-provoking effects. This has resulted in the identification of substantial numbers of substances associated to some degree with tumor production in animals or with mutagenic effects in tissue culture tests. The ensuing dilemma, namely, that of assessing the relevance of environmental agents in man, is broached more fully in Chapter 15.

A relationship between the successful identification of human tumor viruses and the manner in which they were first studied is apparent. Viruses such as EBV and HSV-2, concerning which a number of observational studies were conducted in man, are now—at least to some degree—considered significant human viral carcinogens. On the other hand, the RNA C-type viruses, which came to attention as animal carcinogens in the laboratory, are no longer regarded as likely human carcinogens.

This suggests, as will be noted again, that despite the obvious technical advantages of experimentation in laboratory animals, the identification of carcinogens relevant to man is most likely to come from observations on man. This conclusion holds, we believe, despite the variability in experimental conditions and the imprecision in measurements that can be made on human subjects.

Immunologic studies also appear promising in the assessment of potential human carcinogenic agents. As already noted in respect to HSV-2, both cell-mediated and humoral responses are of interest. Furthermore, because various human population groups differ markedly in their susceptibility to particular neoplasms, it is essential to control for known or suspected factors that may confound assessments of carcinogenic risks, namely, cigarette smoking habits, socioeconomic factors, occupational exposures, dietary idiosyncracies, airborne contaminant exposures, other diseases (e.g., hepatitis), and exposures to ionizing radiation, polluted water, and the like.

Counteracting the Carcinogenicity of Agents The effectiveness of carcinogens may also be minimized by directly counteracting their carcinogenicity in some fashion. Thus, one might attempt to terminate cigarette consumption, develop safer cigarettes, reduce occupational exposures, redesign equipment to shield from radiation, and, in general, develop systematic consumer protection policies. For example, under an "assigned marketing system for consumer protection" (AMSCOP), new products containing possible carcinogens would be released into a given market area of the United States in such fashion that the dates of introduction could be correlated rapidly with changes in specific cancer incidence patterns in the area. The existence of such a system would, for example, have identified the congenital malformations due to thalidomide much more rapidly than actually occurred. In similar fashion, epidemiologic studies on the long-term effects of chronically administered drugs, such as insulin, contraceptive pills, diuretics, aspirin, digitalis, laxatives, and so on, should be undertaken in selected population groups that have been chronically exposed.

Minimizing the Risks of Developing Cancer

Although efforts to control cancer have, until now, emphasized environmental agents and the means for reducing their effectiveness, this approach ignores the classic concept of the *epidemiologic triad* in the pathogenesis of disease. Rather than cancers being initiated simply by the interaction of an exogenous agent with a specific cellular site, most—if not all—human cancers result from the action of carcinogenic agents in susceptible human hosts under "environmental" conditions favorable to the neoplastic outcome. In view of this, a rational cancer control program should place as much emphasis on modifying individuals to minimize their cancer risks as upon efforts to reduce the effectiveness of the carcinogenic agents themselves. Unfortunately, little progress has been made in this arena, perhaps because of the relative lack of attention received.

Immunopotentiation On the basis of experiences with the infectious diseases, possibilities for enhancing the effectiveness of human immune responses to carcinogenic challenge may be considered. Antigenic substances, such as blood group antigens, embryonal antigens, membrane antigens, viral antigens, and so on, are present in a variety of human cancers. The question is whether any of these can be exploited for the production of vaccines against cancer. In the laboratory, animals have been successfully vaccinated against the effects of experimental oncogenic viruses, but not against naturally occurring neoplasms.

With respect to the herpes variety of DNA viruses, there have been many efforts to develop vaccines against EBV, a presumed agent of Burkitt's lymphoma, as well as against herpetic viruses believed responsible for cervical cancer and perhaps nasopharyngeal cancer. While thousands of Americans have flown to Germany at great expense for vaccination against HSV-2, no significant clinical remissions have been reported, nor is there any evidence that the procedure immunizes against subsequent risk of cancer. There are, in fact, substantial reasons why these kinds of vaccine cannot be effective. Persons infected with herpes genitalis retain a level of HSV-2 antibodies throughout the remainder of their lives, the titer increasing somewhat with each clinical exacerbation and then diminishing. Thus, in viral infections characterized by alternations of latency and clinical recrudescence, such as those caused by the genital herpesvirus, humoral immunity would not be expected to exert much of an effect. Whether cell-mediated immune mechanisms can be evoked remains to be seen.

An interesting possibility for vaccination against cancer derives from the long observed "antagonism" between pulmonary tuberculosis and cancer. As far back as 1926, mice resistant to the tubercle bacillus failed to develop cancers when injected with mixtures of cancer cells and living mycobacteria (Centanni and Rezzesi, 1926). In 1901, a therapeutic trial involving the injection of bovine mycobacteria into cancer patients was undertaken (Loeffler, 1901). Recently, it has been shown that products of the tubercle bacillus as well as of *Bacillus Calmette-Guerin* (BCG) not only enhanced the activity of the reticuloendothelial system and its capacity for antibody production but also increased natural resistance to infection in general (Old and Clarke, 1959).

The complete inhibition of ascites tumor growth has been observed at the site of inoculation in guinea pigs immunized intradermally with living BCG (Zbar, Bernstein, and Rapp, 1971). The inhibition was mediated by the host during a delayed hypersensitivity-type immunologic response to the infecting organism. The participation of the host's immune system is essential for this reaction, because BCG has no effect on the viability of tumor cells in vitro and because guinea pigs with impaired immune defenses are unable to suppress tumor growth in the presence of BCG.

These experimental findings have their clinical counterpart in a number of significant investigations on human populations. Morton et al. (1970), for example, treated 12 patients with advanced malignant melanoma as well as skeletal and soft tissue sarcomas by direct intranodular injection with BCG. Tumor regression of the injected nodules up to 30 months in duration was noted. In addition, the therapeutic results correlated well with the patients' immunologic competence at the onset of immunotherapy. All patients who could be sensitized to dinitrochlorobenzene or to tuberculin developed a fourfold rise in antibody titer and had a positive response to immunotherapy, in contrast with patients who could not be sensitized and who failed to respond to the BCG.

Morton and his colleagues also noted a correlation between antitumor antibody titer and the progression of cancer. Thus, patients who developed recurrent disease demonstrated progressive declines in their antitumor antibody titer. A possible explanation for this is that the antibodies are produced at a relatively constant rate but are constantly absorbed from the circulation by the growing tumor mass. Therefore, removal of the tumor would result in an increase in the titer of antibodies, whereas regrowth of the tumor would be accompanied by a reduced titer. A second explanation for these findings might be specific immunosuppression by the growing tumor, which would account for declining antibody titer in patients with recurrent disease. Morton et al. could find no evidence to support the latter hypothesis. Active immunization with BCG and autologous tumor cells induced a heightened immune response against the tumor antigens. These results suggest that immunotherapy can become an important adjunct to cancer treatment in the future.

A growing awareness of the possible role of cell-mediated immunity in cancer and the rediscovery of Freud's observation that living mycobacteria are excellent stimulants of a delayed hypersensitivity response (Levy, Mahaley, and Day, 1972) have led to an increasing number of studies on the value of BCG in the treatment of leukemia, melanoma, sarcoma, and other tumors. The basis of the apparent therapeutic response is incompletely understood. Levy and his colleagues presented evidence for a serum factor that blocks the cell-mediated antitumor immunity in melanoma patients (Levy, Mahaley, and Day, 1972). Furthermore, Sparks et al. (1973) have recently reported clinical complications of BCG immunotherapy that might mitigate against its widespread use.

Of at least equal importance to the clinical application of BCG immunotherapy in cancer patients is the possibility that prior vaccination in childhood with BCG may reduce the subsequent risk of neoplasia. Scattered reports in the literature indicate this may be the case. The death rate from leukemia was found to be one-half as common among BCG-vaccinated as among nonvaccinated persons below age 15 in the province of Quebec, Canada (Davignon et al., 1970, 1971). This conclusion was reached on the basis of a statistical evaluation of mortality among children whose vaccinations were recorded in the Central BCG Record of the Dominion. No differences in mortality rates due to accidents were noted in the two populations. The authors concluded that "BCG appears to act through proliferation of immunocommited cells, particularly reticuloendothelial cells. . . . It remains to be seen whether . . . the lower incidence of leukemia in persons vaccinated with BCG is actually due to non-specific stimulation of immunity" (Davignon et al., 1971).

These findings of Davignon et al. were subjected to criticism by Kinlen and Pike (1971), who derived estimates of leukemia mortality rates in areas of Canada and Scotland where BCG vaccinations were presumably either common or rare and concluded that no association with BCG inoculation existed. However, their calculations were based upon a number of estimated figures over which the investigators had little or no control. For example, their calculated age specific leukemia death rates ignored immigration and emigration of children to and from the areas of interest. In addition, their rates for Glasgow were based largely upon linear interpolations between two censuses. Despite this, however, their own statistics reveal that children below age 15 in Quebec did, in fact, experience leukemia death rates lower than children in the rest of Canada. Essentially the same finding is apparent in their statistics for Glasgow, where BCG had been administered, as compared with the rest of Scotland, where it had not.

Some confirmation of a possible association between prior BCG vaccination and reduced leukemia mortality is seen in the findings of Rosenthal et al. (1972). Utilizing the records of the maternity division of Cook County Hospital where BCG vaccination had been employed, it was noted that between 1964 and 1969 only one death from leukemia was recorded among 54,414 vaccinated black infants below the age of 7 years as compared with 21 deaths among 172,986 similar, although unvaccinated, children. This difference is statistically significant and suggested to the authors "the value of BCG vaccinations in preventing leukemia in children." The investigators qualified their conclusion by noting that "since this is a retrospective study, no firm conclusions can be drawn."

More recently, a report has been published concerning the use of combination therapy with BCG and transfer factor as a treatment for Hodgkin's disease (Medical News Item, 1974). In this study there appeared to be a direct association between a strongly positive reaction to purified protein derivative (PPD) and a favorable clinical course. An early, but authoritative, review of the possible role of immunization against *Mycobacterium tuberculosis* and cancer resistance is that of Mackaness (1964). Mackaness pointed out that the resistance developed by mice during infection with *M. tuberculosis* was not exclusively directed against the infecting organism. Rather, the resistant host manifested two conditions, namely, "a state of immunological reactivity of the host and the presence of the specific microbial antigens to which the host has become reactive. When these two co-exist in the tissue the host is found to be non-specifically resistant." Mackaness suggested that tumor resistance "may be due to an interaction of antigen and a specific antibody adsorbed to the surface of host macrophages and that the antibody involved in the reaction is possibly identical with the antibody that confers the state of delayed-type hypersensitivity" (Mackaness, 1964).

Our laboratory at the University of Maryland is currently undertaking an investigation of the association between antecedent tuberculosis and subsequent cancer risk in humans. A cohort of some 17,000 confirmed tuberculosis cases, diagnosed between 1946 and 1960 in Baltimore City, is being followed prospectively through time to death or survival with or without cancer as of a recent date. Observed cancer risks are being compared with those expected for the general population of the same age, sex, and race. Additional analyses will focus upon cancer risk according to clinical severity and extent of tuberculosis, with adjustment for smoking habits. The results of this study may add to our basic understanding of the biologic relationships between tuberculosis and cancer. Should an association be confirmed, this could lead to consideration of BCG vaccination or tuberculin inoculation of children as a primary preventative for cancer of particular sites.

By these and other means, one may hope to stimulate specific or nonspecific host resistance to cancer incidence, recurrence, or metastasis. The traditional means for accomplishing this—if the infectious disease analogy holds—includes active immunization with tumor antigens, passive immunization with humoral antibodies, and adoptive immunization with cytotoxic lymphocytes, as well as immunopotentiation with BCG and other antigenic substances.

Metabolic and Genetic Modifications Besides reducing cancer risk through potentiation of immune responses, a number of other approaches, both theoretical and practical, are possible. For example, most, if not all, carcinogenic substances must undergo metabolic degradation to produce their effects. The carcinogenic outcomes are largely a function of the degree to which the substances are metabolized. Bladder cancer is rather easily induced by β-naphthylamine in dogs, less so in mice, and least of all in rabbits that can scarcely, if at all, metabolize this carcinogen.

Thus, if the existing metabolic pathways for known or suspected carcinogens could somehow be modified, their carcinogenicity could be reduced. Furthermore, since both human and animal hosts have the capacity to inactivate and excrete some carcinogens by enzymatic degradation, this suggests another potential method for reducing individual cancer risk, that is, by perhaps inducing the inactivating enzymes by means of drugs or dietary factors.

Related to this is another possibility, namely, modifying the host's genetic constitution or gene expression. Methods for the selective excision or substitution of genes involved in carcinogenesis by restriction endonuclease techniques, among others, may soon become possible. Short of actually modifying the genetic constitution, one might hope to modify gene expression through effects on single "repressors" or "activators" within the genetic material.

Early Detection   Among the methods for modifying individuals to minimize their cancer risk, perhaps the most readily available is the detection and elimination of precancerous lesions. The classic example is cervical carcinoma in situ, which is generally destined to become invasive unless treated. In similar fashion, an unknown proportion of cervical dysplasias also progresses to carcinoma if untreated. The challenge of detecting and eliminating such lesions, utilizing present-day technology, is great, but quite surmountable. Exfoliative cytology provides a valid, accurate, reliable, and inexpensive means for accomplishing this in a manner generally acceptable to both patients and physicians.

When the Pap test became widely available in the 1950s, optimism prevailed that mortality from cervical cancer might eventually be reduced to negligible proportions, if not eliminated altogether. Twenty-five years and numerous field trials later, opinions on the matter are now divided, with some experts contending that this objective is unattainable, at least in populations at large. This judgment, in our opinion, is unsubstantiated and premature at best.

Statistics from the well-known cervical cancer screening program of British Columbia are often cited in support of the pessimistic view (Table 13). Of interest here is that women who never underwent cytologic screening experienced cervical cancer risks between 7 and 10 times greater than those of previously screened women; and that the latter seemed to be exposed to a persistent, although low, level of clinical invasive cancer. These data have been interpreted to suggest that "the maximum possible benefit to a population from cytologic screening is a reduction of clinical disease to about one-

Table 13.   Effect of cytologic screening on cervical cancer in British Columbia, 1961–1971

| Year | Invasive cervical cancer (incidence/100,000) | |
	Screened	Unscreened
1961	4.1	29.3
1962	4.3	21.0
1963	4.7	29.5
1964	4.6	27.8
1965	4.2	28.8
1966	4.8	28.6
1967	5.4	33.4
1968	4.4	36.5
1969	3.4	51.4
1970	4.9	46.5
1971	4.7	51.0

Source: Knowelden and Phillips, 1974.

seventh its previous rate and that a voluntary program can probably not exceed this by very much" (Knowelden and Phillips, 1974).

Such inferences may be unwarranted, because the screened population *in fact* consisted of a variety of women who underwent Pap testing one or more times since the initiation of the British Columbia screening program. Thus, a number of women contributing to the persistent cancer rate among screened patients underwent testing once many years ago and have not since benefited from periodic evaluation. Cervical cancer prevalence in this group might very well have fallen if a higher proportion of the subjects could have been induced to undertake periodic screening examinations.

The most convincing evidence to validate the efficacy of periodic Pap testing for the prevention of invasive cervical cancer would come from the results of large population-based cytologic surveys encompassing the periodic screening of all or most eligible women in a defined geographic area over a fairly prolonged period of time, perhaps 7 or 8 years. In order to mount such a study, it would be desirable for the total population of eligible women in the area to be identified at the onset. The first and subsequent screening rounds should reach at least 90% or more of the eligible subjects, and each round should be completed within a few months. Women moving out of the study area should be monitored, and women moving in should be excluded. Nonrespondents should be contacted personally to maximize the participation rate. Finally, standardized methods for cytologic testing (scrapes, smears, swabs of exocervical, endocervical, or vaginal pool specimens) should be employed and diagnostic consistency ensured by centralized review of all specimens.

In view of these desiderata, it is not surprising that studies of this type have not yet been undertaken. In the most ambitious of the United States screening surveys conducted in Memphis, Tennessee, some years ago, the target population was never identified (Kaiser et al., 1960). Instead, the number of women in the community was estimated by interpolation of census data, and participation was solicited indirectly through newspaper advertisements, broadcasts, and the like. It was estimated that approximately 68% of the eligible white women and 57% of the eligible black women were screened at the first round. Less than 45% of the eligible population returned for the second round. Barely 20% participated in the third screening, and less than 8% in the fourth.

Effectiveness of Cancer Screening Because the large majority of Memphis women at risk of cervical cancer were not screened more than once, it does not seem reasonable to make inferences from the Memphis survey about the efficacy of cytologic screening in preventing mortality from cervical cancer. Unfortunately, none of the other major screening programs undertaken in the United States was more successful (Kessler and Aurelian, 1975). Because of the inherent methodologic difficulties, all the surveys have suffered from inadequate response rates and lack of effective follow-up or regular rescreening of subjects. Accordingly, this approach is unlikely to prevent mortality from cervical cancer.

Can the approach be modified? We shall attempt to answer this question after examining our own statistics on cervical cancer mortality and incidence. These were generated by means of a comprehensive epidemiologic study encompassing essentially all histopathologically diagnosed cases of invasive and intraepithelial cervical cancer diagnosed in metropolitan Baltimore, Maryland, between 1950 and 1975. Data sources included all pathology reports, hospital records, and relevant gynecologic, surgical, and radiology records, as well as a complete search for requisite death certificates.

The data revealed a significant decline in mortality from squamous carcinoma of the cervix uteri, a decline to rates slightly lower than one-half those obtaining as recently as the early 1950s. The pattern was manifest has repeatedly been shown to be approximately twice that of whites. The decline in death rates among both racial groups was essentially the same in magnitude, suggesting that nonwhite women benefited proportionally as did whites, despite their inherently higher risk of the disease and irrespective of the putative cause or causes (Table 14).

Our statistics suggest that the cervical cancer death rate began to decline first among women of ages 40–49 years, both white and nonwhite, that is, among those suffering the highest à priori risk of cervical neoplasia. Such trends strongly suggest an increasing impact of exfoliative cytologic

Table 14. Time trends in mortality from cervical cancer

Race	Place	Time period	Average annual mortality rates per 100,000 females by specific age group (years)[a]						
			Total[b]	20–29	30–39	40–49	50–59	60–69	70+
White	United States	1950–1951	9.6	1.0	6.6	17.7	24.3	28.6	33.4
		1955–1956	8.8	1.1	6.6	15.3	22.0	26.1	32.4
		1960–1961	7.8	0.8	5.8	13.6	19.4	23.1	29.4
		1965–1966	6.5	0.8	4.9	11.5	15.6	19.1	25.0
		1970–1971	5.0	0.5	3.5	8.6	12.0	14.8	19.9
	Baltimore, Maryland	1950–1954	12.2	(2.4)	13.3	24.0	29.1	36.2	27.8
		1955–1959	9.7	(1.4)	10.7	18.9	24.5	25.2	32.0
		1960–1964	9.5	(3.4)	(11.2)	17.8	25.9	17.1	26.4
		1965–1969	7.1	(1.1)	(2.9)	17.9	16.1	21.6	20.3
		1970–1974	6.5	(0.0)	(5.7)	(15.4)	17.5	(15.3)	(15.5)
Nonwhite	United States	1950–1951	22.0	3.2	18.7	43.1	60.0	57.4	56.4
		1955–1956	23.4	3.2	19.0	41.1	62.3	70.2	62.6
		1960–1964	19.7	2.3	15.9	34.5	49.5	64.7	57.6
		1965–1966	17.7	2.1	14.6	28.9	40.4	59.8	58.4
		1970–1971	13.1	1.5	8.9	22.3	31.6	41.2	49.4
	Baltimore, Maryland	1950–1954	22.4	(4.4)	(19.2)	50.1	66.3	(38.4)	(76.9)
		1955–1959	23.5	(0.9)	(18.9)	48.1	65.4	76.8	(53.2)
		1960–1964	23.5	(2.3)	20.1	31.0	69.0	82.3	(63.3)
		1965–1969	16.5	(0.0)	(12.1)	35.6	45.2	(36.0)	(57.6)
		1970–1974	13.6	(2.7)	(10.2)	20.9	27.5	45.9	59.5

Source: Kessler, 1974. Baltimore rates for 1974 derived from unpublished statistics of the Baltimore Department of Health, 1976.
[a] Rates for specific age groups based on an average of fewer than five deaths per year given in parentheses.
[b] Rates adjusted to total U.S. population, 1950.

testing and, to a lesser extent, colposcopy in the early detection of invasive and preinvasive cervical disease. That the decline in cervical cancer mortality is not primarily attributable to improvements in treatment modality or responsiveness is suggested by the stability of relative survival rates among patients with invasive cervical cancer since the 1950s (Table 15).

The incidence of newly diagnosed invasive cervical cancer began to decline for the first time in the late 1960s. As had been observed a decade earlier for mortality, the incidence trend was similar in white and nonwhite women, suggesting that both groups benefited equally from increased access to Pap testing. By way of contrast, the incidence of newly diagnosed in situ carcinoma of the cervix has risen markedly in all women since the late 1950s, that is, long before mortality or incidence of invasive cervical cancer had substantially declined (Table 16). The five- to tenfold increase in intraepithelial carcinoma rates must be related to the greatly augmented exfoliative cytoscreening that characterized this period of time. Another factor is the increasing tendency of physicians to classify essentially similar lesions as carcinoma in situ rather than as severe dysplasia. Also contributing to the trend, in our opinion, is the promiscuity-associated epidemic spread of herpes genitalis infections which have been reported in many parts of the country and abroad.

Table 15. Time trends in survival from cervical cancer by stage of disease: whites in the United States, treated and untreated

| Stage | Time | Percentage of patients in this stage[a] | Relative survival rate (percent) | | | |
			3-year	5-year	10-year	15-year
Localized	1940–1949	46	70	64	58	54
	1950–1959	50	82	77	72	70
	1960–1964	50	83	77		
	1965–1969	45	83	78		
	1970–1971	44				
Regional	1940–1949	37	44	37	31	30
	1950–1959	34	54	47	41	36
	1960–1964	37	50	43		
	1965–1969	43	53	44		
	1970–1971	43				
All stages	1940–1949	100	53	47	42	39
	1950–1959	100	64	59	54	52
	1960–1964	100	63	57		
	1965–1969	100	63	56		
	1970–1971	100				

Source: Axtell, Cutler, and Myers, 1972, and Axtell and Myers, 1975.
[a] Patients whose disease was of indeterminate state are included under "All stages."

Table 16.   Time trends in cervical cancer incidence, 1950–1969 (Baltimore women under age 60)

Race	Time period	Total[b]	By specific age group (years)[a]			
			20–29	30–39	40–49	50–59
		Invasive cancer				
White	1950–1954	14.6	(6.9)	29.6	41.2	37.0
	1955–1959	14.1	(7.3)	30.0	33.6	39.3
	1960–1964	16.6	(7.4)	34.2	47.2	40.9
	1965–1969	13.1	(5.6)	24.7	42.8	27.8
Nonwhite	1950–1954	27.4	6.2	35.6	91.6	90.5
	1955–1959	32.4	11.9	59.3	87.6	101.4
	1960–1964	28.2	9.2	50.9	73.4	92.0
	1965–1969	21.9	7.6	35.6	53.1	82.4
		In situ cancer				
White	1950–1954	5.0	(5.6)	15.9	(8.4)	(5.6)
	1955–1959	11.9	17.4	33.4	27.5	(5.9)
	1960–1964	18.9	30.0	53.5	34.7	15.5
	1965–1969	31.1	51.9	99.0	46.2	21.7
Nonwhite	1950–1954	9.7	12.4	23.7	20.8	12.1
	1955–1959	24.0	51.9	63.4	34.2	13.1
	1960–1964	29.9	49.7	98.8	39.5	20.3
	1965–1969	40.0	82.8	110.5	60.5	24.8

Source: Kessler, 1974.

[a] Rates based on average of fewer than five cases per year given in parentheses.

[b] Rates adjusted to total U.S. population, 1950.

A significant change in the stage at diagnosis of cervical neoplasia has taken place since the 1950s. At that time, approximately one-third of the cases were diagnosed in stage 0, that is, carcinoma in situ. Fifteen years later the proportion rose to approximately three-fourths (Table 17). While this trend is manifest in women of all ages, the greatest beneficiaries have apparently been those in the youngest age groups. Similar trends are apparent among both white and nonwhite women, although the proportion of stage 0 lesions achieved by the latter is somewhat lower. This suggests that screening has been somewhat less effective among nonwhites. Our analysis also revealed that, while social class had no effect among whites, nonwhite women of a low social class attained a considerably lower proportion of cases detected in stage 0 than did their counterparts of higher socioeconomic standing.

Mortality from cervical carcinoma is thus preventable for women undergoing periodic health examinations that include regular cytologic screening under direct visualization. The unresolved problem concerns the means of offering such preventive services—or an adequate substitute for them—to all women at risk in the community.

Table 17.   Time trends in stage at diagnosis of incident cervical cancer (Baltimore women under age 60)

Race	Time	No. of cases	Percent of cases in given clinical stage				
			0	I	II	III	IV
White	1950–1954	449	34.6	23.6	20.1	14.6	7.1
	1955–1959	498	52.8	21.2	14.1	7.6	4.3
	1960–1964	545	63.7	13.5	10.9	9.2	2.6
	1965–1969	540	75.1	8.4	9.4	3.9	3.3
Nonwhite	1950–1954	268	37.0	21.3	17.1	19.4	5.2
	1955–1959	432	49.1	24.9	12.5	9.7	3.7
	1960–1964	501	57.8	18.9	13.2	7.0	3.1
	1965–1969	587	71.1	12.5	7.1	6.7	2.5

Source: Kessler, 1974.

Numerous efforts have been and are still being made to extend Pap testing to women who are not regularly seen by their gynecologists or family physicians. Nevertheless, a certain number of women remain unscreened and probably account for much of the persistent incidence of, and mortality from, cervical cancer in American communities. In all likelihood, non-pregnant, nonwhite women of low socioeconomic status and elderly white women of all classes are those most likely to elude timely cervical cancer detection. Given the existing medical care system in this country, it is difficult to conceive how this group might be identified and screened.

For the future, one might speculate about the possibility of building a universal screening program into the national health insurance program, if and when this program becomes law. For instance, annual or biennial Pap testing might be covered, and letters sent or other follow-up procedures undertaken for each adult female who has not been credited with such a test in the previous 3 or 4 years. The existence of a centralized data bank for serving the insurance program would also make it possible to ensure adequate follow-up for all women with nonnegative Pap test results. Home visits to such patients, as well as to nonrespondents or nonparticipants in other categories by public health nurses or other ancillary medical personnel capable of obtaining a cervical specimen could also be considered, although the costs might prove prohibitive.

Even under optimal circumstances, Pap testing is associated with a small but definite false-negative rate, perhaps on the order of 5% for invasive and 10% for in situ lesions (Graham, Sotto, and Paloucek, 1962). The variability is a function of 1) the number of neoplastic cells shed, 2) localization of the scrape or swab, 3) adequacy of specimen fixation, and 4) characteristics of the women being screened (age, timing of the cycle, hormone balance, menopausal status, and so on).

Self-Screening To circumvent some of the difficulties associated with communitywide Pap testing, techniques have been devised to permit the collection of cytologic specimens by the women themselves. George Papanicolaou first employed a self-administered technique for this purpose, saying, "An intelligent woman can easily be taught to prepare her own smears" (Papanicolaou and Traut, 1943).

The glass pipettes and rubber bulbs of Papanicolaou's laboratory have been replaced by single-unit plastic vaginal irrigation pipettes, most predominantly those developed by Davis in the early 1960s (Davis, 1962). The pipette contains an irrigating and cell preservative solution. In use, it is uncapped, inserted by the woman, squeezed, released, and recapped. It may then be carried or mailed without refrigeration to the laboratory, where the sample is resuspended, centrifuged, and examined microscopically. Two advantages of the irrigation pipette technique are that the sample 1) may be obtained in privacy by the woman herself, and 2) is likely to include exfoliated cells from all parts of the cervix. A possible significant disadvantage is that relatively fewer cells are obtained than from a scraping or swabbing under direct visualization.

Comparable data on the validity of vaginal irrigation and cervical scrapes in detecting cervical neoplasms are scarce. The pipettes have sometimes been evaluated by individuals having little or no experience in their use, as contrasted with their expertise in evaluting the classical Pap smear. In some studies the irrigation tests were performed by physicians; in others, the pipettes were dispensed to patients with printed (but no oral) instructions. Cytotechnologists trained to read Pap smears were sometimes assigned to read the microscopically distinctive irrigation smears. To some extent this may account for the discrepancies in reported false-negative rates associated with the irrigation method. These range from a high of 39% to a low of 0% (Kessler and Aurelian, 1975). As already indicated, false-negative rates for the cervical scrape tend to be lower, although not invariably so. Furthermore, a number of cervical cancers negative on scrape have been detected through vaginal irrigation.

Vaginal irrigation specimens, being cells suspensions, are probably more adaptable to automated screening than Pap smears. Various configurations of scanning microscopes and computers have been designed for the analysis of exfoliated cells, both scraped and suspended. Some are linked to photometers that differentiate between cells of varying optical density. Others incorporate fluorescence photometry, which provides simultaneous measurements of two optical properties of the cells— fluorescence and light absorption or scatter.

Self-administered techniques appear to offer a feasible solution to the problem of periodically screening populations remote from medical centers and pathology laboratories. In the United States, these techniques might be considered for the screening of presumably normal women who, for one reason or another, refuse to appear for periodic examination. In addition, women whose smears are cytologically nonnegative and who do not return for diagnostic confirmation might be monitored temporarily through the mail by means of the self-administered test.

Although the cervical scrape is probably more valid and reliable for screening, especially when performed by a physician under direct visualization of the vaginal vault, there are circumstances in which the self-administered irrigation technique might prove advantageous. Experience has shown that response rates in community Pap testing programs have rarely exceeded 50% or so, overall. In marked contrast is the experience with self-administered vaginal irrigation, where response rates of 90% or higher are not uncommon (Kessler et al., 1974).

The significantly higher acceptance rate for vaginal irrigation, as compared with Pap testing among participants in screening programs, largely compensates for the inferior validity of the pipette. This is illustrated by the theoretical examples in Tables 18 and 19. In the laboratory, that is, once the cytologic specimen has been obtained, the two techniques differ primarily, if at all, in the rate at which they yield false-negative results. Ignoring the complementary (in this case, less important) problem of false positivity, the test validity of the two techniques is assumed to be 90% and 60%, respectively. These figures probably unduly favor the scrape and minimize the true validity of irrigation. In any event, out of every 1,000 women whose specimens actually reach the laboratory, 900 would be effectively screened by the scrape and only 600 by irrigation. The absolute advantage of the scrape here is 30%; its relative advantage is 50%.

Assuming the given rates of test validity, what would happen to the effectiveness of the screening programs in light of the different acceptance

Table 18.   Exfoliative cytology by scrape and irrigation: Estimate of effectiveness in the laboratory

Item	Scrape[a]	Irrigation
Target population	All women scraped	All women irrigated
Test acceptance	~100%	~100%
Test validity[b]	~90%	~60%
Test effectiveness	~90%	~60%
Women effectively screened/1000	900	600

Source: Kessler, 1976.

[a] Advantage of scrape—absolute: 300/1000 = 30%; relative: 300/600 = 50%.

[b] Estimated as complement of false-negative rate.

Table 19. Exfoliative cytology by scrape and irrigation: Estimate of effectiveness in the community

Item	Scrape	Irrigation[a]
Target population	All adult women	All adult women
Test acceptance	~50%	~90%
Test validity[b]	~90%	~60%
Test effectiveness	~45%	~54%
Women effectively screened/1000	450	540

Source: Kessler, 1976.

[a] Advantage of irrigation—absolute: 90/1000 = 9%; relative: 90/450 = 20%.

[b] Estimated as complement of false-negative rate.

levels for the two methods *in the field*, namely, 50% versus 90%? Because of the reluctance of women to appear for Pap testing, only 450 out of the 1,000 sought would be effectively screened. In contrast, irrigation would effectively screen 540 of the target population. The absolute advantage of irrigation in this case is 9%, with a 20% relative advantage.

These figures suggest that cervical scraping remains the best method for detecting early cervical neoplasia among women who can be induced to present themselves for periodic cytologic screening. On the other hand, self-administered methods might be preferred for other types of women.

Other Approaches Another promising method for detecting precancerous cervical lesions would be based on Aurelian's AG-4 and AG-e antigens, described above. Employed in conjunction with regular exfoliative cytologic testing, the sensitivity and specificity of the combined screening method may well prove to exceed that of either the cytologic or immunologic techniques alone. Clinical trials designed to investigate this possibility are now in progress.

Cancer risks could also be reduced by determining the basis for individual differences in susceptibility to cancer and taking appropriate actions related thereto. Thus, although 90% of lung carcinomas are attributable to cigarette smoking, the majority of smokers—even heavy smokers—will never incur a risk of this neoplasm. These individuals are protected by host factors of one type or another, while others, similarly exposed, succumb. A knowledge of the genetic, hormonal, immunologic, or psychosocial factors underlying these differences in susceptibility may eventually make it possible to improve the effectiveness of cancer control programs in the United States. To be sure, knowledge acquired with respect to a pathogenic process may prove inadequate for translation into operational terms. For example, while hereditary predisposition to osteogenic sarcoma, Wilm's tumor, retinoblastoma, and other childhood cancers is recognized, no effective mechanisms for reducing risk or for specifically identifying those at high risk have yet been developed. The same is true for cancer precursors such as intestinal polyposis and xeroderma pigmentosum.

Preventing the Transformation of Normal Cells

Assume that the means to reduce the effectiveness of external agents or to improve human host defenses against cancer prove inadequate. A crucial objective in cancer control would then be to prevent the transformation of normal cells into cancer-forming cells. This might be achieved by elucidating the genetic factors responsible for individual differences in cancer susceptibility. Acquisition of knowledge concerning the epigenetic basis for species differences in cancer, the effects of nutrition on tumor susceptibility, and factors influencing cell proliferation would also be helpful. With respect to the latter, cancer promoters and cocarcinogens, as well as age, hormones, diet, and other factors, affect cell proliferation. The process also appears to be impaired by amino acid deficiency and in diabetes mellitus. We have, for example, observed a significant reduction in the risk of cancer among male diabetics (Kessler, 1970). Species differences in cancer susceptibility are sometimes due to differences in metabolic activation or inactivation of chemical carcinogens, as noted above. They may also stem from species differences in patterns of excretion, capacity for DNA repair, and immunologic competence.

Immunologic surveillance probably plays an important role in preventing the malignant degeneration of cancer precursors but may also be important in preventing the transformation of normal cells. Thus, increasing our knowledge about immunologic mechanisms may not only make it possible to reduce cancer risks in susceptible individuals but may even open the door to the prevention of potentially dangerous cellular transformations. The elucidation of these mechanisms would require the acquisition of new information concerning the nature of the genes responsible for controlling immune responses to preneoplastic antigens.

These may be nonspecific, such as in the sex-linked agamma-globulinemic state where antibodies are absent and where the immune response is simply abolished. On the other hand, specific "immune response" genes (Ir) may possibly exist, and, for example, control human immunologic responses in leukemia. A related question concerns the respective roles of cellular (T cell) and humoral (B cell) components in the immune response to cancer in man.

The relationship of alterations in cell surfaces and membranes to human cancer also needs elucidation if it is to be exploited as a possible means of preventing malignant transformation. Tumor cells have largely escaped from host cell regulatory mechanisms and changes in cell surface membranes are characteristic of the process. An important issue is whether these changes are secondary to the carcinogenic process or of primary etiologic significance to it. There would be great value in determining whether, in specific cancers, there occur specific changes in the cell surface respecting biochemical constituents, physicochemical structure, permeability, rates of synthesis and degradation, social behavior of the tumor cells, and tumor-specific surface antigens.

The means to prevent cell transformations will ultimately be achieved when the mechanisms of normal cell differentiation and dedifferentiation are fully understood. One would like to know how normal cells acquire their differentiated character, what events are necessary to prepare a cell for replication, whether the dedifferentiation occurring when normal cells are transferred to tissue culture predisposes them to transformation, and whether methods can be found to induce precancerous cells to redifferentiate, to kill them, or to block their progression.

If transformation cannot be prevented, then an additional objective in cancer control might be to prevent the development of frank cancer from the transformed cells. To accomplish this would obviously require basic knowledge that does not yet exist. For example, factors affecting interactions between cancer cells and adjacent normal tissue—as this might affect tumor growth—need elucidation. These interactions might involve local immune responses, local vascular responses (e.g., angiogenic factors), and direct cell-to-cell transformation, as well as a search for normal tissue factors that influence metastasis.

Preventing the Development of
Cancer from Transformed Cells

Once the cellular transformation has taken place, an objective of cancer control might be to interfere with tumor development. For example, methods might be devised to induce quiescent microtumors to divide, thereby rendering them more susceptible to antitumor drugs and possibly to antibodies, Whether the application of mathematical models to the carcinogenic process could generate useful new information here is moot. However, models relating to the action of chemotherapeutic agents in cancer have already proved useful and may be more so in the future.

Another possible method for preventing the development of cancer from transformed cells would involve the direction and elimination of neoplastic microfoci. To some extent, the relevant methods exist and are already in use for the early detection of cervical neoplasms or preneoplastic conditions such as cervical dysplasia. Analogous methods are in use—although proving somewhat less effective—in cancers of the urinary bladder, lung, and oral pharynx. Methods need to be devised for transporting detectable substances to the neoplastic microfoci for diagnosis. For example, work is in progress to conjugate specific low energy gamma emitters with specific antitumor antibody molecules to help pinpoint neoplastic microfoci. Specific beta emittors could be conjugated with antibody to deliver a lethal dose to the tumor. This would be analogous to the action of iodine-131, which localizes in thyroid cancers and helps to destroy them.

Assessing Cancer Risks in Individuals and Populations

An essential element in any cancer control program should be the assessment of cancer risks in individuals and population groups of interest. Predictors of high and low cancer risk by specific site need to be developed. Patients who have been irradiated, those with endocrine abnormalities, immune deficiencies, or precancerous conditions such as ulcerative colitis and cystic mastitis would be of special concern. In addition, individuals who have already had a tumor run a greater than average risk of developing a second primary neoplasm. However, because these known high risk groups constitute only a small proportion of those who will subsequently develop cancer, other relevant population groups need to be identified and followed. These might include occupational cohorts, those known to be otherwise heavily exposed to cigarettes or other carcinogens, and the like.

Biochemical markers are needed for the identification of cancer-associated or precancerous states. AG-4, already discussed, may constitute such a marker for those cervical atypias that are destined to transform. With respect to bladder papillomas, we have been attempting to develop discriminants based on a combination of histopathologic and epidemiologic factors for the identification of patients whose lesions are highly likely to progress to invasion. Biologic markers would also be highly desirable for identifying those at highest risk of cancer among patients with Down's syndrome, chronic cystic mastitis, multiple polyposis, pernicious anemia, ulcerative colitis, hemochromatosis, von Recklinghausen's neurofibromatosis, xeroderma pigmentosum, and other preneoplastic states.

The improvement of existing screening tests and diagnostic methods would also make it possible to more effectively evaluate cancer risks in individuals and population groups. Validity, accuracy, reliability, yield, cost, and acceptability are the criteria deemed appropriate for assessing such improvements (Kessler, 1978). Prognostic factors are another essential element in any consideration relating to cancer control. In any given type of tumor, the clinical prognosis may be affected by constitutional factors, immune status, concomitant nonneoplastic diseases, endocrinologic state, psychological factors, as well as diet and certain characteristics of the tumor itself. The development and exploitation of more reliable prognostic indicators would strengthen cancer control at the level of secondary prevention.

Curing or Controlling Cancers in Man

Once a frank cancer has actually developed, cure or clinical control becomes the primary objective. One would hope to achieve this through improvements in surgery, radiotherapy, chemotherapy, or perhaps immunotherapy. Surgery is, of course, the most effective treatment for many neoplasms, although radiotherapy is used in perhaps 40% of cancer patients, either alone or in combination with other modalities of treatment. Chemotherapy is based upon exploitation of differences between normal and malignant cells in respect to their nutritional requirements, metabolic pathways, enzymes, and so on. Any or all of these might be modified in order to realize therapeutic improvements of one kind or another.

Possible avenues for improving immunotherapy would resemble those used to stimulate host resistance to cancer incidence, that is, active immunization with antigenic preparations, passive immunization with specific antitumor antibodies, as well as nonspecific enhancement of the immune responses of patients to their tumors.

Rehabilitating the Cancer Patient

A final objective in cancer control concerns improving the rehabilitation of patients whose cancers have developed and progressed. One would hope to return them to their activities of daily living as soon as possible, to palliate them to the extent possible, and to deal effectively with any associated psychosocial problems. This form of "tertiary prevention" is to be distinguished from the "secondary prevention" of metastases. Secondary prevention, in turn, is to be distinguished from "primary prevention" of the initial neoplastic process, that is, the end most devoutly to be pursued.

Benefits Versus Risks in Cancer Control

In 1963, the Health Insurance Plan of Greater New York (HIP) initiated a controlled clinical trial designed to answer the question, "Does periodic breast cancer screening with mammography and clinical examination result in a reduction in mortality from breast cancer in the female population?" (Shapiro, Strax, and Venet, 1971). The results of the study, which did not permit separate assessments of the two screening techniques, indicated that differences in mortality experience between the screened and unscreened study subjects were concentrated among those of ages 50 to 59 years, with little if any benefits accruing to younger women.

In 1973, a Breast Cancer Detection Demonstration Program (BCDDP) was jointly undertaken by the American Cancer Society and the National Cancer Institute. A total of approximately 280,000 women between the ages of 35 and 74 years—representing the first 10,000 volunteers to appear at each of 28 medical centers across the country—were enrolled in a program calling for annual history taking, physical examination, and mammography screening. During the previous year, a committee of the National Academy of Sciences reviewed evidence on the biologic effects of ionizing radiation and warned that a finite number of breast cancers could be induced by even very low doses of diagnostic radiation if the absence of a threshold dose were assumed (Advisory Committee on the Biological Effects of Ionizing Radiation, 1972).

The HIP study findings, as well as published data on radiation carcinogenesis, were later reviewed by Bailar who concluded that "the routine use of mammography in screening asymptomatic women may eventually take almost as many lives as it saves" (Bailar, 1976). The statement concerned the apparent risks and benefits of radiologic screening in women under 50 years of age, of whom many thousands had enrolled in the BCDDP project. Shortly thereafter, the National Cancer Institute and the American Cancer Society announced that they "cannot recommend the routine use of mammography in screening asymptomatic women of ages 35–50 . . . at this time" (Medical News Item, 1976). The result was a major disruption in the BCDDP project that affected the participation of older women, as well as those under 50, because of a reluctance to expose themselves to potentially carcinogenic radiation.

The complexities of weighing benefits and risks in cancer control are exemplified by the issue of mammographic screening for breast cancer. Eight elements in the decision-making process are discussed below.

1. *Estimating the degree of risk*   Considerable experimental evidence showing that ionizing radiation can cause breast cancer has been published. In extrapolating the results of these studies to humans, Bailar (1976) suggests that four conditions be met: 1) the subjects should not have other diseases related to breast cancer, 2) the radiation doses should be low and repeated at long intervals of time, 3) the types of radiation and energy levels should resemble those used in human mammography, and 4) the radiologic exposures should be limited to the breast and adjacent structures. In his review of the published experimental studies, Bailar concluded that none met all of these conditions. Nevertheless, evidence on the carcinogenic effects of radiation in certain animal species is substantial.

2. *Generalizing from the results of clinical studies*   The incidence of breast cancer is substantially higher among tuberculous women repeatedly fluoroscoped during artificial pneumothorax treatment than among controls (Myrden and Hiltz, 1969). Females exposed to the atomic bombings of Hiroshima and Nagasaki also experienced increased risks of this neoplasm (Wanebo, Johnson, and Sato, 1968).

Furthermore, women x-rayed for postpartum mastitis appear to incur a greater risk of breast cancer than expected (Bross and Blumenson, 1976).

In none of these studies were Bailar's conditions met. The issue could have been resolved by the Breast Cancer Detection Demonstration Program if controls had been selected, or if the cohort of 280,000 had been randomized into screened and unscreened groups. Unfortunately, neither was the case.

3. *Extrapolation of dose effects*   In the published clinical studies, radiation exposures of the subjects tended to be substantially higher than those of healthy screenees. Thus, whereas the average dose to the skin in the HIP study was 7.7 rads, women undergoing repeated fluoroscopy because of artificial pneumothorax therapy are exposed to doses on the order of *150 times greater* (Lester, 1977). Furthermore, with present-day technology it is possible to produce adequate mammographs with skin dose exposures of as little as 0.3 rads, that is, involving *25 times less* radiation than that utilized in the HIP study. The average radiation exposure to women participating in the BCDDP Project has been reduced to 1.2 rads, with a range of 0.2 to 2.5.

These figures suggest that cancer control policies cannot always be established on the basis of studies, albeit competent ones, conducted in earlier years under different sets of prevailing conditions. The broader issues of radiogenic thresholds and the like render animal-to-man or therapeutic radiation-to-diagnostic radiation extrapolations tenuous indeed.

4. *Biases inherent in outcome assessments*   If an asymptomatic woman is screened for cancer, the procedure is likely to advance the time at which her neoplasm would otherwise be detected without in any way affecting its course. This *lead time bias* produces an artifactual increase in the apparent duration of survival among screened cancer patients—a duration which, in fact, may be no greater than that among the unscreened. In screening programs, there is also a much greater likelihood of detecting cancers that are indolent rather than rapidly growing. This is because slow growing neoplasms are more likely to remain clinically asymptomatic than virulent ones that may progress rapidly to death before screening is possible. This *length bias* can usually not be controlled except in the unusual circumstance in which comparable asymptomatic subjects are randomly allocated to screened and nonscreened statuses and followed over prolonged periods of time.

5. *The "definitive" study*   The HIP study is commonly referred to as a unique investigation. It has, in fact, never been replicated. While in one sense this may be a source of pride, in another sense it creates a serious problem. In seeking answers to crucial questions such as those related

to the effectiveness of cancer control measures, should decisions be based upon single studies, however well designed? One wonders why, in the 16 years since the initiation of the HIP study, no comparable endeavor has ever been supported by either federal or private funds. The reason cannot lie in the large size and high cost of the HIP study alone because a number of clinical trials related to the control of other chronic diseases have since been undertaken.

The situation is such as to leave one in the position of having to recommend national policies on mammography for women under age 50 on the basis of studies conducted years ago under radiologic and other conditions substantially different from those existing today. The unfortunate failure to include controls in the BCDDP project already alluded to means that this large study cannot shed additional light on the question.

6. *Other considerations in risk assessment*   Since the risk of breast cancer in subjects who have undergone mammography is related in part to radiation dose, the risk versus benefit equation will obviously vary over time according to prevailing radiologic practices. Thus, as new mammographic equipment reduces exposures, the risks of screening will decline vis-à-vis the benefits. The equation may also change when women at known high risks to breast cancer are selected for screening. For example, women with chronic cystic mastitis or first degree family histories of breast cancer incur substantially increased probabilities of developing breast cancer; to them the hazards of radiogenic screening are relatively insignificant. This situation would contrast with programs in which participants are largely asymptomatic low risk women, especially those at the younger ages.

Lester (1977) has suggested a flexible policy in which mammography would not normally be performed on women under 35 years of age. One screening would be done in the 35–40-year age period, to serve as a baseline against which subsequent mammographic changes possibly indicative of mammary cancer might be measured in later years. Women of ages 50 years and older would receive an annual mammographic examination. The formula provides for a reduction in the frequency of screening among women low in risk factors and in those with prior negative breast mammographs.

Thier (1977) has recommended the regular screening of women over 50, with mammography among those between 40–49 years of age being restricted to women in the highest risk categories.

7. *The "contamination effect" in cancer control*   Despite these well-articulated judgments by experts on the desirability of hierarchical and selective mammographic screening programs, the operational difficul-

ties are formidable. Foremost among these is the difficulty of convincing the majority of women in one age category to undergo a screening procedure that has been deemed hazardous to the health of women in other age categories. The adverse impact of this "contamination effect" is maximal in the public health arena, that is, with respect to community-based screening programs. At the same time, there is a deterrent effect on cancer screening in the private sector as well, because women attended by their own physicians are likely to read and be influenced by what they see and hear. This situation is apt to render a second, and urgently needed, clinical trial on the effectiveness of mammography difficult, if not impossible, to accomplish.

With respect to cancer control at the level of secondary prevention, clinical trials to evaluate the relative effectiveness of surgical modalities provide illuminating examples of the problems encountered. A major one stems from the tendency of surgeons to rely upon methods taught to and employed by them. This tradition runs counter to the rationale of controlled clinical trials, that is, the randomization of patients into specified treatment groups. The consequence is that participating physicians often exclude from study protocol significant numbers of otherwise eligible patients, thus creating problems of patient selectivity and bias. These and other difficulties experienced in the conduct of controlled clinical trials in breast cancer have been admirably summarized by Fisher (1973).

8. *Benefits as a function of costs*   From the HIP study data it is possible to estimate that mammography may reduce the number of breast cancer deaths by perhaps 10% below expectation. If the overall lifetime risk of breast cancer is 7%, then a well-designed mammographic screening program should save 10% of 7%, or 0.7%, of the women screened. In other words, one would have to invest the requisite personnel, time, and other resources in examining 993 healthy women in order to detect seven with early breast cancer. This reduces to 143 normal screenees per breast cancer detected.

Looked at in this fashion, a community-based mammographic screening program might seem expensive because the costs of examining 143 healthy women would have to be deducted from the benefits resulting from one early breast cancer detection. Another way to look at costs, however, is in terms of the benefits achieved by the entire population screened. Each woman who has been screened and found normal is, in a real sense, benefiting from the procedure. Thus, if the total cost of the screening program can be divided among 1,000 women as beneficiaries rather than the seven, calculated per capita costs will fall precipitously. The difference between the two methods of calculating costs may be crucial in mobilizing public and political support for a cancer control program.

Another type of cost needs to be considered in respect to screening procedures entailing substantial numbers of false-positive diagnoses. This is the cost of frightening substantial numbers of healthy persons unnecessarily and impelling them to undergo additional procedures before a definitive diagnosis is reached. While it has not been studied extensively, the false-negative rate in mammography is believed to be relatively small. In other screening modalities (e.g., exfoliative cytology), the false-positive findings are more common and therefore more deserving of attention.

The Pap Test, Still Unvalidated

In recent years, the validity of the Pap test as an effective screen for cervical cancer has come under increasing inquiry. It has been argued that cervical cancer death rates began falling long before the widespread introduction of the Pap test in the 1950s and that the costs of annual screening for cervical cancer are high in comparison with the rather small number of lives saved (Marx, 1979). The Connecticut Division of the American Cancer Society, for example, has estimated that each case of cervical cancer detected by screening in that state in 1974 cost in excess of $3,300. Furthermore, the rate at which cervical neoplasia progresses from its earliest stages to invasion is acknowledged to be very slow, often involving decades of time.

These points, among others, have led to recommendations that cytologic examinations less frequent than once a year would be adequate. A consensus of sorts has been reached with respect to the need for two or three Pap tests within the first year or two of screening to reduce the false-positive rate, followed by less frequent testing thereafter. It is also agreed that high risk women—prostitutes and those infected by genital herpesvirus or showing evidence of AG-4 antibodies—should be screened more often. The same holds true for women with previous marginal or abnormal Pap tests.

The statistics on Pap testing in the United States are somewhat deceptive. They reveal that more than 56 million tests were taken in 1974, of which only 13.5 million represented women being screened for the first time in 1 or 2 years (Marx, 1979). The large majority of these tests involved multiple smears on the same women, that is, those with dysplasias or other cytologic abnormalities in need of attention. The Pap testing of such women should not be considered screening but rather a component part of their diagnostic regimen.

Another factor contributing to costs is the fact that, in every country, a certain number of women, for one reason or another, elude regular exfoliative cytologic testing, both public and private, while others are screened excessively without reference to need. The challenge is to reach those unscreened women who are at high risk and to reduce the unnecessary testing of others.

We recently had an opportunity to evaluate the characteristics of women who respond to Pap test screening campaigns. A free Pap test program was inaugurated by a voluntary health agency in a Maryland county. Appeals for participation were made primarily through local newspapers, television, and radio, as well as local community organizations. Despite these efforts, screenees turned out to be far more educated, of considerably higher socioeconomic status and otherwise less in need of a Pap test than the women of the county as a whole. In contrast with all county residents, for example, only about 7% of the respondents had never had a previous Pap test and all but 22% had had their last test within the previous 24 months. All but 15% could name the private physician to whom they wished the results of the test to be sent (Kessler, 1978).

These findings suggest that new methods must be developed for the screening of high risk women who are most at need. The self-administered cytodiagnostic technique may prove more acceptable to women out of the mainstream who do not have a gynecologist, who dislike the disrobing and physical manipulations associated with classical Pap testing, or who simply cannot spend sufficient time to make the necessary appointment or clinic visit.

Of all the major neoplasms, cervical cancer appears to be the one that best meets the accepted criteria for the suitability of a mass screening test, namely, 1) it is an important health problem; 2) its pathogenesis, including development from latent to overt disease, is well established; 3) it traverses a recognizable latent or early symptomatic state; 4) suitable screening tests are available; 5) Pap testing is acceptable to most target populations; 6) well-accepted treatments for cervical cancer are available; and 7) pathologists are in agreement on the various preinvasive stages of the disease (Kessler, 1978).

What is currently lacking is strong epidemiologic evidence on the effectiveness of cytologic screening in reducing mortality from cervical cancer. This need could be addressed by conducting a randomized clinical trial in which one group of previously unscreened women were periodically Pap tested while a second served as controls. To secure the requisite numbers of subjects, the study would probably have to be conducted in one of the less developed countries where relatively few women are presently being screened.

Priorities in Cancer Control

As in essentially all areas of public interest, funds and resources for cancer control activities are limited, and priorities must be fixed. But how, by whom, and on what basis? Cancer control agencies, supported by public funds and accountable to the Congress or state legislatures, tend to favor action programs of high visibility. Federal research funding agencies, on the other hand, seek to renew their budgets each year on the basis of the quality of research supported by them. Preference sometimes appears to be given to projects that address the lay public's concerns rather than those deemed important by the scientific community.

Research scientists today find themselves caught on the horns of a dilemma, namely, the desire to pursue the most promising research leads and the need to survive by generating grant support. The latter need is best accomplished by responding to government requests for research in specified areas, irrespective of one's scientific preferences; the former invokes a more intellectual—and therefore sometimes less practical—calling. A solution to the problem must take account of the competing needs of all interested parties: the government, the biomedical community, and the lay public.

A somewhat more empirical and less structured cancer control program might prove to be more effective at a time when the questions to be asked are many and the answers are few. A less structured program would entail fewer long-term financial commitments to projects specified by government officials and a renewed emphasis on competitive, peer-reviewed grants submitted by the academic community. When, for example, a promising new advance in cancer chemotherapy appears likely, its development can be supported. The impressive therapeutic advances in leukemia, choriocarcinoma, and Burkitt's lymphoma were encouraged in this fashion. In addition to research and development, funds should be allocated for evaluation and decision making in cancer control. Thus, questions relating to the effectiveness of CT scanning in the detection of brain tumors, mammography in breast cancer, and exfoliative cytology in cervical cancer can—once and for all—be answered.

Such goals cannot be achieved overnight. They mandate the recruitment into biomedicine and the subsequent support of a new generation of young and well-trained individuals whose minds can be unleashed in the scientific service of the nation. All too often recent graduates in biomedicine tend to seek the safe confines of a research team within which to pursue financial security, academic tenure, and (sometimes only incidentally) opportunities for independent research.

After joining a research team, the cancer scientist is often locked into a system that does not or cannot permit the intellectual freedom and latitude to pursue his or her own scientific interests, however promising, at the expense of the institutional interests. Members of such teams may discover that a cancer center, in accepting a five or a 10 million dollar grant, has encumbered itself with a myriad of constraints, including a prepackaged and sometimes unimaginative cancer research program.

This situation contrasts with that of not so many years ago, when young people opting for careers in cancer research would join a university department and be encouraged to develop their own scientific interests in whatever aspects of the cancer problem they felt they could make a contribution. It was probably this open and freewheeling academic system that encouraged personal initiative and led to the assumption of world leadership in medicine and bioscience by the United States in recent decades. This is quite different from systems elsewhere in which professors are surrounded by sycophants and in which governments themselves not only make the operational decisions but set the scientific priorities as well.

In addition to generating new ideas in cancer control, hundreds, or perhaps thousands, of old ideas are in need of being resolved. Is obesity related to neoplasia of the breast, endometrium, and gallbladder? What is the basis for the association between alcohol and upper respiratory and gastrointestinal cancers? Are the arsenicals naturally present in food carcinogenic in man? Are the factors responsible for nasopharyngeal cancer in Chinese the same. as those that are operative among nickel and metal refinery workers? Can fortification of bread with iron and B vitamins reduce the risk of thyroid and hypopharyngeal cancers? How are gastric ulcers related to stomach cancer, gallstones to gallbladder cancer, and diabetes mellitus and pancreatitis to pancreatic cancer? Can asbestos alone, independent of cigarette smoking, cause mesothelioma? Does circumcision per se protect against penile cancer? Are ovarian cysts precancerous? Do condyloma acuminata predispose to vulvar cancer? Are only the genetically predisposed susceptible to sunlight-induced melanomas? Can hereditary retinoblastomas be distinguished from those that are not hereditary? Can cytogenetic studies contribute to the detection of individuals at high risk of leukemia and other neoplasms? Is Hodgkin's disease infectious?

These and a myriad of other questions remain to be resolved before cancer in humans can be effectively controlled. An effective public policy would provide the means for setting priorities among the many possible research initiatives, if only because sufficient funds will never be available for scientists to pursue them all. Decisions respecting the allocation of resources to specific operational control programs will continue to be based largely on the perceived needs of the general public and their elected representatives.

REFERENCES

Advisory Committee on the Biological Effects of Ionizing Radiation 1972. The Effects on Populations of Exposure to Low Levels of Ionizing Radiation (BEIR Report). National Academy of Sciences, National Research Council, Washington, D.C.
Agricola, G. 1556. De Re Metallica, Basel.

52   Kessler

Aurelian, L., Schumann, B., Marcus, R. L., and Davis, H. J. 1973. Antibody to
    HSV-2 induced tumor-specific antigens in serums from patients with cervical
    carcinoma. Science 181:161–164.
Aurelian, L., Strnad, B. C., and Smith, M.F. 1977. Immunodiagnostic potential of a
    virus-coded, tumor-associated antigen (AG-4) in cervical cancer. Cancer
    39:1834–1849.
Axtell, L. M., Cutler, S. J., and Myers, M. H. 1972. End Results in Cancer, Report
    No. 4. U.S. Government Printing Office, U.S. Department of Health, Education,
    and Welfare, Publication No. (NIH) 73-272, Washington, D.C.
Axtell, L. M., and Myers, M. H. 1975. Recent trends in survival of cancer patients.
    1960–1971. U.S. Department of Health, Education, and Welfare, Publication No.
    (NIH) 75-767, Washington, D.C.
Bailar, John C., III 1976. Mammography: A contrary view. Ann. Intern. Med.
    84:77–84.
Bailar, John C., III, King, H., and Mason, M. J. 1964. Cancer rates and risks. U.S.
    Government Printing Office, U.S. Public Health Service Publication No. 1148,
    Washington, D.C.
Bross, I. D. J., and Blumenson, L. 1976. Screening random asymptomatic women
    under 50 by annual mammographies: Does it make sense? J. Surg. Oncol.
    8:437–445.
Butlin, H. T. 1892. Three lectures on cancer of the scrotum in chimney sweeps and
    others. Br. Med. J. 1:1341; 2:66.
Centanni, E., and Rezzesi, F. 1926. Studio Sperimentale Sull'antagonismo fra tuber-
    culosi e cancro. Riv. Med. 42:195–200.
Davignon, L., Lemonde, P., Robillard, P., and Frappier, A. 1970. B. C. G. vaccina-
    tion and leukemia mortality. Lancet 2:638.
Davignon, L., Lemonde, P., St-Pierre, J., and Frappier, A. 1971. B. C. G. vaccina-
    tion and leukemia mortality. Lancet 1:80–81.
Davis, H. J. 1962. The irrigation smear: Accuracy in detection of cervical cancer.
    Acta Cytol. 6:459–467.
Fisher, B. 1973. Cooperative clinical trials in primary breast cancer: A critical
    appraisal. Cancer 31:1271–1286.
Golberg, L. 1975. Safety evaluation concepts. J. Assoc. Off. Anal. Chem.
    58:635–644.
Gold, P., Wilson, T., Romero, R., Shuster, J., and Freedman, O. 1973. Immunology
    and cancer: Further evaluation of the radioimmunoassay for carcinoembryonic
    antigen of the human digestive system as an adjunct to cancer diagnosis. Dis.
    Colon Rectum 16:358–365.
Graham, J. B., Sotto, L. S. J., and Paloucek, F. P. 1962. Carcinoma of the Cervix.
    W. B. Saunders Company, Philadelphia.
Herbst, A. L., Poskanzer, D. C., Robboy, S. J., Friedlander, L., and Scully, R. E.
    1975. Prenatal exposure to stilbestrol: A prospective comparison of exposed
    female offspring with unexposed controls. N. Engl. J. Med. 292:334–339.
Hieger, I. 1949. Chemical carcinogenesis: Review. Br. J. Ind. Med. 6:1–23.
Kaiser, R. F., Erickson, C. C., Everett, B. E., Jr., Gilliam, A. G., Graves, L. M.,
    Walton, M., and Sprunt, D. H. 1960. Initial effect of communitywide cytologic
    screening on clinical stage of cervical cancer detected in an entire community.
    Results of Memphis-Shelby County, Tennessee Study. J. Natl. Cancer Inst.
    25:863–881.

Kennaway, E. L. 1924. Formation of cancer-producing substance from isoprene (2-methyl-butadiene). J. Path. Bacteriol. 27:233–238.

Kennaway, E. L. 1925. Experiments on cancer-producing substances. Br. Med. J. 2:1–4.

Kennaway, E. L., and Hieger, I. 1930. Carcinogenic substances and their fluorescence spectra. Br. Med. J. 1:1044–1046.

Kessler, I. I. 1970. Cancer mortality among diabetics. J. Natl. Cancer Inst. 44:673–686.

Kessler, I. I. 1974. Cervical cancer epidemiology in historical perspective J. Reprod. Med. 12:172–184.

Kessler, I. I. 1976. Mortality from cervical cancer: Can it be prevented now? Compr. Ther. 2:38–47.

Kessler, I. I. 1978. Case finding and mass screening in the early detection of disease. In: Tice's Practice of Medicine, vol. 1, ch. 22. Harper & Row, Hagerstown, Md.

Kessler, I. I., and Aurelian, L. 1975. Uterine cervix cancer. In: Schottenfeld, D. (ed.), Cancer Epidemiology and Prevention: Current Concepts, ch. 11. Charles C Thomas, Springfield, Ill.

Kessler, I. I., Kulcar, Z., Rawls, W. E., Smerdel, S., Strnad, M., and Lilienfeld, A. M. 1974. Cervical cancer in Yugoslavia. I. Antibodies to genital herpesvirus in cases and controls. J. Natl. Cancer Inst. 52:369–376.

Kinlen, L. J., and Pike, M. C. 1971. B. C. G. vaccination and leukemia: Evidence of vital statistics. Lancet 2:389–402.

Knowelden, J., and Phillips, A. J. (eds.) 1974. An evaluation of cancer control measures, vol. 16. UICC Technical Report Series, Geneva.

Lester, R. G. 1977. Risk versus benefit in mammography. Diagn. Radiol. 124:1–6.

Leuenberger, S. G. 1912. Die unter dem Einfluss der synthetischen Farbenindustrie beobachtete Geschwulstentwicklung. Beitr Z Klin Chir., Tübing. 80:208–316.

Levin, David L., Devesa, S. S., Godwin, J. D., and Silverman, D. T. 1974. Cancer rates and risks, 2nd edition. U.S. Government Printing Office, U.S. Department of Health, Education, and Welfare, Publication No. (NIH) 75–691, Washington, D.C.

Levy, N. L., Mahaley, M. S., Jr., and Day, E. D. 1972. Serum-mediated blocking of cell-mediated anti-tumor immunity in a melanoma patient: Association with BCG immunotherapy and clinical deterioration. Intl. J. Cancer 10:244–248.

Lilienfeld, Abraham M., Levin, M. L., and Kessler, I. I. 1972. Cancer in the United States. Vital and Health Statistics Monographs, American Public Health Association, Harvard University Press, Cambridge, Mass.

Loeffler, F. 1901. Einer Neue Behandlungsmethode des Karzinoms. Deutsche med. Wchnschr 27:725–726.

Mackaness, G. B. 1964. The immunological basis of acquired cellular resistance. J. Exp. Med. 120:105–120.

Martland, H. S., and Humphries, R. E. 1929. Osteogenic sarcoma in dial painters using luminous paint. Arch. Pathol. 7:406–417.

Marx, J. 1979. The annual Pap smear: An idea whose time has gone? Science 205:177–178.

Medical News Item. 1974. B. C. G. transfer factor and Hodgkin's disease. JAMA 227:131–133.

Medical News Item. 1976. JAMA 236:1223.

Morton, D. L., Eilber, F. R., Joseph, W. L., Wood, W. C., Trahan, E., and Ketcham, A. S. 1970. Immunological factors in human sarcomas and melanomas: A rational basis for immunotherapy. Ann. Surg. 172:740–749.

Myrden, J. A., and Hiltz, J. E. 1969. Breast cancer following multiple fluoroscopies during artificial pneumothorax treatment of pulmonary tuberculosis. Can. Med. Assoc. J. 100:1032–1034.

National Institutes of Health. 1974. Digest of scientific recommendations for the National Cancer Program. U.S. Department of Health, Education, and Welfare, Publication No. 74-570, Washington, D.C.

National Institutes of Health. 1974. National Cancer Program Operational Plan FY 1976–1980. U.S. Department of Health, Education, and Welfare, Publication No. 75-777, Washington, D.C.

Office of Technology Assessment. 1977. Cancer testing technology and saccharin. U.S. Government Printing Office, Washington, D.C.

Old, L. J., and Clarke, D. A. 1959. Effect of *Bacillus Calmette-Guérin* infection on transplanted tumours in the mouse. Nature 184:291–292.

Papanicolaou, G. N., and Traut, H. F. 1943. Diagnosis of uterine cancer by the vaginal smear. The Commonwealth Fund, New York.

Pott, P. 1775. Chirurgical Observations Relative to the Cataract, the Polypus of the Nose, the Cancer of the Scrotum, the Different Kinds of Ruptures, and the Mortification of the Toes and Feet. Hawes, Clarke and Collins, London.

Rehn, L. 1895. Blasengeschwülste bei Fuchsin-Arbeitern. Arch. Klin Chir. 50:588–600.

Rosenthal, S. R., Crispen, R. G., Thorne, M. G., Piekarski, N., Raisys, N., and Rettig, P. G. 1972. B. C. G. vaccination and leukemia mortality. JAMA 222:1543–1544.

Rostoski, O., Saupe, E., and Schmorl, G. 1926. Die Bergkrankheit der Erzbergleute in Schneeberg in Sachsen ("Schneeberger Lungenkrebs") Ztschr. f. Krebsforsch., Berl., 23:360–384.

Segi, M., and Kurihara, M. 1972. Cancer Mortality for Selected Sites in 24 Countries, no. 6 (1966–1967), Japan Cancer Society, Nagoya, Japan.

Shapiro, S., Strax, P., and Venet, L. 1971. Periodic breast cancer screening in reducing mortality from breast cancer. JAMA 215:1777–1785.

Southam, A. H., and Wilson, S. R. 1922. Cancer of the Scrotum. Br. Med. J. 2:971–973.

Sparks, F. C., Silverstein, M. J., Hunt, J. S., Haskell, C. M., Pilch, Y. H., and Morton, D. L. 1973. Complications of BCG immunotherapy in patients with cancer. N. Engl. J. Med. 289:827–830.

Strnad, B. C., and Aurelian, L. 1978. Proteins of Herpesvirus Type 2, III: Isolation and Immunologic Characterization of a Large Molecular Weight Viral Protein. Virology 87:401–415.

Süss, R., Kinzel, V., and Scribner, J. D. 1973. Cancer, Experiments and Concepts. Springer Verlag, New York.

Thier, S. O. 1977. Breast cancer screening: A view from outside the controversy. N. Engl. J. Med. 297:1064–1065.

Von Frieben, O. 1902. Demonstration Eines Cancroid des Rechten Handruckens, Das Sich Nach Langdaurender Einwirkung von Roentgenstrahlen Entwickelt Hatte. Fortschr. Roentgenstr. 6:106.

Von Volkmann, R. 1875. Beiträge Chirurgie, Breitkopf und Härtel, Leipzig.

Wagner, J. C., Sleggs, C. A., and Marchand, P. 1960. Diffuse pleural mesothelioma and asbestos exposure in the North Western Cape Province. Br. J. Ind. Med. 17:260–271.

Wanebo, C. K., Johnson, K. G., and Sato, K. 1968. Breast cancer after exposure to the atomic bombings of Hiroshima and Nagasaki. N. Engl. J. Med. 279:667–671.

Yamagiwa, K., and Itchikawa, K. 1918. Pathogenesis of Carcinoma. J. Cancer Res. 3:1.

Zbar, B., Bernstein, I. D., and Rapp, H. J. 1971. Suppression of tumor growth at the site of infection with living *Bacillus Calmette-Guèrin*. J. Natl. Cancer Inst. 46:831–839.

2

Prospects for Cancer Control through Diagnosis and Screening

Nathaniel I. Berlin

In principle, there are three ways of controlling disease. The first is by pre-vention, a method that generally requires knowledge of the cause. The second is effective treatment. For the neoplastic diseases, this would be defined in terms of a high cure rate, a low toxicity, and ready availability, preferably at low cost. The third method, which applies particularly although not exclusively to cancer, is to achieve a diagnosis of the disease at a stage in which the available therapy is effective.

What are the prospects for cancer control through diagnostic means? Our discussion can best begin with a brief and somewhat simplistic review of what might be called the biology of cancer. There are three stages in the evolution of solid tumors. Not considered here are the relatively infrequent lymphomas and leukemias that cannot be classified in this manner.

CANCER STAGES

In Stage I, every transformed cell is confined to the organ of origin. In Stage II, the cancer has spread to regional lymph nodes. In Stage III, there are distant metastases, most commonly in the lungs, liver, brain, and bone, but with no organ totally exempt. This is a simple staging system, possibly the simplest that can be devised. More complex systems have been developed by the American Joint Committee for Cancer Staging and End Results Reporting and by the International Union Against Cancer. These classification systems, were, however, developed for other purposes.

This work was supported in part by a grant from the National Cancer Institute CA-15145.

The simple three-stage system has several implications in the design of programs for either the diagnosis or the treatment of cancer. In order for this system to be useful in cancer control, one must have some idea about how much time a given patient spends in a certain stage. Such knowledge is necessary for each organ site and for the more common cancers of each organ. Figure 1 presents a schematic representation of the three cancer stages in terms of tumor size, metastasis, symptoms, and diagnosability.

There is good reason to believe that, for most cancers, the first stage may last for several years from the initial transformation event. Stage I is depicted as long and Stage II as relatively short; that is, once the tumor has spread to the regional lymph nodes, it has likely spread elsewhere. This is certainly true for breast cancer. For example, in 75% of the cases in which the disease has spread to regional nodes, there is evidence of distant metastases (Fisher, et al., 1975). Stage III is considerably more variable.

The duration of each stage varies widely from one tumor type to another. Some variation may exist within given tumor types as well, although this is probably not as great. For example, the interval between the

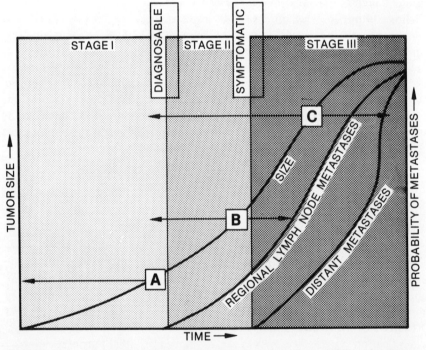

Figure 1.   Schematic representation of the growth of a tumor, the probability of metastases, and when a tumor is diagnosable or symptomatic, by clinical stage.

peak incidence of carcinoma *in situ* and invasive cancer of the uterine cervix may be on the order of 10 years. Thus Stage I is likely to last for 10 years or so (Galvin and De Linde, 1949). Saccomanno it al. (1965) offer data consistent with the suggestion that for carcinoma of the lung Stage I may be of several years' duration. The data reveal that, while some smokers have cancer cells in their sputum, years often elapse before the cancer itself can be localized.

Today, perhaps two-thirds of all cancers are diagnosed in Stage III rather than in the more treatable Stages I and II. After making three assumptions, it is not difficult to calculate how long it should take for a cancer to become diagnosable or clinically evident through the production of symptoms. The required assumptions are: 1) that cancer cells are of a fixed average volume, 2) that there is a constant generation time, and 3) that there is a division of each daughter cell.

These simplifying assumptions probably apply well to the early phases of most neoplasms, but become progressively less appropriate as the cancers become larger. With tumor growth, the generation time may increase, and more importantly, the interval between cell divisions becomes so long that some daughter cells may not divide at all. The net effect is to slow down the rate of tumor growth. For example, assuming a 2-month generation time and a cell with a volume 10 times that of a red cell, it can be calculated that 3 ½ years would elapse before the tumor achieves a diameter of 1 cm. For most cancers, this is the lower size limit for tumors that can be diagnosed. Under the same assumptions, the tumor mass would attain a volume of 1 liter in another 22 months.

The probability of metastases is depicted in Figure 1. Symptoms tend to occur late, and some cancers can be diagnosed before the occurrence of symptoms. The goal of cancer control through diagnostic means is to make the diagnosis before metastasis has occurred, that is, in Stage I.

Figure 1 also demonstrates that the proportion of a cancer's biologic life span that is known to the patient and to the physician is small in relation to the total life span of the cancer. This is of great significance in cancer control because of the implication that cancers remain confined to the organ of origin for long periods of time. This provides a rigorous basis for the definition of "early diagnosis" in terms of tumors in Stage I. The proof that a diagnosis has in fact been made "early" would require long-term follow-up because this definition implies that there are no metastases. Therefore, if the cancer is removed, the patient should experience a normal life expectancy. It is evident that the demonstration of early diagnosis can be made only in a group of patients, not in individual patients.

The therapeutic consequence of the detection of a tumor in Stage I is that, if it can be located, removal would prove truly curative. This could also apply to patients in Stage II, when removal of all cancer cells is technically possible. However, for Stage III cancers, some form of systemic therapy is necessary for cure, the only caveat being that the etiologic agent of the tumor does not cause a second neoplasm. Bilaterality and multicentricity of lesions are common in carcinoma of the breast and possibly for carcinoma of the lung. It must also be recognized that if one removes every last cancer cell, a cure will result, but that, at the same time, relatively few cures have been obtained in the treatment of clinically diagnosed metastatic tumors.

Chemotherapists currently evaluate their results in terms of remissions, complete or partial. Complete remissions are usually defined by the absence of residual tumor. I would like to suggest, as others have done, that we consider patients "cured" when their survival becomes equivalent to that of the normal population. This approach cannot be applied to individual cancer patients but can be utilized for populations of patients and matching controls.

Given our present knowledge concerning the biology of cancer and the current status of cancer treatment modalities, cancer control through diagnostic means is theoretically possible if methods can be found and systems developed to detect malignancies before metastasis has occurred.

CANCER DIAGNOSIS

The research efforts undertaken by the National Cancer Institute in cancer diagnosis have been considerably more modest that those related to the etiology or to the development of drugs for treatment. At the same time, over the past quarter of a century, the American Cancer Society has sponsored programs advocating early diagnosis and publicizing "early warning signals." Unfortunately, the well-known early warning signals of cancer more often than not occur late in the course of the disease. As a matter of fact, it can be estimated that approximately two-thirds of cancer patients at the time of their definitive initial treatment have metastatic disease.

The probability of metastases at the time of diagnosis for seven common neoplasms is shown in Table 1. The curves were derived from the relative survival rates, i.e., the ratio of patients alive with cancer at time t compared to those alive in a matched control population at time t.

At some point in time the rate of change in both populations becomes the same and the relative survival curve becomes horizontal (Figure 2). From this it is possible to determine what fraction of the cancer population has normal survival characteristics. This group can be assumed to be free of metastases at the time of the initial diagnosis and treatment. The fraction

Table 1. Probability of metastases at time of
diagnosis

Organ site	Probability (percent)
Pancreas	99
Lung	93
Prostate	69
Large bowel	59
Breast	52
Uterine cervix	47
Uterine corpus	32

RELATIVE SURVIVAL =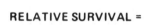

% PATIENTS WITH CANCER
SURVIVING AT TIME t
―――――――――――――――――――
% SURVIVING IN A COMPARABLE
(MATCHED) POPULATION WITHOUT
CANCER AT TIME t

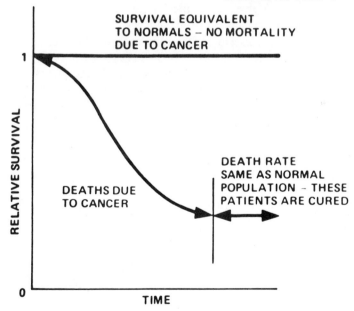

Figure 2. Schematic representation of the survival of a population of cancer patients relative
to that of a matched normal population.

ranges from a low of 32% for uterine corpus to a high of 99% for pancreas cancer. This is sometimes not appreciated, because in most patients micrometastases cannot be diagnosed by current techniques. The evidence for their existence is that months or years after the removal of the primary neoplasm distant metastases become apparent. These metastases were present all along, although unrecognized, and in fact were unrecognizable by current diagnostic techniques, short of multiple "shotgun" biopsies of many organs.

The diagnostic process itself can be divided into three stages. The first stage is screening in order to identify those in the population with a high probability of cancer. It is hoped that those screened will not yet have metastatic disease. Screening programs are also undertaken to identify those symptomatic individuals who have not yet visited a physician. This may be a large group. A second stage in the process is to ascertain the presence or absence of cancer in the high risk screenees and the third stage is to estimate the extent of the disease. On the basis of such information, a treatment plan can be developed and a prognosis made.

Determination of the population at risk is an essential component of cancer control. For practical purposes the population at risk may be regarded as females over the age of 40 and males over the age of 45. There is one exception, namely, that females over 21 should be considered at risk for cervical cancer. Cigarette smokers and some industrial workers constitute relatively unique high risk groups for particular cancers (e.g., lung) which occur predominantly among them. In large measure the population at risk is defined in Table 2, which shows the ages at which screening should be initiated, by organ site. This was determined as the age at which the age-specific incidence begins to take a sharp upward turn. Ninety percent or more of the tumors in these organs will occur above the age given in Table 2.

Four organ sites account for 52% of all cancers (Table 3). They are the breast, bowel, lung, and uterus. Another six organs are the site of 23% of

Table 2.   Age at which cancer site-specific screening should begin[a]

Cancer site	Age (years)
Uterine cervix	20
Breast	35–40
Lung (males)	45
(females)	55
Bowel	50
Uterine corpus	50
Bladder	55
Prostate	60

[a] Ninety percent or more of the tumors at the given cancer site occur at or above the given age.

Table 3.   Relative frequency of cancer by organ site

Organ site	Relative frequency (percent)
Large bowel	14.0
Uterus (cervical and corpus)	13.1
Breast	12.9
Lung	12.0
Prostate	7.4
Bladder	4.0
Stomach	3.3
Pancreas	2.9
Lymphoma	2.9
Ovary	2.4
All others	25.1

the neoplasms, while the remaining 25% are divided among a wide variety of organs in the body. From these figures it is apparent that the breast, lung, bowel, uterus, and prostate are those organs that should be most intensively screened.

SCREENING TESTS

How can one practice cancer control through diagnostic means in a population? This must obviously be done through screening tests. These tests should be simple, relatively inexpensive, suitable for automation or execution by paramedical personnel, and deliverable to large population groups. The screening tests need not yield a definitive answer because this is the objective of diagnostic tests. The latter are also employed to determine the extent of disease and hence to serve as a basis for prognosis.

Before screening tests are used they must be evaluated critically. Evaluation may take place at various levels but the most important is the following: If a test for cancer of a given organ is applied to a population, will it result in a reduction in mortality from that cancer, and if so, in how much of a reduction? I believe that this type of evaluation can best be done in a randomized controlled clinical trial, in which some patients are given the test while others are allowed to follow their usual pattern of obtaining medical care.

To date, no screening program has yet matched these criteria. The Health Insurance Plan (HIP) study of Shapiro et al. (1973) for carcinoma of the breast was designed to assess the mortality reduction attributable to screening and to evaluate the response rates of the women who were offered the test. Only 20,000 out of the 30,000 women offered the examination responded, and only 14,000 of these women completed the entire screening protocol. There is as yet no comparable study on the effectiveness of screening for carcinoma of the cervix by means of the Pap test. It is widely believed that the Pap test has reduced mortality from carcinoma of the cervix, although some question this. Certainly, it must be acknowledged that mortality from uterine cancer began to decline before the Pap test was introduced. Furthermore, not many women have had more than a single Pap test. One is justified perhaps, in suggesting that the Pap test has reduced cervical cancer mortality, but the extent of this reduction is at present difficult to determine.

Screening tests can be evaluated in terms of the absolute numbers of cancer cases they detect compared with numbers predicted on the assumption of no screening. They can also be assessed, in a less precise fashion, in terms of the stage at which the cancer is detected, that is, how large the tumor is and whether the cancer has spread to the lymph nodes or beyond. Screening programs can be rated in terms of sensitivity and specificity; that is, how many who have cancer are identified, and how many who do not have cancer are correctly so designated.

Before screening tests can be advocated for use on a large scale, other significant questions require resolution. The most important of these, given a valid screening test, concerns the frequency of the screening examinations. Very little is presently known about this, and we must await the development of theories and the design of studies to test them.

To some extent the answers will depend upon the end points used. I am indebted to Dr. Michael Schwartz of the Michigan Cancer Research Foundation for emphasizing alternative end points. One end point is increased life expectancy in the screened population, and another is the proportion of patients cured, or those attaining normal life expectancy. Intensive and successful screening for disease that occurs at a young age would necessarily result in a higher percentage increase in life expectancy than would a comparable program in an older age group.

Some idea of the complexities in determining the optimum frequency of screening can be gained from the following sequence. If one starts with the assumption that an individual has cancer and applies a screening test, then ideally the test should be positive. Technical errors may occur and the test result may be negative, or the test itself may not be sufficiently sensitive and thus read negative. If one repeats the test after a short interval and the technical errors are eliminated, the reading may be positive. But in some instances the test may still lack sufficient sensitivity and the result would still be negative. At some later date the test will become positive. It is not known precisely when during the clinical course of a given cancer a screening test becomes positive. This will, of course, vary with the test and the cancer. Tests based on exfoliative cytology have the capacity to become positive very early;

carcinoembryonic antigen (CEA) on the other hand, becomes positive too late for successful treatment in most instances of colon cancer.

Given the answers to the scientific questions, a variety of societal questions remains. Since these involve expenditures of one kind or another, they can be considered in terms of cost benefit ratios. How can a screening test be applied to all or most individuals in a population? Who benefits? How can all those over the age of 40 be enrolled? What methods can be used to maintain their participation?

Such questions cannot yet be fully answered. They will be answered in part if third party carriers are willing to pay for screening examinations. In part the answers will come from the development of lifetime record systems and from the maintenance of records in data banks of one sort or another. The techniques for creating and maintaining such record files exist; access to them can be as close as the nearest telephone.

Implementing an effective diagnostic cancer control program may be expensive, but if the diagnostic efforts can, in fact, accomplish for other solid tumors what has already been done for breast cancer and what is probably about to be done for lung cancer, then an organized program becomes both desirable and feasible.

A brief summary of screening tests is perhaps in order. Screens can be classified as either cytologic or chemical tests. The screens presently used for lung cancer include sputum cytology and x-rays. A test based on aryl hydrocarbon hydroxylase inducibility in lymphocytes, which is aimed at identifying the high risk group within the smoking population, is in development. Screens for breast cancer include physical examination, x-rays, and thermography; cytologic and ultrasound techniques are also being developed. For bowel cancer there is a test for occult blood, the digital rectal examination, and sigmoidoscopy, while a cytologic approach is being explored. For uterine cervix cancer detection, "do it yourself" kits should be evaluated as supplements or alternatives in given situations to Pap tests. The rectal examination is a traditional screening technique for prostate cancer, although ultrasound may prove to be of value.

If new detection methods, whether immunologic or serologic, that screen cancers earlier in their biologic life can be developed, then an even greater reduction in mortality is possible.

CONCLUSIONS

The following is a summary of the highlights in this chapter.

1. The biologic life of most cancers is such that there is probably a long period (Stage I) preceding the development of metastases.

2. Stage I is more often than not asymptomatic.
3. Currently, two out of every three patients have metastases at the time of diagnosis, but in most patients these are not recognized. Symptoms are, therefore, a late manifestation of cancer.
4. To reduce cancer mortality through screening we must search for cancer in asymptomatic individuals.
5. The population at risk of cancer is large.
6. There is no simple screening test now available.
7. The optimum frequency of screening intervals is not presently known.
8. Once adequate screening programs are instituted, compliance by the population at risk will become a major consideration in planning cancer control programs.
9. Current screening techniques can probably reduce cancer mortality; they have been shown to do so for breast cancer.
10. A screening program is one method for reducing cancer mortality. Until and if other approaches succeed, the necessary research underlying the development of diagnostic cancer control programs should be supported.

REFERENCES

Fisher, B., Slack, N., Katrych, P., and Wolmark, N. 1975. Ten year follow-up. Results of patients with carcinoma of the breast in a cooperative clinical trial evaluating surgical adjuvant chemotherapy. Surg. Gynecol. Obstet. 140:528–534.
Galvin, G. A. and Te Linde, R. W. 1949. The present day status of noninvasive cervical carcinoma. Am. J. Obst. Gynecol. 57:15–36.
Goldman, L. B. 1963. Early Cancer. Grune & Stratton, New York.
Mass Health Examinations. 1971. World Health Organizations, New York.
O'Donnell, W. E., Day, E., and Venet, L. 1962. Early detection and diagnosis of cancer. C. V. Mosby Company, St. Louis, Mo.
Proceedings of the National Conference on Advances in Cancer Management. Part II: Detection and Diagnosis. 1976. Cancer. January. [The papers in the supplement provide an excellent summary of this subject area.].
Saccomanno, G., Saunders, R. P., Archer, V. E., Auerbach, O., Ruschner, M., and Beckler, P. A. 1965. Cancer of the lung: The cytology of sputum prior to the development of carcinoma. Acta Cytol. 9:413–423.
Screening in Medical Care. 1968. Oxford University Press, New York.
Shapiro, S., Strax, P., Venet, L., and Venet, M. 1973. Changes in five-year breast cancer mortality in a breast cancer screening program, pp. 663–678. Presented at the Seventh National Cancer Conference. Lippincott Company, Philadelphia.
Wilson, J. M. G., and Jungner, G. 1968. Principles and practice of screening for disease. World Health Organization, New York.

3
Possibilities and Limitations in Screening for Cancer

William Pomerance[1]

At this particular point in our knowledge of cancer, the best prospects of perhaps saving lives and certainly prolonging lives are by the detection of early disease. Despite all the propaganda that has existed about the signs and symptoms of cancer, we know that early cancer is totally asymptomatic. Symptoms that occur in association with early cancer are usually coincidental and generally unrelated to the disease itself. Some early lesions that are relatively slow growing but still conform to the criteria for the definition of early cancer do occasionally produce symptoms.

How does one go about the task of detecting early cancer in populations? Since the concern is for asymptomatic patients, it would seem that entire populations should be screened. This is an obvious impossibility for many reasons. Another approach would be to attempt to identify groups that are at high risk for the development of cancer. Once this is accomplished, then, when such people are screened, the proportion of patients detected with cancer will be acceptably larger.

Screening methods are designed to identify among asymptomatic individuals at some increased risk of developing cancer of a particular site those with a high probability of actually having cancer. Some limitations to screening in cancer control are obvious. For example, since breast cancer occurs with relative infrequency below age 35, it would not be advisable to screen women below this age. Since the incidence curve begins to rise sharply after this age, these older women represent groups that are at considerable risk. There is an age factor of risk in lung cancer, but when this is combined with another high risk factor, such as heavy smoking, we

---

[1] Deceased.

67

then have a group of individuals who fit the definition of high risk quite well. When we subject such a group to a screening program, we have the possibility of detecting an appreciable number of early cancers.

REQUISITES FOR SCREENING METHODS

All screening methods in use should lead to the identification of early cancers, defined as those lacking metastatic involvement of the regional lymph nodes. The rationale for using metastic involvement rather than size of lesion as the basis for defining the stage of a cancer is that, while there often is a relationship between size and involvement of lymph nodes, there need not be. If the lymph nodes are not involved, there is the possibility of surgical excision or eradication by radiation therapy. The extent of the lesion is thus defined by the same criteria as those used in the diagnosis. Important caveats regarding lymph node involvement include consideration of the number removed and the number of microscopic sections of each node which are examined.

In order to be usable, screening mechanisms must fit certain specifications (Table 1). The mechanisms must be readily applicable to large numbers; if not, they obviously would not constitute a feasible approach to the screening of populations. The personnel, the equipment, and the facilities must be readily available and accessible to the target population. Furthermore, the mechanisms used must be fairly simple; the simpler, the more readily applicable.

It is desirable that paramedical personnel be employed in the screening programs. As more is learned about cancer screening, it becomes increasingly apparent that paramedical personnel can contribute significantly both in general medical care and in the specific application of the screening mechanisms in the detection of early cancer. In the National Cancer Institute/American Cancer Society (NCI/ACS) Breast Cancer Detection Demonstration Projects, for example, the examinations were initially performed by general surgeons, each of whom was responsible for 2 to 4 hours of work per week unless they were too busily occupied with their private practices or were undertaking surgery in the operating room. Occa-

Table 1.   Requirements of screening mechanisms

1. Readily applicable to large numbers
2. Fairly simple
3. Applicable by paramedical personnel
4. Acceptable to the population
5. Carrying a very small risk
6. Low rate of false positives
7. Infrequency of false negatives
8. Relatively inexpensive (cost-benefit ratio)

sionally, groups of medical residents in training were assigned to the Breast Cancer Clinic for a period of 2 weeks; this, too, is obviously far from an ideal approach.

Screening by nurse technicians or radiology technicians who have been taught breast examination can make a tremendous difference. This approach is more advantageous than any of the other approaches to physical examination of the breast. Of course, a physician who applies himself or herself as diligently as a nurse technician to the task of examining the breast would do at least as well.

This aspect of screening is important; it should be extended to other screening tasks as well. For example, it is becoming clear that paramedical personnel may be able to screen mammograms and thermograms. In general, such individuals can be employed in very much the same way as cytology technicians who screen exfoliative smears. In fact, much of the screening process can be accomplished by paramedical personnel. One might go so far as to suggest that any screening procedures that are applied should have the potential of being performed by paramedical personnel.

It is very important that the screening process be acceptable to the target population. One may have a very good screening method, but if it is not acceptable to the screenees, it loses its utility as a cancer control modality. A good example is the proctosigmoidoscopic or colonoscopic examination, which is becoming more readily available in various clinics around the country. The fact that these methods are not generally accepted by the population makes them undesirable. A further desideratum for screening mechanisms applied to large populations is that they should carry a very small individual risk. This problem is shortly alluded to with special consideration of the risks associated with mammography as conducted by the Breast Cancer Detection Demonstration Projects.

So far as efficacy is concerned, some false-positives in cancer screening are acceptable. The unresolved issue is to clearly define the level that would be acceptable. For example, the statement has been made that if we could use thermography as a primary screening mechanism in the detection of early breast cancer, it would be acceptable even with a false-positive rate as high as 50%, since this would reduce the radiation hazards of mammography by one-half. The screening mechanisms employed in our Breast Cancer Detection Demonstration Projects include a history and physical examination, mammography, and to some extent, thermography (the latter limited to an experimental trial). These methods yield a false-positive rate of 1.5%, if we describe a false-positive as a biopsied patient who does not have cancer. Whether this is a technically acceptable percentage or not is difficult to say, but it certainly has been accepted by many investigators. Cytologic screening as conducted in the three-institution Lung Cancer Screening Study has yielded no false-positives.

False-negatives should also be infrequent. With reference again to the Breast Cancer Detection Demonstration Projects, we can demonstrate fairly conclusively that false-negatives amount to approximately 10%. False-negatives with regard to breast cancer in the screening centers are defined rather broadly. They include any cancer occurring within 1 year of the time of a screening that did not specifically indicate the need for a biopsy.

Another screening requisite in the research setting becomes significant only as the magnitude of the studies increases, that is, the program should be relatively inexpensive. Cost-benefit ratios must eventually be considered, if only to avoid unacceptable burdens on the national or local economy.

We have not represented here all possible requirements of screening programs. Others are known and still others are being developed. As screening methods are studied more intensively, it becomes apparent that some of the frequently stated dogmas need modification. Suggestions have been made that early colon cancer be screened on the basis of blood detection in the stool. This method has been in use for some time. Whether it is effective or not we do not know; we are just now undertaking a study to answer this question. The particular method used is a modification of the Guaiac test, called the "hemocult test," which has been reported to have a very high percentage (5%) of false-positives, generally due to the ingestion of animal meats. However, this limitation may be inconsequential because it would require the ingestion of 1 kilogram of beef per day to produce a positive result in the stool. Such an intake level would be unusual even in the American diet. With the ingestion of less than ½ kilogram of meat, a false-positive result is rarely obtained. It is now known that the false-positive test is due only to hemoglobin, that is, to the blood in the meat rather than to the myoglobin of the beef tissue itself.

TYPES OF SCREENING METHODS

A variety of screening methods are outlined in Table 2. Individuals at higher than average risk for specific cancers may be identified on the basis of selected items in their medical history. These include family history, reproductive history, dietary history, occupational history, smoking history, and so on. Physical examination has limited but definite significance in the detection of early cancer. Such areas as the breast and the body orifices offer the best opportunities for physical detection. Cytologic examination is important in terms of exfoliated cells. While first applied in screening for cervical cancer, the method has potential for cancer screening in many other areas of the human body, including, and with a high degree of efficacy, the esophagus, stomach, pancreas, colon, upper and lower respiratory tracts, and urinary bladder. We must be ingenious enough to devise appropriate methods that are scientifically valid and yet relatively simple and accepta-

Table 2.   Screening methods

1. History
2. Physical examination
3. Cytologic
     Exfoliative
     Circulating
4. Imaging
     X-ray (transmission)
     Isotopic (emission and transmission)
     Ultrasound
     Thermography
5. Visualization
     Endoscopy
6. Chemical
     Hormones
     Proteins
     Enzymes
7. Immunologic
     Serologic
     Cell-mediated

ble. Circulating studies have not yet demonstrated their practical value, but their potential significance should also not be ignored.

With regard to x-ray imaging by means of the usual x-ray transmission, many modifications are possible for screening. The electrostatic method, for example, may replace the silver halide method with some improvement in imaging, as well as with savings in costs and perhaps a reduction in radiation exposure. Isotopes have also demonstrated their usefulness, more significantly for some neoplasms than for others. This is an area that needs more intensive research and is, in fact, being explored as a very promising approach to cancer control. However, at this point in time there does not seem to be any cancer site where isotopes have proved to be significant in the detection of early lesions.

Ultrasound as an imaging technique has been available for a relatively short period of time. It has not been explored as much as it should be as a screening tool, and with technologic improvements, it could prove its worth in the future as an important screening method. One possible target of ultrasound today is the detection of pancreas cancer. At present, the accuracy of pancreatic cancer diagnosis as demonstrated by surgical exploration is probably well below 50%, and in most institutions, below 33%. In the short period of time that investigators have been involved with ultrasound, they have improved the technique to the extent that the patient with cancer of the pancreas can be identified with approximately 70% accuracy. These technical improvements have been such that ultrasound may now be the method most often employed in the detection of pancreatic cancer.

The theoretical basis for thermography as a screening technique is that the increased rate of cell division in cancer is associated with an increase in metabolic rate and a consequent increase in blood supply that produces more heat. The evidence for this is not clear-cut and some cancers may, in fact, not be associated with increased heat production. Another problem is that very early cancers may produce so little increase in heat as to be unrecognizable. For example, in our Breast Cancer Detection Demonstration Projects more than 50% of the cancers detected had a normal thermogram. To some extent this may be due to inexpert reading; in part it may stem from faulty technique or perhaps from limitations of the equipment. Certainly we must address ourselves to the cancer control potential of this nonhazardous, noninvasive breast-screening modality. As with ultrasound, we are still in the process of learning more about thermography, a potential cancer-screening device which may not yet be ready for full-scale application.

Endoscopy is an approach that is not yet recognized as a screening method, although it has been used as such. Proctosigmoidoscopy and laryngoscopy, primarily of the indirect type, have also been recommended. The fiberoptic flexible endoscopes which are now available promise accessibility to almost any area of the body, and we look forward to the increasing prominence of endoscopy not only in the initial screening for cancer but also in the evaluating of the screening result as well as in the definitive diagnosis. In lung cancer, bronchoscopy is an absolute necessity for localizing radiographically visualized tumors. This is probably also true of pancreatic cancer, where cannulation of the pancreatic duct is made possible by endoscopy, and of colon cancer, where colonoscopy can detect lesions occasionally missed by barium enemas.

Two other approaches to cancer screening, chemical and immunologic, may become widely available at some time in the near future. We are certainly encouraged by the success of the human chorionic gonadotropin (HCG) test for screening hydatidiform moles and choriocarcinoma. Whether other tests will prove useful to the same extent is still unknown, but a major effort is being expended in the identification of hormones, protamines, or enzymes in the urine, serum, or other body fluids which are associated with the existence of cancer. The enzyme approach may be the most promising because it could indicate the existence of a genetic defect associated with cancer. The immunologic effort is of more recent initiation, but it is being intensively explored.

Incidently, these tests should not be regarded as mutually exclusive. There is no reason why they could not be used in combination. In fact, some combinations are already in use, although not so much for screening as for monitoring the clinical course of a neoplasm.

A combination of hormonal, immunologic, and protamine determinations has been employed to monitor treated breast cancer. There is a strong likelihood that such combinations can be used for monitoring other cancers as well. With refinement of these tests to render them more sensitive, we can look forward to the day when they will become useful screening mechanisms; they could certainly be the screening mechanisms of choice.

THE BREAST CANCER DETECTION DEMONSTRATION PROJECTS

It might be helpful at this point to examine some preliminary results from the Breast Cancer Detection Demonstration Projects, conducted under the combined auspices of the National Cancer Institute and the American Cancer Society. Two hundred seventy thousand women between the ages of 35 and 74 have been enrolled in 27 different clinical centers throughout the United States. At this writing, all the subjects have undergone initial screening.

Although the data from the initial screening are still largely unedited and with the pathology only partially reviewed, it may be worthwhile to consider some findings from the screening of the first 224,000 women. Among them some "abnormality" was observed on mammographic examination in 29%, on thermographic examination in 22%, and on physical examination in 11%. If we remove the overlap that exists among some of the women, we may note that 42% were identified as other than negative in their screening. That these findings are not necessarily clinically significant is indicated by the fact that only 3.8% of the total screenees were recommended for biopsy and that only about one-half of those so recommended were actually biopsied after further screening by the responsible physicians. The validity of this screening procedure is demonstrated by the fact that, despite the use of a very broad definition of interval cancer, only 10% of the possibly extant cancers are missed by this screen.

If we look at the cancers identified by the screen, it may be seen that only 8% of the women did not have a mammographic abnormality, whereas 46% lacked a physical abnormality, and 50% a thermographic one. Evaluating these figures somewhat differently, it can be concluded that at least 46% of the cancers would not have been detected if mammography had not been used in the screening effort. Applying the same logic to the physical examination, at least 8% of the cancers would have been missed had this modality been omitted. It should also be noted that while in a considerable number of cancers the findings were deemed benign by both physical examination and mammography, biopsy was nevertheless recommended. Perhaps thermography contributed to the decision for biopsy in some of these cases.

As an indication of the "early" stage of the disease being recognized by screening, we note that the percentage of positive nodes approximates 23%. This is far below the figure of 55% that is usually quoted for women admitted for breast biopsy to general hospitals. While the Health Insurance Plan of Greater New York (HIP) study failed to show any benefit to women screened between the ages of 40 and 49 years, approximately 27% of the women in whom cancers were detected in the Breast Cancer Detection Demonstration Projects were between 35 and 49 years of age. Furthermore, only 27% of the women with cancer in this age group had positive nodes, an indication that these women probably enjoyed a better prognosis than they would have without the screening.

The major beneficiaries of screening in the HIP study were those women detected by mammography alone. Since more than 45% of the cancers detected in the Breast Cancer Detection Demonstration Projects are in this category, one would anticipate a considerably improved survival rate. It can also be assumed that mammographic screening has technically improved in the years since the HIP study was performed, and that the difficulties presented by the premenopausal dense breast have, in the main, been overcome.

REDUCING RADIATION RISKS

Let us now consider the problem of ionizing radiation risks entailed in mammography. It should be noted that radiation dosage per mammographic examination (at least in the Breast Cancer Detection Demonstration Projects) has been reduced to approximately one-fifth to one-tenth of the dosage delivered in the earlier HIP study. Efforts are currently being made to further reduce this dosage. Some of the possible approaches to dosage reduction are listed in Table 3. One may hope that, as a result of these efforts, the dosage may eventually be reduced to one-tenth of the dose being delivered today.

LIMITATIONS AND BENEFITS OF SCREENING

Before concluding, we should consider the limitations of screening and its benefits (Table 4). Nonacceptance of screening is an obvious problem that must be borne in mind. Pap smears have been used for about 30 years and we can say little more than that approximately 78% of the population has been screened at least once, with fewer than 50% screened more than once. Nonavailability refers to some of the aspects discussed previously. In addition, we may simply not have screening methods for some of the cancer sites of interest. However, if we assiduously address ourselves to these problems,

Table 3.   Approaches to dosage reduction

Energy source	Smaller focal spot tubes; heavy ion beams
Collimators	To reduce scatter, improve contrast and resolution
Filters	Increase filtration, without sacrifice of resolution
Detectors	To improve efficiency of photon capture; better filmscreen matching; new filmscreen combinations; ionography-electrostatic process
Computerization	To identify smaller density differences
Reconstruction	To allow smaller doses of radiation
Periodicity	Will biennial screening be as effective as annual screening?
Reduced number of images	Will one film (image) be as effective as two films (images)?

there is no site for which screening to determine the existence of early cancer is ruled out. The excessive hazards of screening have already been referred to. The physical status of the patient is often such that we may not be able to apply the screen. In some cases (e.g., a patient close to death because of his or her cardiac status), screening for cancer is not even indicated.

If we cannot identify groups at high risk of neoplasia, cancer control efforts will fail because the total population will be too large to screen. Therefore, cancer risk assessment on the basis of genetic, familial, hormonal, chemical, and other environmental factors is necessary to identify the truly high risk groups. We must continue to develop new screening mechanisms and to improve existing ones in order to facilitate the early diagnosis of cancer.

Table 4.   Limitations of screening and its benefits

1. Nonacceptance of screening modalities
2. Nonavailability of screening modalities
3. Excessive hazards of screening modalities
4. Physical status of the screenee
5. Failure to identify high risk group
6. Nonidentification of screening mechanism leading to early diagnosis
7. Nonacceptance of treatment for early disease

Finally, the treatment for early cancer must be acceptable and not too massive. We should ask ourselves what we would do if we were able to identify small and early pancreatic cancer. What could we do for the patient that would still render his or her life subsequent to treatment as acceptable and manageable as possible? Our approach to screening must therefore also consider improvements in therapy to make the screening process as a whole acceptable and useful to the potential patient.

CONCLUSIONS

We have tried to suggest that screening is a vital part of the total approach to the problem of cancer. In the absence of effective preventive measures, screening and therapy are all that remain. At this point in time the promise of improving survival and prolonging life is not too great, except for early stage disease. With a reasoned approach to the selection of screening methods, their application and their improvement, it should be possible to recognize early cancer sufficiently well to achieve an acceptable level of cancer control.

Part II
Theoretical Considerations

4

Decision Making in Cancer Screening by Risk Factor Analysis

Anita K. Bahn, Prakash L. Grover,
and Daniel G. Miller

Evidence on the effectiveness of screening for cancer has been considered by other contributors to this volume. Although in general, patients diagnosed with a localized tumor appear to experience longer survival than those diagnosed at a regionalized stage (American Cancer Society, 1975; Axtell, Cutler, and Myers, 1972; Sutnick et al., 1976), it would be inappropriate to infer from this that early detection necessarily leads to increased survival. As discussed later, the observed increase in length of life may be wholly or partly artifactual (Bailar 1976; Zelen and Feinleib, 1969).

This leads us to conclude that pilot evaluation studies must precede any substantial investment in cancer-screening programs. Such was not done with multiphasic health-screening or periodic health examination programs. In the nearly 40 years that these activities have been in vogue, they have been accepted more on faith in preventive medicine than on demonstrated effectiveness. Knox (1974) considered the available evidence and concluded that "until further information becomes available, we must take it that demonstrable primary health benefits of multiphasic screening are quite small and that, although they are probably real, even this is open to some doubt."

We associate ourselves with the "snails" of Sackett and Holland (1975), who contend that "screening like any other health maneuver, may do more harm than good and must meet scientific as well as political criteria before it is implemented." On the other hand, we cannot agree with

This work has been supported by the Fanny E. Rippel Foundation and by NIH grant no. CA-23321.

79

Cairns' (1975) view that "since screening programs seem to be of limited use and too expensive, we are left *only* with the prevention of cancer by seeking out and eradicating its causes." Such conclusions are based upon the results of existing approaches to cancer screening with which we are in disagreement.

TRADITIONAL CANCER-SCREENING PROGRAMS

The traditional programs can be faulted conceptually, methodologically, and with respect to resource allocation. Conceptually, they tend to be rigid and invariant in design. Entire adult populations are assumed to be at equal risk of developing cancer, and consequently all screenees are prescribed the identical battery of tests and rescreening schedules. Furthermore, the programs are often oriented exclusively toward cancer detection and treatment; prevention is ignored or minimized.

The reality, however, is that the characteristics of cancer call for different approaches. For example, it has been estimated that approximately 80% of all cancers are caused by environmental factors (Higginson, 1975), including some that might be amenable to prevention through education and motivation. Furthermore, each type of cancer has a unique but low incidence rate. Such characteristics emphasize the need for selective screening, effective health education to change cancer-causing habits, and self-surveillance for cancer monitored under medical guidance.

Methodologically, existing screening programs may be faulted for their emphasis on one or two sites, a segmental approach that creates logistic and financial disincentives against participation. In addition, overskilled persons (physicians) have been employed as the routine screeners. Finally, the follow-up of screenees has often been inadequate.

The problem of resource allocation follows from the conceptual and methodologic drawbacks described above. It is not feasible to allocate the manpower and other resources required for screening the adult population of the United States by means of the traditional methods. These limitations, added to the low yield of such screening programs, result in an inordinately high cost-effectiveness ratio.

AN ALTERNATIVE: THE RISK FACTOR APPROACH TO SCREENING

Recognizing that the existing design of cancer-screening programs is ill-conceived, expensive, and therefore infeasible, a new program has been devised using the risk factor approach. This program, termed CANSCREEN, was developed jointly by the Fox Chase Cancer Center, Philadelphia, and the Preventive Medicine Institute–Strang Clinic, New

York. After pilot testing of the project in both cities during 1974, the Philadelphia clinic opened in March 1975 and the New York clinic opened in July 1975. Currently, the program is in operation in the American Oncologic Hospital of Fox Chase Cancer Center, the Preventive Medicine Institute–Strang Clinic, the Evanston Hospital of the Northwestern University Medical School, and five other clinics. The centers are coordinated by the Central Program located at Fox Chase Cancer Center where the data from all centers are pooled for analysis.

The objective of the CANSCREEN program is the achievement of a cost-benefit ratio low enough to make cancer screening of a large proportion of the adult population practical.

CANSCREEN is a multisite screening program that aims at sorting the population on the basis of risk factors. Persons at high risk are screened more intensively and frequently. Thus, "the population at large receives simple and inexpensive tests while expensive, time-consuming or more frequent screening procedures are reserved for the relatively few persons identified at high risk" (Sutnick et al., 1976). A risk factor is defined as any environmental, personal, social, familial, or biologic characteristic that, on the basis of available knowledge, predisposes an individual to a higher probability of developing cancer of a particular site than the general population. Thus, an individual may be at higher risk because of a demographic characteristic (age, sex, race, or socioeconomic status), exposure to a carcinogen at work, family history of cancer, a personal habit such as smoking, or a condition that is a precursor to malignancy.

The conceptual development of CANSCREEN and the early attempts at validation of instruments and procedures have been documented elsewhere (Sutnick et al., 1976) and are referred to later in this chapter. Below, the essential features of the current program are described.

1. *Multisite screening*   The program screens 11 potential cancer sites:
    a. Skin
    b. Mouth and throat
    c. Larynx
    d. Thyroid
    e. Lung
    f. Stomach
    g. Kidney and urinary bladder
    h. Large intestine and rectum
    i. Cervix and uterus
    j. Breast
    k. Prostate and testicle

    Site selection was based on United States data prepared for each of the major cancer sites (e.g., cancer of the breast, as in Table 1). The prin-

Table 1.   Data reference sheet for cancer of the breast

I.   Justification for Screening

	Female
A. Incidence rate/100,000	75.5
Mortality rate/100,000	27.9

B.   Benefit of early diagnosis
1.   10-year RSR (localized disease) 73%
2.   Difference in 10-year RSR, localized versus nonlocalized disease 36%
3.   Cases diagnosed in localized stage 45%

II. Early Diagnosis

Procedure	Pt. Acceptance	Risk	Sensitivity	Specificity
Breast self-exam	good	low	fair	poor
Palpation	good	low	fair	fair
Mammography	good	low	fair	fair
Cytology (when nipple discharge present)	good	low	fair	fair

III. Risk Factor Analysis

	.01%	0.1%	0.2%
A. By age[a]	25–34	45–54	55–64

B.   By symptoms
1.   Breast pain, unrelated to menses
2.   Nipple discharge

C.   By signs
1.   Breast mass or lump
2.   Change in breast size
3.   Nipple or skin retraction
4.   Breast skin changes
5.   Axillary masses

D.   By Family History
1.   Cancer of breast in mother, sister, and aunt

E.   By Past Medical History
1.   Nulliparous, age 35
2.   Cystic mastopathy
3.   Endometrial cancer
4.   Breast cancer

F.   By environmental history[b]

[a] Age group within which the incidence is .01%, 0.1%, and 0.2%, respectively.
[b] Japanese rate one-fifth that of rate in United States; risk lowest in women who have borne and nursed several children.

cipal criteria in selecting a site for screening were: 1) relatively high incidence, 2) effectiveness of early detection, and 3) accessibility of the site to inspection by the examiner. Cancer of the lung was included mainly for purposes of primary prevention (counseling against smoking) and because of its relatively high incidence, even though the second and third selection criteria are not satisfied in this case.

2. *Risk factor approach using a self-administered health history question-naire*   Because the risk factors were identified from etiologic studies, they necessarily reflect the current state of the art. Several of the studies were, in fact, based on nonrepresentative or small samples. Further-more, only those risk factors were included that could be elicited by means of a self-administered questionnaire or through a clinical exami-nation.

3. *Use of a nurse examiner*   Although a consultant physician is available on call, the major responsibility for selective clinical examination is delegated to a specially trained nurse examiner. The examiner validates the positive history and symptoms recorded in the questionnaire, elicits other symptoms, and performs a routine examination limited to the following areas:
   a. Skin
   b. Head (oral cavity)
   c. Lymph nodes
   d. Breasts
   e. Pelvis
   f. Testes and prostate
   g. Rectum (digital)
   h. Blood pressure

   The nurse also takes a Pap smear if called for by risk factor analysis, plays a key educational role in instructing screenees on how to reduce cancer risks and to be alert to signs and symptoms, instructs in breast self-examination, and recommends proctoscopy or mammography where indicated by decision logic. In the Philadelphia CANSCREEN clinic, the nurse examiner is being trained for proctoscopy. She currently performs proctoscopies under the supervision of a physician.

4. *Predetermined decision logic*   The cumulative patient record forms the basis for screening decisions. This record includes: 1) the self-reported and validated medical history and compilation of risk factors from the questionnaire, 2) the physical examination findings, and 3) data from routine laboratory examination (microhematocrit, urine albumin-blood dip stick, and three fecal hemoccult slides brought in by each screenee at the time of the clinic examination after a 3-day special diet). These data serve as inputs for a decision logic called a *decision matrix*, which serves as a sequential protocol established for each cancer site to be screened. The matrix is an innovative tool that serves as a screenee record of all of the above data, and based upon these inputs, permits the nurse (and counselor) to give special advice to each screenee.

   An example of a decision matrix for cancer of the skin is presented in Figure 1. To the left of the matrix itself are listed the specific items in the questionnaire that relate to skin cancer. These are divided into five categories:

Category A—symptoms likely to be associated with cancer of this site but not validatable within the scope of the screening clinic

Category B—signs and symptoms reported by the patient and subject to screening validation

Category C—risk factors for that site, such as a family history of cancer of that site or, as in skin cancer, that the patient is fair skinned and therefore sunburns easily

Category D—a patient history of cancer of that site

Category E—no positive findings

Positive responses from the questionnaire are checked in the Q column; when validated by the examiner, in the E column; and when validated by an interviewer for special study purposes, positive responses are checked in the I column. Potentially, a screenee could respond positively to none, one, or more than one of the questions in these categories (A, B, C, and D), thus accounting for 15 possible combinations (e.g., A, AB, BCD). If the screenee does not respond positively to any of the questions, then Category E, "No positive findings," is checked. The 16 combinations of categories form the rows of the decision matrix. In Figure 1, the response for the screenee is classified in row C because he is fair skinned.

The results of the clinic examination and laboratory procedures are recorded under one of three categories corresponding to the columns of the matrix: 1) No Suspicious Findings (NSF); 2) Findings of Increased Risk (FIR); and 3) Findings Suspicious of Cancer or Other Diseases (SCOD). Thus, based on the physical and laboratory data, the examiner chooses the appropriate column of the matrix, with SCOD overruling FIR if both are checked. In the case illustrated in Figure 1, there were no suspicious physical or laboratory findings (NSF) and the subject was therefore classified in the "NSF" column.

The nexus of row and column contains numbers corresponding to a list of advice rules (Table 2). For the screenee of Figure 1, the advice rules for row C column NSF are number 11 (prescribing an examination every 3 years pending additional information from subsequent annual questionnaires or other sources) and numbers 7 and 10 (prescribing specific risk factor advice, e.g., guarding against excessive sun exposure). The matrix can be overruled by the nurse examiner where this is necessary in his or her judgment.

At the conclusion of the examination, a comprehensive summary of the recommendations for all the screened cancer sites is made for

Skin   1

| A | | Q | I | E |

Bleeding or changed mole in past
6 months   1 └──┴──┴──┘

| B |

Unhealed sore for 1 month or more   2 └──┴──┴──┘

Skin changes due to X-ray treatment   3 └──┴──┴──┘

Old severe burn scars   4 └──┴──┴──┘

| C |

Fair-skinned, easily sunburned   5 └──┴──┴──┘

| D |

Pt. hx. skin cancer   6 └──┴──┴──┘

| E |

No positive responses   └──┴──┴──┘

ED: _____

_____

Examiner's
Notes: _____

	NSF	FIR	SCOD
A	1	7/10/1	1/7/10
AB	1/10	7/10/1	1/7/10
AC	7/10/1	7/10/1	1/7/10
AD	1/7/10	1/7/10	1/7/10
ABC	7/10/1	7/10/1	1/7/10
ABD	1/7/10	1/7/10	1/7/10
ACD	1/7/10	1/7/10	1/7/10
ABCD	2/7/10	2/7/10	2/7/10
B	11	7/10/12	1/7/10
BC	*12 7/10/11	7/10/12	1/7/10
BD	3/7/10	3/7/10	2/7/10
BCD	3/7/10	3/7/10	2/7/10
C	*12 7/10-11	7/10/12	1/7/10
CD	3/7/10	3/7/10	2/7/10
D	3/7/10	3/7/10	2/7/10
E	11	7/10/12	1/7/10

* Advice rule 12 applies
  only when exposed to
  carcinogens

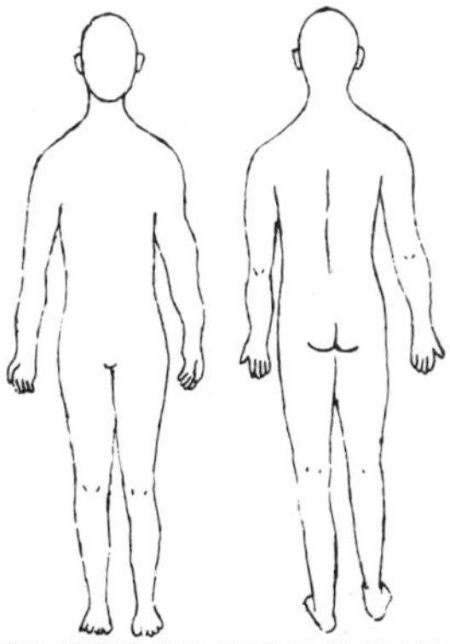

1. ☐ Matrix overruled

FINDINGS:
2. ☐ NOT EXAMINED

3. ☐ NSF 4. ☐ Other: _____

FIR:
5. ☐ Solar keratosis
6. ☐ Radiation skin changes
7. ☐ Old severe burn scar
8. ☐ _____

SCOD:
Nevus:
9. ☐ Soles 10. ☐ Palm
11. ☐ Genitals
12. ☐ Areas of irritation:

13. ☐ Bldg. nevus 14. ☐ Chgd. nevus
15. ☐ Sore/ulcer 16. ☐ Skin tumor
17. ☐ Irritation/inflammation
18. ☐ _____
19. ☐ See diagram

| RE: Examine skin |

Figure 1.   Decision matrix: skin cancer. (Matrix reprinted by permission.)

Table 2.   Advice rules

Referral
1. Refer to physician or specialty clinic for evaluation of new finding(s)/symptom(s) within 1 week, then (12).
2. Initiate immediate follow-up with physician or specialty clinic for evaluation of finding(s)/symptom(s) related to patient history, then (12).
3. Initiate or continue follow-up for patient history with physician or specialty clinic, then (12).

Additional Procedures
4. Order complete urinalysis.
   If positive, then (1) or (2) in case of patient history of kidney or bladder cancer.
   If negative, then follow advice in NSF column.
5. Order proctosigmoidoscopy, unless done within the last year. If findings are abnormal, then (1), or (2) in case of patient history of colorectal cancer.
   If findings normal, then (11) if age 45, (12) if over age 45, or (3) in case of patient history of colorectal cancer.
6. Order mammogram, unless done within the last year (even if patient is followed by a physician but has not had a mammogram). If findings are suspicious, then (1) or (2) in case of patient history of breast cancer. If findings normal, then (12) and reevaluate need for mammography, or (3) in case of patient history of breast cancer.

Education
7. Advise protection from sun exposure.
8. Advise smoking cessation.
9. Advise moderation or cessation of alcohol intake.
10. Advise of increased risk, watch for warning signs, take appropriate protective measures.

Return Visit
11. Reexamine 3 years after initial visit, pending additional information from the annual Health History Questionnaire or other sources.
12. Reexamine annually.
13. Annual hemoccult slide test.
    If positive, then (1).
    If negative, then (11).
14. Negative Pap smear for 2 consecutive years, then reexamine in 3 years.
15. Annual Pap smear, and reexamine in 2 years.
16. Annual Pap smear, and reexamine in 3 years.

---

each screenee. In consultation with the screenee, the health counselor then designs a health plan based on his or her risk profile.

5. *Health counseling*   Studies have revealed that as much as three-fourths of the medical advice given during a clinic visit is *not* completely understood or remembered by the patient (Davis, 1966) and that one-half or fewer of patients comply with their prescribed regimens (Francis,

Korsch, and Morris, 1969; Podell and Gary, 1976). For this reason, the CANSCREEN program includes a health counselor whose responsibility is to bridge the apparent gap in communication between health provider and consumer and thereby ensure compliance.

The health counselor reinforces the advice given by the nurse examiner and discusses ways in which the screenee can minimize his or her chances of developing cancer. Research findings in health education (Grover et al., 1976) have also been incorporated in our program to ensure maximal participation, commitment, and compliance. The counselor and the screenee jointly develop a personal health plan for the screenee and affix their signatures to it as a symbol of commitment. Included in the health plan is an agreement that the counselor will monitor the screenee's progress through periodic contacts.

6. *Follow-up*   The follow-up phase of CANSCREEN consists of three distinct, although interrelated, aspects: 1) physician contact, 2) compliance with recommendations, and 3) periodic screening.

The type of physician contact afforded a given screenee depends upon the findings. In general, the results of the examination are mailed to each screenee's personal physician or other medical designee. If the findings suggest increased risk (FIR) or suspicion of cancer or other diseases (SCOD), the screenee is, in addition, advised to visit the physician for additional tests or evaluations. The physician contacts serve not only to facilitate the entry of the screenee into the regular health care system for requisite diagnostic or medical care, but also to establish a relationship between the physicians and the CANSCREEN program such that all information concerning the screenee's cancer risks and experience may be exchanged.

Follow-up contacts are made by the CANSCREEN health counselor to ascertain whether screenees have complied with the suggested physician referrals and to encourage them to follow advice concerning breast self-examination. For example, if the recommended health plan included behavior changes concerning a reduction in risks caused by smoking, alcohol intake, or exposure to solar radiation, the counselor encourages and tries to ensure compliance with the plan.

Follow-up also includes rescreening, the frequency of which is determined on the basis of risk factor analysis. At present, screenees classified as low risk are advised to be examined once every 3 years, while those assessed at high risk are screened annually. In any case, each screenee is requested to complete an annual health history questionnaire.

An overview of the CANSCREEN program process is presented in Figure 2.

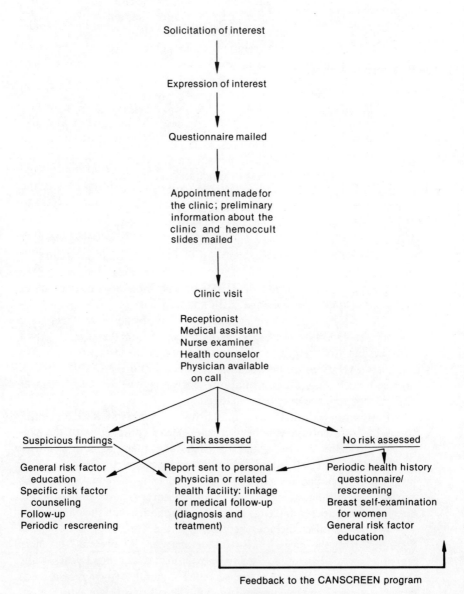

Figure 2.   An overview of the CANSCREEN program.

EPIDEMIOLOGIC CONSIDERATIONS

Our approach to screening and primary prevention, described above, should logically be cost-effective and efficient. Let us now discuss a number of epidemiologic issues arising from such a model.

The Risk Factor Approach

Common sense suggests that populations with the highest prevalence of cancer are the appropriate target groups for mass screening. This is because the yield of cancer cases detected increases with the prevalence and also because the predictive value of a positive test also increases with the prevalence of the cancer in the population (Figure 3).

Two factors may account for the higher prevalence of undetected cancer in one population as compared with another: 1) differences in the true incidence of the cancer, and 2) differences in the population's access to medical diagnosis.

Differences in age-specific incidence rates between populations may reflect a wide variety of known and unknown risk factors. Those reported in

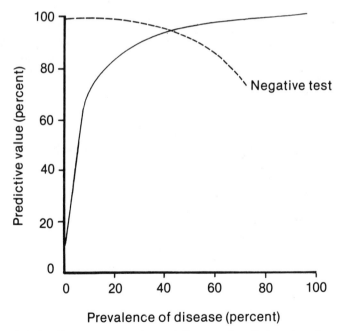

Figure 3.   Relationships between prevalence of disease and predictive value of screening test. Source: Mausner and Bahn: *Epidemiology, An Introductory Text*. W. B. Saunders, Philadelphia, 1974.

the literature include, for various cancer sites: socioeconomic status, occupational and environmental exposures, smoking, excessive use of alcohol, other life-style factors, ethnicity, genetic, and familial tendencies; and certain predisposing medical conditions. Those specific risk factors (and their associated cancer sites) that have been incorporated into our risk factor approach, or are being considered for such use, are listed in Tables 3 and 4.

Age is the predominant demographic host characteristic associated with increased cancer incidence. Age, sex, and socioeconomic status provide a prescreening strategy for selecting target populations. It should be noted, however, that there may be conflicting risk levels for different cancer sites in a given population. For example, a low socioeconomic group will tend to have a relatively high incidence of cervical cancer but a relatively low incidence of breast cancer. Certain industrial groups with known exposures to cancer hazards may also provide foci for targeted screening programs.

The quality and extent of medical care utilized by a population are a function not only of the existing medical facilities but also of the social and cultural mores that influence one's perceptions of cancer and the seeking of medical services. To the extent that those in the lower socioeconomic classes are hard to reach, it would seem that mass screening programs should be directed specifically to them as one of the groups in need. Traditionally hard-to-reach groups, however, must not only have easy access to screening programs but also be motivated to utilize them. The converse also applies: the "worried well," who tend to be overscreened, should not be unduly sought.

Table 3.   Risk factors for given cancers currently used in the CANSCREEN program[a]

Smoking (lung, oropharynx, larynx, kidney, bladder)
Alcohol (oropharynx, larynx)
Fair color (skin)
Familial aggregation (breast, colon, stomach, uterus)
Intercourse before age 18 (cervix)
Nulliparous (uterus, ovary, breast)
Mouth irritation (oral)
Nulliparous before age 35 (breast)
X-ray treatment neck (thyroid)
Predisposing diseases: pernicious anemia, gastric ulcer, gastrointestinal polyps, ulcerative colitis, repeated prostate infections, venereal disease, undescended testicles

[a] Excluding clinical symptoms and signs.

Table 4.   Risk factors for given cancers under consideration for use in the
CANSCREEN program

Late age at menarche (breast)
Use of reserpine (breast)
Infertility (breast)
Obesity (breast)
Number of sex partners (cervix, prostate)
Uncircumcised male partner (cervix)
Obesity, hypertension, diabetes (uterus)
Estrogen replacement (uterus)
Oral contraceptive use (?) (breast)
Chewing tobacco (oropharynx, larynx)
Specific occupational exposures (lung, bladder, etc.)
Additional predisposing diseases: fibrocystic disease of breast, Hashimoto's
    thyroiditis, gastritis, regional ileitis, kidney stones
Cancer of other sites

Risk Factor Selection and Evaluation

Risk factors other than those related to demographic characteristics cannot usually be determined except through direct questioning of the individuals themselves. We have devoted considerable thought to the selection of risk factors to be ascertained in the CANSCREEN program. Our principal concerns include: 1) the feasibility of eliciting the required risk factor information, 2) the magnitude of each risk factor, 3) the risk factor's estimated etiologic fraction, and 4) the interaction of the risk factors with each other and with the clinical symptoms.

A major consideration in selecting a risk factor is the feasibility of eliciting the requisite information from the screenee by means of a self-administered questionnaire. This approach is necessary because it is not possible for us to conduct routine checks of medical records related to risk information.

When a subject is queried on his or her family history of cancer, even among immediate blood relatives, specific cancers may be recalled with greater certainty than others. For example, while breast carcinoma in a relative is unlikely to be confused with other neoplasms, several different primary types might be recalled as "cancer of the abdomen." Some of these ambiguities can be clarified by the examiner, but the names of congenital diseases are unlikely to be familiar to most screenees.

Risk factors relating to occupational exposure are of increasing importance, as evidenced by recent reports of potential carcinogenic hazards in the workplace (Bahn et al., 1976a). Unfortunately, the relevant exposures are often elicited with great difficulty by workers being asked to recall job histories and exposures dating back some 15 to 30 years (i.e., the usual period of cancer induction). Workers may recollect only the trade names of substances to which they were exposed. Furthermore, the list of potential hazards is becoming quite long. Thus, better methods of eliciting occupational information in adequate detail need to be developed. Perhaps workers should begin to keep their own personal job history-exposure records.

There are also potential problems with self-reporting of "stigmatizing" risk factors. For example, the number of sexual partners and one's age at first intercourse bear a positive relationship to the risk of cervical cancer. However, questions designed to elicit such information may suffer inadequate response rates as in the Maryland Medicaid Study described below. In a similar fashion, could one expect individuals to report truthfully on their alcohol consumption and smoking history at a time when they have been sensitized to the carcinogenic potential of these self-inflicted environmental hazards?

With respect to the question of the magnitude of the risk associated with a suspect factor, we believe that the relative risk should be at least 3.0 to be operationally useful. More modest relative risks would seem to be of little value in decision making on prescriptive screening.

Risk factors under consideration for population screening often have different levels of significance at different ages. For example, familial aggregation in breast cancer is believed to be far more important for premenopausal than postmenopausal women (Anderson, 1972; Craig, Comstock, and Geiser, 1974; Robbins and Berg, 1964).

Another important consideration in screening strategy is the etiologic fraction or population attributable risk proportion of cancer associated with a specified factor. The etiologic fraction reflects not only the relative risk but also the percentage of the population exposed to the factor in question. Not only is cigarette smoking a factor associated with a high relative risk (10 or more) for lung cancer, but it also accounts for 80%–85% of all lung cancers in males of certain age groups (Lilienfeld, 1976) because a high proportion of these men smoke.

Certain occupational exposures are associated with a high relative risk of nasal sinus or other cancers, but at the same time the attributable risk or etiologic fraction and the absolute risk are small (Cole and Goldman, 1975). Numerical values for the etiologic fraction of various risk factors are usually not available from the clinical literature and often cannot be estimated because the prevalence of the characteristic in the general population has never been determined. Theoretically, of course, the required figures could be estimated from values of control patients in well-designed retrospective case control studies.

The magnitude of the etiologic fraction depends, as already noted, on the target population. Thus, for example, certain carcinogenic exposures would be associated with much higher etiologic fractions in industrial cohorts than in the general population.

Besides considering etiologic fractions, the cancer screener must also take account of genetic conditions, such as familial multiple polyposis of the colon, and ulcerative colitis. These greatly increase an individual's risk of developing particular cancers. However, these as well as most other known risk factors, account for only a small proportion of the adult cancer burden. Cigarette smoking is the outstanding exception.

While the research literature provides some numerical values for individual risk factors in cancer, it is quite sparse with respect to the relation of one risk factor to another. In planning a screening program, one would like to know whether the risk factors are independent (e.g., additive) or correlated, and what sort of interaction, if any, exists between them. With respect to cervical cancer, for example, the relevant questions would include whether "low socioeconomic status" and "many sex partners" are duplicative, additive, or multiplicatively related to each other as risk factors.

Cofactor relationships may also exist. For example, studies suggest that asbestos is an important risk factor for lung cancer only in conjunction with cigarette smoking (Selikoff and Hammond, 1975). The combination of cigarette smoking and asbestos exposure results in a relative risk of nearly 100 as compared with 10 for smokers not exposed to asbestos. A synergistic relationship also appears to exist between uranium mining and smoking (Lundin et al., 1969).

The absence of adequate measures of correlation and interaction for many potential risk factors has necessitated the establishment of a pragmatic decision rule in CANSCREEN: The presence of any one risk factor for a specific cancer site raises a signal, but the strength of the signal is not increased if more than one risk factor is present. Of course, it may be anticipated that our prospective study of screenees, as well as the research of others, will eventually make it possible to quantify the individual risk factors and their interactions.

Another practical question is how to combine risk factors with clinical symptoms in an "index of suspicion." Given a characteristic or an exposure associated with a high relative risk for a specific cancer, an even greater alarm would be justified if symptoms suggestive of that cancer are also present. The issue is complicated by the problem of nonspecific symptoms. For example, combination of an ubiquitous high risk factor such as cigarette smoking with an ubiquitous symptom such as coughing may result in a large number of persons being subjected to needless screening tests for a cancer of low incidence for which medical treatment can as yet accomplish relatively little.

At present, our decision rule (matrix logic) is based on a simple linear model. The combination of one or more risk factors, plus one or more clinical symptoms and/or a positive family history, results in an action rule of a higher level than if the symptom(s) or the history were not present. Ideally, one would prefer a more elaborate model based on the number of risk factors, the intensity and duration of exposure, and the number of symptoms and their severity. Unfortunately, the present state of our knowledge precludes this approach.

In summary, the limitations in our approach to risk factor analysis include: 1) a lack of precise measures of reliability in the ascertainment of risk factors, 2) assignment of equal weight to all risk factors, regardless of the magnitude of their associated relative risks, and 3) the simplistic combination of risk factors, clinical symptoms, and family histories without taking into account interactions among them, if any.

Most of these limitations result from the current state of our knowledge concerning risk factors. Follow-up data from the CANSCREEN program will contribute new evidence about known risk factors, the nature of multiple risk factor relationships, and perhaps clues to new risk factors (e.g., occupational).

Although some risk factors, such as genetic characteristics or life-style may not be effectively modifiable for the primary prevention of cancer at present, their identification can contribute to the secondary prevention or early detection of malignant disease.

Validity and Reliability of Instruments and Procedures

The Questionnaire   Each element of the CANSCREEN program must be as reliable and valid as possible, if the program is to succeed. Perhaps no instrument is more important than the self-administered questionnaire. Its questions concerning the respondent's medical history, risk factor exposures, and clinical symptoms must be clear, unambiguous, and understandable to persons of varying education levels and social backgrounds. Earlier papers have summarized the steps taken in field testing the questionnaire among a thousand white and black persons sampled from the Medicaid rolls of rural and suburban areas in Maryland (Halpern et al., 1975; Bahn et al., 1976b) as well as the results of testing different versions of the questionnaire (Sutnick et al., 1976). A third version of the questionnaire is now being used. All positive and relevant negative responses are requeried by the nurse examiner; any inconsistencies are noted on the matrix record. We are also planning a study to validate a random sample of all negative responses on a routine basis.

Where difficulties inhere in particular questions, for which a "yes" response indicates certain symptoms or risk factors, our policy is to address further probing questions to the respondent to ensure specificity of responses. Also troublesome, as noted previously, are the ubiquitous non-specific chronic symptoms and other reported clinical signs or symptoms that cannot be validated by the examiner. These factors can increase the "false-positive" rate in screening surveys.

Nurse Examination   The validity of physical examinations performed by nurses is a subject with far-reaching implications for the practice of health care delivery. It may be argued that a skilled nurse who has been trained by an oncologist for specific screening tasks and has repeatedly performed these tasks with consultant backup, is more proficient than the typical general medical practitioner. Indeed, the usefulness of physician extenders (nurse examiners and nurse practitioners) in performing delineated clinical functions has been demonstrated in several studies (Greenfield et al., 1974; Miller, 1976; Sackett and Holland, 1975; Taller and Feldman, 1974).

Based on the results of these studies, we have carefully selected and trained nurses to perform the CANSCREEN examinations. Of considerable utility are the algorithms of advice rules for further tests and the frequency of screening. These rules facilitate a standardized approach that tends to reduce internurse and interclinic variability. For purposes of quality control, the supervising physician reviews all charts in which the decision matrix has been overruled by the nurse. In addition, a physician is always available to provide consultations when the nurse cannot make a definitive judgment.

The Decision Matrix   The experimental basis for our utilization of risk factors in the decision matrix has been discussed. Periodic investigation of the outcomes of these decisions in terms of false-negatives and false-positives will gradually improve the data base and the decision process itself.

For this reason, among others, it is necessary to follow up all screenees, not only for the direct benefits to the patients themselves, but also to validate and improve our decision rules. Screenees reported "suspicious for cancer" as well as those reported "*not* suspicious for cancer" are followed up. The first group is followed through diagnostic tests to the final outcomes of disease, death, or the absence of disease. The second group is followed routinely, by means of a mailed annual questionnaire, and is rescreened no less than once every 3 years, depending upon the individual risk profiles and subsequent observed changes.

Consider, however, the complexity of determining the validity of the decision "no need for further investigation at this time." Should one classify the case as a "false-negative" if 6 months later a cancer specifically screened for is diagnosed? Perhaps this was not a "missed" cancer at all but, rather, the consequence of the screenee's heightened awareness of a new "lump" or other sign or symptom resulting in early self-referral. Should an arbitrary postscreening period be established to classify the "false-negatives" more systematically?

We believe that the "validating period" for false-negativity should vary with the specific type of cancer, in recognition of the distinctive natural histories of the different neoplasms. For example, uterine cervical cancers are typically slow growing, while others tend to develop very rapidly. Unfortunately, because so little is known about the natural history of most cancers, it is difficult to establish such time periods with any degree of assurance. Accordingly, we record all observations relating to the natural history of the neoplasm for each individual case in our program. In the analysis, we intend to investigate the effect of different time period limitations upon the observed percentages of false-negatives and true-negatives.

Follow-up to ascertain the false-positive rate is also necessary. The level of false-positives, however, must be kept reasonably low because of the psychological trauma to the subjects and the cost of unnecessary diagnostic procedures. The follow-up of cases classified as "probably positive" represents less of an evaluative problem in these terms than the follow-up of individuals presumed negative.

Evaluation Outcomes   Let us assume that all elements of the system are functioning well and that a multisite screening program for targeted high risk populations can be carried out at a moderate cost, utilizing a self-administered questionnaire, nurse examiners, risk factor analyses, and decision matrices. What criteria should be established for evaluating the program? More specifically, what statistics should be collected to determine whether or not the objectives of the program, including cost-effectiveness, have been fulfilled? What biases must be avoided or taken into account in interpreting the results? We shall address these questions from the perspectives of secondary prevention and primary prevention.

Secondary Prevention   The criterion utilized most often in evaluating screening programs is the *yield*. How many cancers does the program detect that would normally pass undetected? Among the first 724 screenees who went through the CANSCREEN program at our Philadelphia clinic, seven basal cell carcinomas and six cancers of other sites were detected. This is a significantly larger number than one would expect on the basis of national incidence data. Of course, inferences about the effectiveness of a program should also take into account the difference that such early detection makes in the prognosis of the patients.

Early detection, or secondary prevention, is aimed at prolonging the survival as well as the quality of life of cancer patients. However, observed survival time from diagnosis to death is confounded by the well-known phenomenon of *lead time bias* (Bailar, 1976; Shapiro, Goldberg, and Hutchison, 1974; Zelen and Feinleib, 1969). Thus, screening may result only in the earlier diagnosis of a cancer with an already unalterable course. In other words, even though the patient is observed for a prolonged time period, the ordained time of death is not forestalled by the screening process.

Length bias is another artifact of screening. It derives from the fact that slow growing, indolent tumors with good prognoses are more likely to be detected by screening than fast growing tumors with poor prognoses. The latter, because of their short duration from onset to symptomatic stage, will reach medical diagnosis sooner and are thus less likely to be identified in a screening program.

The problem of *selection bias* must also be considered. In general, we do not know how individuals select themselves for participation in a screening program. Symptomatic subjects may be overselected who, in the absence of the program, might have visited their physicians for diagnosis and treatment. Selective factors may act in other unknown ways as well.

In view of the above, an increase in observed survival time per se is not an adequate criterion for evaluating the outcomes of screening programs. The best measure of the effectiveness of secondary prevention is a reduction in age-specific mortality rates among screenees as compared with controls.

Primary Prevention   A second objective of CANSCREEN is primary prevention, that is, a reduction of the cancer incidence rate, through individual health counseling or prescriptive screening, and by treatment of in situ and premalignant lesions.

The evaluation of health education and counseling is complex and largely beyond the scope of this chapter. However, if counseling is successful, one would expect an eventual decrease in the incidence of specific cancers such as those associated with smoking, excessive use of alcoholic beverages, and exposure to the sun. In the short run, evidence obtained by the health counselor of the screenee's compliance with risk factor reduction must suffice as a measure of success. Preliminary data on the extent of compliance by screenees in our Philadelphia clinic are summarized in Table 5.

When "premalignant" lesions are detected, questions arise concerning their probability of becoming malignant as well as the advisability of surgical removal. One would hypothesize that if such lesions (e.g., colonic polyps) are discovered and removed, a reduction in the incidence of cancer of that site would be expected. However, in the absence of a self-designed test of the hypothesis, what should be done? Is it ethical to advise surgical

Table 5.   Degree of screenees' compliance with their health plan: Philadelphia
clinic, August 1975 to January 1976 ($N = 446^a$)

	Complied (%)	Partially complied (%)	Not complied (%)	Total (%)
Breast self-examination ($N = 227$)	82	14	4	100
Smoking ($N = 174$)	52	33	15	100
Alcohol consumption	56	12	32	100

[a] 446 = Number of compliance episodes. The actual number of screenees to whom these data relate is less than 446.

removal of all "premalignant" lesions? Surely, it may even be questioned whether the health system can handle the demands placed on surgical personnel and other resources resulting from such a policy.

There are also the as yet unanswered questions concerning the natural history of in situ lesions. While some lesions will certainly progress to malignancy, others will undoubtedly regress without therapeutic intervention. Intraepithelial lesions of the cervix uteri are an example.

At the same time, certain diagnostic procedures may be associated with an increased cancer incidence. For example, the risk-benefit of radiation hazards associated with repeated mammographies among asymptomatic low risk women below 50 years of age has of late been debated rather intensely. (Bailar, 1976). The result has been a recommendation by the National Cancer Institute and the American Cancer Society against such procedures (American Medical News, 1976). The CANSCREEN program has been following a rule of selective rather than universal mammographic screening, both for the reasons cited above and because of cost considerations.

To adequately evaluate the contribution of screening in the primary and secondary prevention of cancer, appropriate control populations of nonscreened subjects are needed. This issue, its inherent problems, and a possible compromise solution are addressed in the next section.

Control Populations   It is not enough to ascertain the feasibility and validity of a screening activity, its yield, and the cost. The most important question is: *Does the program make a difference?* In order to answer this question, a control population is necessary.

To minimize the problems of self-selection and other biases referred to earlier, a randomized trial along the lines of the Health Insurance Plan of Greater New York (HIP) study of breast cancer screening (Shapiro, Strax, and Venet, 1967) would be highly desirable. How might such a trial be carried out, with due consideration for the ethical issues? A model that would permit evaluation of the CANSCREEN program as a whole, as well as its questionnaire and clinical examination procedures, is presented in Figure 4.

The approach begins with the identification of a large Reference Population, such as industrial or prepaid medical groups of selected ages. The proposed trial is then explained to all members, and those who agree to participate constitute the Study Group. Some information must also be ob-

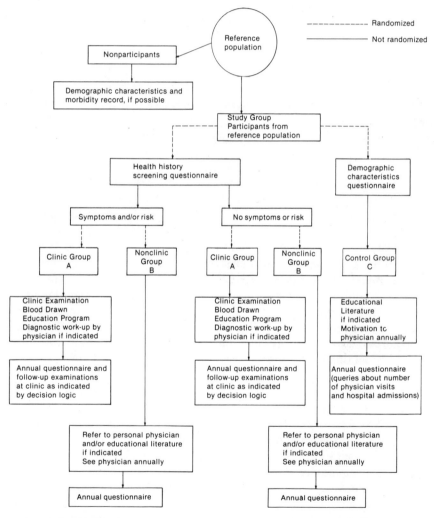

Figure 4.   Model for a randomized controlled trial of a multisite cancer detection program.

tained about the nonparticipants, especially with regard to their demographic characteristics and health status before and during the screening trial.

To test the screening value of the questionnaire per se, a Control Group (C) is selected at random from among the participants. Group C is administered an abbreviated questionnaire related to demographic questions and selected risk factors, such as smoking history. No information about clinical symptoms should be elicited because this would then necessitate, for ethical reasons, the provision of specific intervention advice, visits to a physician, and so on. Thereafter, an annual follow-up questionnaire concerned with hospital admissions and cancer diagnoses would be administered, both for information gathering and to help maintain contact with the group. In addition, it would be appropriate to provide the control subjects with educational material about cancer and the risks of smoking and to generally advise them to see their physician promptly for symptoms or signs of cancer and for annual check-ups.

The remaining participants would be asked to complete the entire CANSCREEN questionnaire, including details on risk factors, medical history, and clinical symptoms. Based upon their questionnaire responses, the screenees would be classified into two strata: 1) those with symptoms and/or risk factors, and 2) those without these characteristics. Each stratum would then be divided randomly, one-half constituting Clinic Group A and the other half Nonclinic Group B.

The Group A screenees would be requested to participate in the full CANSCREEN program including clinical examination, while Nonclinic Group B subjects would be referred to their personal physicians or merely receive health educational literature, depending on their questionnaire responses. Both groups would be followed annually, Group A in accordance with the information collected and the decision matrix rules, and Group B in accordance with their responses on the annual questionnaires alone.

It should be emphasized that an annual follow-up of individuals in all three groups (A, B, and C) is necessary to ensure the completeness of the outcome information. Comparing outcomes of Clinic Group A and Nonclinic Group B subjects would assist in assessing the advantage, if any, of the CANSCREEN clinic versus referral to a personal physician for appropriate health management. Comparing the Nonclinic Group B with Control Group C would permit evaluation of the CANSCREEN questionnaire alone, as a community outreach tool in the early detection of cancer.

The outcome criteria referred to would be employed in program evaluation and cost-effectiveness measurement. One should, of course, consider all the problems associated with prospective studies, including the large numbers of persons to be followed over long periods of time, the effect of secular changes in medical practice and in public attitudes, as well as selective attrition at various stages of the trials. Notwithstanding all of these problems, however, the approach provides the basis for a sound evaluation of mass screening programs for cancer.

An alternative control selection procedure, in circumstances in which a randomized trial is not feasible, might involve the selection as a control of another demographically comparable population not undergoing screening. Baseline measurements of cancer incidence and mortality would be made on this control population and on the study population before and after the initiation of screening in the latter group. Such a design might prove feasible where entire communities are co-opted for study, for example, where one rural community served by a primary health care screening center is contrasted with another community of similar characteristics but without such a center, serving as the control (Kessler and Levin, 1970).

CONCLUSIONS

The conceptual foundations and major characteristics of a multisite cancer screening program, CANSCREEN, have been described. The program is designed for the periodic screening of large populations using a risk factor approach, with selective application of screening tests and other procedures to those persons determined to be at high risk for developing cancer of a given site. Health education with respect to risk factors is integrated with the program, which is aimed at primary prevention wherever possible. The method largely involves helping people to carry out self-surveillance through early recognition of signs and symptoms.

Early results suggest that the program has the potential to be cost-effective, and that it meets the criteria of yield and patient compliance. It is recognized that the program must ultimately be evaluated in terms of length and quality of survival from cancer. A randomized controlled trial is proposed to estimate these parameters.

REFERENCES

American Cancer Society. 1975. Cancer statistics, 1975—25-year cancer survey. CA 25:2–21.
American Medical News. 1976. Mammography use supported. Am. Med. News 19(45):20.
Anderson, D. B. 1972. A genetic study of human breast cancer. J. Natl. Cancer Inst. 48:1029–1034.
Axtell, L. M., Cutler, S. J., Myers, M. H. 1972. End Results in Cancer, Report No. 4. U.S. Government Printing Office, U.S. Department of Health, Education, and Welfare, Publication No. (NIH) 73-272, Washington, D.C.

Bahn, A., Rosenweike, I., Hermann, N., Grover, P., Stillman, J., and O'Leary, K. 1976a. Melanoma after exposure to PCB. (Letter to Editor). N. Engl. J. Med. 295:450.

Bahn, A., Sevada, E., Sommers, D., Sutnick, A., Shirley, G., Dean, D., and Miller, D. 1976b. An outreach cancer detection program for medically indigent minority groups: Report of a pilot study. Abstr. Am. Pub. Hlth. Assn. Mtg.

Bailar, J. C., III. 1976. Mammography: A contrary view. Ann. Intern. Med. 84:77–84.

Boyes, D. A. 1969. The British Columbia screening program. Obstet. Gynecol. Surv. 24:1005–1011.

Cairns, J. 1975. The cancer problem. Sci. Am. 233:64–78.

Cole, P., and Goldman, M. B. 1975. Occupation. In: J. Fraumeni, Jr. (ed.), Persons at High Risk of Cancer, An Approach to Cancer Etiology and Control, ch. 11. Academic Press, Inc., New York.

Colley, J. R. T. 1974. Screening for disease: Disease of the lung. Lancet 2:1125–1127.

Craig, T., Comstock, G., and Geiser, P. 1974. The quality of survival in breast cancer: A case-control comparison. Cancer 33:1451–1457.

Davis, M. S. 1966. Variations in patients' compliance with doctors' orders: Analysis of congruence between survey responses and results of empirical investigations. J. Med. Educ. 41:31–54.

Francis, V., Korsch, B. M., and Morris, M. J. 1969. Gaps in doctor-patient communications. N. Engl. J. Med. 280:535–540.

Greenfield, S., Friedland, G., Scifer, S., Rhodes, A., Black, W., and Konaroff, A. 1974. Protocol management of dysuria, urinary frequency and vaginal discharge. Ann. Intern. Med. 81:452–457.

Grover, P. L., Dean, D. H., Livingston, C., Synder, M., and Miller, D. 1976. Evaluating the effect of personalized risk factor education on patient compliance: Some research findings and methodological issues. Presented at the 9th International Health Education Conference, Ottawa, Ontario, August 29–September 4.

Halpern, L., Sommers, D., Bahn, A., Sawada, E., and Sutnick, A. 1975. An outreach cancer detection program for medically indigent groups. Presented at the 8th Annual Meeting of the Society for Epidemiologic Research, Albany, New York.

Higginson, J. 1975. Cancer etiology and prevention. In: J. Fraumeni, Jr. (ed.), Persons at High Risk of Cancer, An Approach to Cancer Etiology and Control, ch. 23. Academic Press, Inc., New York.

Kessler, I., and Levin, M. 1970. The Community as an Epidemiologic Laboratory: A Casebook of Community Studies. The Johns Hopkins Press, Baltimore, Md.

Knox, E. G. 1974. Multiphasic Screening. Lancet 2:1434–1436.

Lilienfeld, A. 1976. Foundations of Epidemiology. Oxford University Press, New York.

Lundin, E., Lloyd, J., Smith, E., Archer, V., and Holaday, D. 1969. Mortality of uranium miners in relation to radiation exposure, hard-rock mining and cigarette smoking—1950 through September, 1967. Health Phys. 16:571–578.

MacGregor, E. J., Fraser, M. E., and Mann, E. 1971. Improved prognosis of cervical cancer due to comprehensive screening. Lancet 1:74–76.

Mausner, J., and Bahn, A. 1974. Epidemiology, An Introductory Text. W. B. Saunders Company, Philadelphia.

Miller, D. G. 1976. What is early diagnosis doing? Cancer. 37:1.

Podell, R. N., and Gary, L. R. 1976. Compliance: A problem in medical management. Am. Family Physician 13:74–80.

Robbins, G. F., and Berg, J. W. 1964. Bilateral primary breast cancers: A perspective clinicopathological study. Cancer. 17:1501–1527.

Sackett, D. L., and Holland, W. W. 1975. Controversy in the detection of disease. Lancet 2:357–359.

Selikoff, I. J., and Hammond, E. C. 1975. Multiple risk factors in environmental cancer. In: J. Fraumeni (ed.), Persons at High Risk of Cancer, An Approach to Cancer Etiology and Control, pp. 467–481. Academic Press, Inc., New York.

Shapiro, S., Goldberg, J., and Hutchison, G. 1974. Lead time in breast cancer detection and implications for periodicity of screening. Am. J. of Epidemiol. 100:357–366.

Shapiro, S., Strax, P., and Venet L. 1967. Periodic breast cancer screening. Arch. Environ. Health 15:547–553.

Shapiro, S., Strax, P., Venet, L., and Venet, W. 1973. Changes in 5-year breast cancer mortality in a breast cancer screening program, pp. 663–678. 7th National Cancer Conference Proceedings, The American Cancer Society.

Sutnick, A. I., Miller, D. C., Samson, B., Dean, D., Kukowski, K., Halpern, L., Jeffrys, C., and Bahn, A. 1976. Population cancer screening. Cancer. 38:325–330.

Taller, S. L., and Feldman, R. 1974. The training and utilization of nurse practitioners in adult health appraisal. Med. Care 12:40–48.

Timonen, S., Nieminen, U., and Kauraniemi, T. 1974. Cervical screening. Lancet 1:401.

Zelen, M., and Feinleib, M. 1969. On the theory of screening for chronic diseases. Biometrika. 56:601–614.

5
Signal Detection Theory in the Early Diagnosis of Cancer

Lee B. Lusted

This chapter concerns the use of a particular analytical tool, Receiver Operating Characteristic (ROC) analysis, in the early diagnosis of cancer. The discussion of the ROC approach is set in a decision analysis context in which the benefit-cost trade-offs of various decisions are considered. It begins with a brief examination of some of the assumptions about cancer screening and diagnosis that underlie attitudes impinging on policy decisions for cancer programs.

The first assumption is that the early detection and diagnosis of cancer is an important end in itself. Perhaps it is the most important goal. The motto is "Earlier is better." However, as some investigators have recently pointed out, the benefits of early detection must not be considered to the exclusion of the risks of the detection or diagnostic procedures. Bailar (1976), in a study of breast cancer detection by mammography, has commented: "A complete analysis of benefits and risks or other costs should include the monetary costs of mammography, the time invested by screenees as well as staff for relatively small return, and the impact on patients of false-positive screening reports, which seem to occur several times as often as the true positives."

A second assumption that follows from the first is that increasingly costly instrumentation and procedures are justified in the hope of finding earlier cancers. This idea is based on an escalation theory that justifies increasing marginal costs to find even earlier and smaller cancers. One would like to find that early cluster of a few cancer cells. This assumption also needs to be subjected to benefit-cost analysis and ethical appraisal.

In examining the various assumptions and the implications for cancer detection and diagnosis, we should try to separate the facts from the values. Facts are facts and values are values. However, in the final stages of the decision process, facts and values merge to guide action.

For the past several years discussions of any length on medical decisions analysis have tended to end in a discussion of values. Value systems
reflect ethical beliefs, and ethical considerations may not receive much
explicit attention by the patient or the physician. The subject of this chapter
is not medical ethics, but it is useful to examine briefly several points on
ethics before the matter of benefit-cost values in the context of cancer diagnosis is considered.

Matters of ethics are related to economics (Fuchs, 1974), especially to
allocation of scarce resources for cancer detection and diagnosis. As
Fletcher (1974) has put the question, "What of what can be done, should be
done; what of what should be done can we afford; and what of what we can
afford are we prepared to pay?" The answer is that we cannot have all the
health or medical care we would like to have. There is an inevitability of
choice. We must choose.

Furthermore, Gustafson (1975) has commented that health seems to be
replacing salvation as the chief end of man. Ill health and finally death are
perceived in certain age groups to be the real enemy.

So the question remains: What priority should be given to development
of instruments and procedures for the earlier detection of cancer, and what
priority should be given to the development and use of earlier therapies?
Should medical specialists in last-ditch remedies continue their unspoken
and undeliberate "conspiracy" with the "American Way of Not Dying" to
give these remedies the greater prominence and a disproportionate claim to
our limited medical and social resources? (Fuchs, 1974).

Scientific review committee members are reminded that they are to
evaluate a research proposal on the basis of scientific merit. But it is difficult to keep separate the facts of scientific merit from value judgments
about the relative social usefulness and cost of the proposal. Many scientists
on such committees are not familiar with decision analysis techniques,
including multiattribute utility-scaling methods. Some coaching in the rudi-
ments of these techniques might help reviewers to sort out and to be more
explicit about the facts versus the values.

ROC analysis in the decision-making context helps to sort out the
probabilities (facts) from the benefit-costs (values) relationships.

CONVENTIONAL ROC METHODS[1]

To begin, consider the situation in which the diagnostic decision maker
must choose between two alternatives: as examples, a particular disease

---

[1] Material in this section is adapted from: Metz, C. E., Starr, S. J., and Lusted, L. B.
1977. Quantitative evaluation of visual detection performance in medicine: ROC analysis and
determination of diagnostic benefit, pp. 220–241. In: G. A. Hay (ed.), Medical Images. John
Wiley & Sons, Inc., London.

may be present or absent, a lesion of a given size may be present or absent, or a disease may be of type A or type B. Two classes of *true states* exist which, for now, we can call *actually positive* and *actually negative*, and two decisions are possible, a *positive* decision (i.e., the decision that the true state is *actually positive*) and a *negative* decision (i.e., the decision that the true state is *actually negative*).

Either decision may be correct or incorrect. Four types of decisions are therefore possible in this situation: a *true-positive* decision (i.e., a *positive* decision for an *actually positive* true state); a *false-positive* decision (i.e., a *positive* decision for an *actually negative* true state); a *true-negative* decision (i.e., a *negative* decision for an *actually negative* true state); and a *false-negative* decision (i.e., a *negative* decision for an *actually positive* true state). All four types of decisions will occur in almost any decision-making situation in the presence of uncertainty, and hence all four types of decisions must be taken into account when measuring (and attempting to specify) decision performance.

Suppose that a physician views a series of images (e.g., radiographs or scintigrams) that are similar except that some of the images are *actually negative* (e.g., are images of normal subjects), while the rest are *actually positive* (e.g., are images of subjects having a certain type of lesion or disease state). Because of statistical fluctuations in the image data (e.g., those attributable to quantum statistics) or in normal anatomical structure or function (e.g., *structured noise* (Revesz, Kundel, and Graber, 1974) caused by neural and/or psychophysical fluctuations internal to the observer (Goodenough and Metz, 1973)), and perhaps because of statistical variations in the form of the lesion or in the manifestation of the disease, the presence or absence of lesion or disease may not always be decided correctly.

The Concept of Confidence Threshold

It is a fundamental assumption of our approach that the observer decides whether or not a lesion, for example, is present by comparing his impression of the image with some *decision criterion* or *confidence threshold*, and by stating that a lesion is present if and only if his confidence that the lesion exists in the image exceeds that threshold. The method by which the observer determines his confidence that the lesion is present is of no concern in applying this approach, although the method used by the observer may influence his ability to detect the lesion. Training and experience would seem to be important factors in determining the skill with which the observer can utilize the image data to form an appropriate estimate of his confidence that a lesion or a disease state is present.

The relative frequencies of the possible correct (*true-positive* and *true-negative*) and incorrect (*false-positive* and *false-negative*) decisions will depend upon the confidence threshold adopted by the observer. The question of what confidence threshold the observer should adopt is discussed later; let it suffice here to say that the degree of apparent *positiveness* the observer requires before he is willing to make a *positive* decision should depend upon both the clinical consequences of the four types of correct and incorrect decisions for the case at hand and also upon the actual frequency of actually positive cases.

Since the underlying detectability of a lesion by an observer does not depend upon the confidence threshold chosen by the observer, however, any useful and complete description of the detectability of lesions (or disease) by a human observer in the presence of uncertainty must take into account the concept of decision threshold.

As a case in point, if an observer is required to detect lesions in two series of images—of the same body part but produced by two different imaging systems, for example—then it may be found that the observer's decisions based upon one series of images yield both *true-positive* and *false-positive* decision frequencies that are greater than those elicited by the other series of images. In order to decide whether the differences in decision frequencies are due to differences in lesion detectability inherent in the two imaging systems, or are due only to the (perhaps unconscious) adoption of different confidence thresholds by the observer, a method of observer performance analysis is required to separate these two factors that influence the relative frequencies of the four types of decisions.

The Conventional ROC Curve

The combination of decision frequencies produced by an observer attempting to detect a given image feature or disease state using a given imaging system depends upon the confidence threshold adopted by the observer. An appropriate confidence threshold depends on the clinical context of the detection problem, and it is extremely difficult to quantitate the confidence threshold a particular observer may adopt. Therefore, it is useful to describe detection performance in terms of the relationship among the various possible decision frequencies that are generated as different confidence thresholds are adopted by the observer, with the values of confidence threshold being implicit, rather than explicit, in the analysis. Receiver Operating Characteristic (ROC) analysis does just this.

At this point it is convenient to establish a convention for notation that will facilitate subsequent discussion. Let s and n represent the two true states *signal actually present* (i.e., *actually positive*) and *noise only actually present* (i.e., *actually negative*), respectively. Let S and N represent the decisions *positive* and *negative*, respectively. Then the conditional probability $P(S/s)$, for example, represents the relative frequency with which actually positive images are decided to be positive in a large number of trials, and $P(S/n)$ represents the relative frequency with which actually negative images are called positive. Similarly, $P(N/s)$ represents the relative frequency with which actually positive images are called negative, and $P(N/n)$ represents the relative frequency with which actually negative images are called negative.

The four conditional probabilities described above are sometimes called the *conditional true-positive probability*, the *conditional false-positive probability*, the *conditional false-negative probability*, and the *conditional true-negative probability*, respectively. One should note that since all actually positive images must be called either positive or negative, $P(S/s) + P(N/s) = 1$, and, similarly, $P(S/n) + P(N/n) = 1$. Thus specification of a combination of conditional true-positive and false-positive probabilities, for

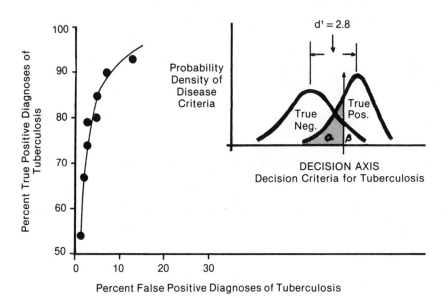

Figure 1. Receiver Operating Characteristic (ROC) curve for the interpretation of chest photofluorograms for the presence of pulmonary tuberculosis. A reciprocal relationship is demonstrated between the percentage of true-positive and the percentage of false-positive diagnosis. Hypothetical population density curves that generated the ROC curve are shown in the upper right diagram. The α and β areas represent false-negative and false-positive diagnoses. d' is an index of detectability and is defined as the mean separation of the two distributions divided by the standard deviation of one distribution. This is written

$$d' = \frac{^mTP - ^mTN}{\sigma}$$

where ^mTP = mean of true-positive population and ^mTN = mean of true-negative population.

example, in fact specifies the conditional probabilities, and hence relative frequencies, of all four types of decisions.

A conventional ROC curve specifies the various trade-offs that are possible among the frequencies of the four types of correct and incorrect decisions as confidence threshold varies in a two-alternative detection experiment by showing the various possible relationships between $P(S/s)$, the conditional true-positive probability, and $P(S/n)$, the conditional false-positive probability. Specifically, the conventional ROC curve is a graph of $P(S/s)$ versus $P(S/n)$. Figure 1 shows a conventional ROC curve for the interpretation of chest photofluorograms for the presence of pulmonary tuberculosis.

ROC curve analysis was first developed for the evaluation of radar signal detectability and was later used to evaluate human detection performance in psychophysics (Green and Swets, 1974). More recently, ROC techniques have been applied to the problems of evaluating diagnostic medical decision-making (Lusted, 1968; McNeil and Adelstein, 1975; McNeil, Keeler, and Adelstein, 1975; McNeil, Varady, Burrows, and Adelstein, 1975) and of evaluating the detectability provided by diagnostic medical imaging systems (Andrus, Hunter, and Bird, 1975; Goodenough, Rossmann, and Lusted, 1972).

ROC ANALYSIS OF BREAST
CANCER DETECTION BY MAMMOGRAPHY

X-ray examination of the breast is used for both diagnostic and screening purposes (Bailar, 1976). As a diagnostic tool, it is used as part of the investigation of breast lesions of unknown nature. It is also employed for periodic screening of general populations, that is, women who are not selected because of a suspicion of breast cancer and who are not known to be at a significantly higher risk of breast cancer than other women of similar age and demographic status.

Most physicians who interpret mammograms seem to make no distinction between use of mammography for screening and for diagnosis. Moreover, most physicians are unaware of the sensitivity and specificity of mammography as a diagnostic test and are not familiar with the effect of disease prevalence on the predictive value of a positive test.

McKeown (1974) has emphasized that ethical considerations of screening are important. Because screening investigations are initiated by doctors rather than patients, he suggests that "it is the medical initiative which creates the obligation which makes a strict validation procedure essential."

In screening for breast cancer among women considered suspect after clinical examination, nearly nine-tenths were found at biopsy not to have the disease (McKeown, 1974). With clinical examination and mammography continued, the proportion who were negative was four-fifths. With the help of ROC analysis and prevalence data, we may see how it is possible that only 20% of women with positive mammograms actually have breast cancer on biopsy or surgery.

Figure 2 (curve A) is an ROC curve for the interpretation of mammograms constructed from the data of Egan (1964). Curve B in the same figure is the ROC curve interpretation performance of nonradiologic personnel (Alcorn and O'Donnell, 1968) Curve B is not of concern in this chapter.

A physician interpretating mammograms could operate at any point along curve A, and, as it has been shown, the physician can change his point of operation by changing his attitude. If he adopts a "better safe than sorry" attitude and calls all suspicious lesions positive, he will move up and

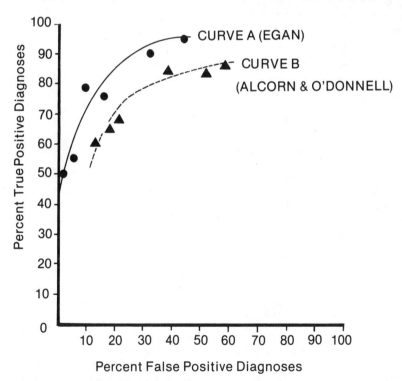

Figure 2.   ROC curves for the interpretation of mammograms. Curve A has been constructed from the data of Egan (1964), and curve B from the data of Alcorn and O'Donnell (1968). Curve A represents interpretation by radiologists, and curve B interpretation by nonradiologic personnel. Curve A, with a larger value for d' than curve B, indicates greater sensitivity of the observers.

right on the curve. This increases the percentage of true-positive results, but it also increases the percentage of false-positive results.

Assume that the physician is operating at a point on the curve that coincides with 90% true-positive and 30% false-positive. Here, sensitivity equals 90% and specificity equals 70%. Using the breast cancer incidence data from the breast cancer screening study conducted by the Health Insurance Plan (HIP) of Greater New York (Shapiro et al., 1972) of approximately 200 per 100,000, a predictive value of a positive mammograph between 1% and 2% has been calculated (Galen and Gambino, 1975). The latter means that, of 100 mammograms positive for disease, 98 would be false-positive and 2 would be true-positive for breast cancer on biopsy. This ROC curve was constructed from studies done several years ago. New film screen systems and xerography have led to better accuracy of interpretation, but ROC curves are not available.

A physician would have to operate at a 90% sensitivity and 90% specificity to obtain a predictive value of positive tests of 10%. As prevalence increases, the predictive value of a positive test increases regardless of the relationship between sensitivity and specificity.

If a population is selected so that its disease prevalence is 2,000 per 100,000 then a 90% sensitivity and a 98% specificity would give a predictive value of a positive test of 50%. That is, for 100 positive mammograms, 50 would be true-positive and 50 would be false-positive for breast cancer.

ROC ANALYSIS, AVERAGE COST, AND AVERAGE NET BENEFIT

Several measures of diagnostic quality may be derived from ROC curves. Metz, Starr, and Lusted (1977) have discussed these measures, and they are therefore not reviewed in detail here. Accuracy, information measure, average cost, and average net benefit are useful measures. Only the latter two are considered below.

Average cost is minimized when the operating point on the ROC curve is chosen such that

$$\frac{dP(S/s)}{dP(S/n)} = \frac{[1 - P(s)]}{P(s)} \times \frac{[C_{FP} - C_{TN}]}{[C_{FN} - C_{TP}]}$$

where C_{FP}, C_{FN}, C_{TP} and C_{TN} are costs of false-positive, false-negative, true-positive, and true-negative decisions, respectively.

Since conventional ROC curves exhibit a monotonically decreasing slope as $P(S/n)$ increases, this expression shows that the optimal operating point is on the lower left portion of the curve, for example, if actually positive cases are rare $[P(s) \ll 1]$ or if the cost of the consequences of a false-positive decision is relatively great.

The *average net benefit* derived from a screening or diagnostic study can be thought of as the reduction in average cost provided by performance of the study. If no significant prior information is available regarding the state of health or disease in a particular case, and if the study is not performed, then one may assume that in many situations no treatment is instituted and thus a *negative* decision is, in effect, made by default. In this case, the average cost of not performing the diagnostic study is

$$\bar{C} \text{ (no study)} = C_{FN} \, P(s) + C_{TN} \, P(n)$$

and the average net benefit, $\overline{NB}$, derived from performing the study is given by

$$\overline{NB} = \bar{C} \text{ (no study)} - \bar{C} \text{ (study)}$$

$$\overline{NB} = [C_{FN} - C_{TP}] \, P(s) \, P(S/s) - [C_{FP} - C_{TN}] \, P(n) \, P(S/n) - \bar{C}$$

The financial costs of breast cancer screening have been studied. In the multiphasic testing program of the Permanente Medical Group, Oakland, California (Collen, 1974), the cost per positive mammogram was $408, and, since only one in five patients were found to show disease on follow-up, the cost of a true-positive was approximately $2,000. In the HIP Study of Greater New York, the annual cost of the mammography program was approximately $1,658,000, or an annual cost of approximately $360,000 for total lives saved.

ROC ANALYSIS OF COLON CANCER DETECTION USING CEA ASSAY: HOW PROBABILITIES APPLY TO THE INDIVIDUAL PATIENT

In discussions about the use of probabilities in medical decisions, physicians often say that probabilities do not apply to the individual patient. There does seem to be some difficulty; that is, it is not intuitively obvious to many people that probabilities can be useful in decisions applied to the unique situation, the unique patient, or the specific set of circumstances that define the $N = 1$ problem (Edward, 1972).

Metz, Hoffer, Lusted, and McCartney (1975, unpublished data) have recently analyzed carcinoembryonic antigen (CEA) assay results by the likelihood ratio approach. Their study demonstrates the usefulness of ROC analysis as applied to the diagnosis of cancer for the individual patient.

In a diagnostic test with a continuous set of value outcomes, the use of a threshold value alone for a positive test ignores the quantitative information provided by the extent to which an individual concentration of values is above threshold. Intuitively, the latter should be related to the degree of certainty concerning the diagnosis.

Table 1.   Likelihood ratios, L, for various serum CEA assay concentrations in colon malignancy[a]

Serum CEA concentration range (ng/ml)	L(colon malignancy; CEA concentration)[b]
0–1.0	0.072 ± 0.072
1.1–2.0	0.59 ± 0.18
2.1–3.0	0.63 ± 0.24
3.1–4.0	0.87 ± 0.49
4.1–5.0	1.00 ± 0.57
5.1–10.0	3.0 ± 1.3
10.1–20.0	11.1 ± 3.0
>20	17.6 ± 6.3

[a] Values computed from data of McCartney and Hoffer (1974) after deletion of cases with interfering medication or previous resection for colon malignancy. Indicated uncertainties are ± 1 estimated standard deviation. For colon malignancy, N = 48; for no colon malignancy, N = 845.

[b] $L(\text{colon malignancy; CEA concentration}) \equiv \dfrac{P(\text{CEA concentration} \mid \text{colon malignancy})}{P(\text{CEA concentration} \mid \text{no colon malignancy})}$

A well-known method that takes quantitative information into account and that has been applied to various problems in medical decision making is the Bayesian approach. Applied to the problem at hand, this method permits calculation of the odds[2] that a particular patient is actually positive, given a CEA concentration within a particular range. The method also requires knowledge of: 1) the prior odds that a case from the population of cases for which assays will be performed is positive before the assay is done, and 2) the probabilities that actually normal and abnormal cases from the population will have CEA concentrations in the range observed. This may be expressed mathematically as follows:

$$\begin{bmatrix} \text{Odds of colon malignancy,} \\ \text{given CEA concentration} \\ \text{in nth range} \end{bmatrix} =$$

$$\begin{bmatrix} \text{Odds of colon} \\ \text{malignancy in} \\ \text{population studied} \end{bmatrix} \times \left\{ \dfrac{\begin{array}{l} \text{Probability of CEA concentration} \\ \text{in nth range for patients} \\ \text{having colon malignancy} \end{array}}{\begin{array}{l} \text{Probability of CEA concentration} \\ \text{in nth range for patients} \\ \text{without colon malignancy} \end{array}} \right\}$$

The second factor on the right is called "the likelihood ratio for CEA concentration in the observed range in colon malignancy" and is the factor

[2] The odds of an event is the ratio of the probability that the event does occur to the probability that it does not occur. The odds of an event, Ω, and the probability of an event, P, are related by the equation: $\Omega = P/(1 - P)$.

by which the prior odds of malignancy are multiplied to yield the posterior odds that apply to the individual patient being tested.

Values for the probabilities of CEA concentrations in various ranges for patients with and without colon malignancy, which are used to calculate the likelihood ratios for the various ranges (Table 1), can be extracted from the data reported by McCartney and Hoffer (1974). The data are plotted as ROC curves in Figures 3A and 3B.

Note that the likelihood ratios in Table 1 show that when CEA concentrations are less than or equal to 5.0 ng/ml, the odds of colon carcinoma in an individual patient are less than or equal to the odds in a normal population.

One can make use of the likelihood ratio to decide whether particular patients should receive further diagnostic studies for colon malignancy. When multiplied by the prior odds of colon malignancy, the likelihood ratio yields the posterior odds in favor of malignancy in an individual patient.

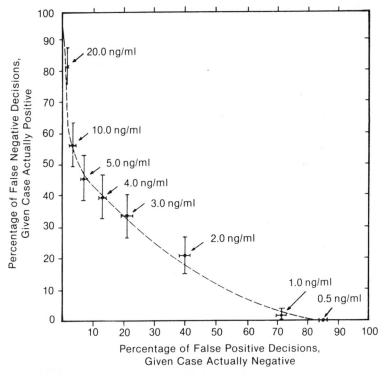

Figure 3A.   ROC curves for the interpretation of CEA assays in colon cancer detection in terms of percentage of false-negative decisions.

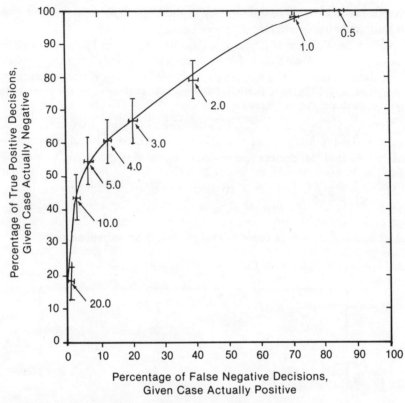

Figure 3B.   ROC curves for the interpretation of CEA assays in colon cancer detection in terms of percentage of false-positive decisions.

Although the likelihood ratios in Table 1 cannot be used to improve the inherent detectability of early colon malignancy by CEA assay, they can enhance the extent to which the CEA assay result can be meaningfully interpreted. The same argument can be applied to any medical diagnostic tests with continuous result outcomes.

CONCLUSIONS

Tests used for the detection or diagnosis of early cancer should be evaluated in reference to their sensitivity and specificity in the context of the prevalence of the disease of interest. ROC analysis is an approach to medical decision making that helps to sort out the trade-offs that are possible among the various types of correct and incorrect decisions. The application of signal detection theory offers useful insights concerning the benefits and costs of cancer detection and their interrelationships in medical, ethical, and economic terms.

REFERENCES

Alcorn, F. S., and O'Donnell, E. 1968. Mammogram screeners: Modified program learning for nonradiologic personnel. Radiology 90:336–338.

Andrus, W. S., Hunter, C. H., and Bird, K. T. 1975. Remote interpretation of chest roentgenograms. Chest 67:463–468.

Bailar, J. C. 1976. Mammography. A contrary view. Ann. Intern. Med. 84:77–84.

Collen, M. F. 1974. Multiphasic testing as a triage to medical care. In: F. J. Ingelfinger, R. V. Ebert, M. Finland, and A. S. Relman (eds.), Controversy in Internal Medicine, Vol. II, pp. 85–91. W. B. Saunders Company, Philadelphia.

Edward, W. 1972. Diagnosis in unique cases. In: J. A. Jacques (ed.), Computer Diagnosis and Diagnostic Methods, pp. 139–151. Charles C Thomas Publisher, Springfield, Ill.

Egan, R. L. 1964. Mammography. Charles C Thomas Publisher, Springfield, Ill.

Fletcher, J. 1974. The Ethics of Genetic Control. Anchor Books, Garden City, N. Y.

Fuchs, V. R. 1974. Who Shall Live? Health, Economics and Social Choice. Basic Books Inc., New York.

Galen, R. S., and Gambino, S. R. 1975. Beyond Normality: The Predictive Value and Efficiency of Medical Diagnoses. John Wiley & Sons, Inc., New York.

Goodenough, D. J., and Metz, C. E. 1973. Implications of a "noisy" observer to data processing techniques. In: C. Raynaud and A. Todd-Pokropek (eds.), Information Processing in Scintigraphy, p. 400. Commissariat a l'Energie Atomique, Orsay, France.

Goodenough, D. J., Rossmann, K., and Lusted, L. B. 1972. Radiographic applications of signal detection theory. Radiology 105:199–200.

Green, D. M., and Swets, J. A. 1974. Signal Detection Theory and Psychophysics. Robert E. Krieger Publishing Company, Huntington, N. J.

Gustafson, J. M. 1975. Forum on medical malpractice. In: Medicine on The Midway, pp. 6–7. The University of Chicago Press, Chicago.

Lusted, L. B. 1968. Introduction to Medical Decision Making. Charles C Thomas Publisher, Springfield, Ill.

McCartney, W. H., and Hoffer, P. B. 1974. The value of carcinoembryonic antigen (CEA) as an adjunct to the radiological color examination in diagnosis of malignancy. Radiology 110:325–328.

McKeown, T. 1974. Unvalidated procedures have no place in screening programs. In: F. J. Ingelfinger, R. V. Ebert, M. Finland, and A. S. Relman (eds.), Controversy in Internal Medicine, pp. 92–98. W. B. Saunders Company, Philadelphia.

McNeil, B. J., and Adelstein, S. J. 1975. Measures of clinical efficacy: The value of case finding in hypertensive renovascular disease. N. Engl. J. Med. 221–226.

McNeil, B. J., Keeler, E., and Adelstein, S. J. 1975. Primer on certain elements of medical decision making. N. Engl. J. Med. 293:211–215.

McNeil, B. J., Varady, P. D., Burrows, B. A., and Adelstein, S. J. 1975. Measures of clinical efficacy: Cost effectiveness calculations in the diagnosis and treatment of hypertensive renovascular disease. N. Engl. J. Med. 293:215–221.

Metz, C. E., Hoffer, P. B., Lusted, L. B., and McCartney, W. H. 1975 (May). Diagnosis of colon malignancy from measurement of serum carcinoembryonic antigen

(CEA): Effects of threshold of abnormality and an alternative approach based upon likelihood ratio estimates. Unpublished manuscript.

Metz, C. E., Starr, S. J., and Lusted, L. B. 1977. Quantitative evaluation of visual detection performance in medicine: ROC analysis and determination of diagnostic benefit, pp. 220–241. In: G. A. Hay (ed.), Medical Images. John Wiley & Sons, Inc., London.

Revesz, G., Kundel, H. L., and Graber, M. A. 1974. The influence of structured noise on the detection of radiologic abnormalities. Invest. Radiol. 9:479–486.

Shapiro, S., Strax, P., Venet, L., and Venet, W. 1972. Changes in 5-year breast cancer mortality in a breast cancer screening program, pp. 663–678. Proceedings of the 7th National Cancer Conference, American Cancer Society, Ind., and National Cancer Institute.

Part III
Diagnostic and Therapeutic Problems

6
Immunodiagnosis of Cancer in Man

Ronald B. Herberman

During the past several years, a rapidly expanding body of research has developed related to the immunodiagnosis of human cancer. Many antigen systems and other promising approaches are being actively investigated. Several distinct clinical applications of immunodiagnostic procedures need to be considered. First, some immunodiagnostic procedures might be useful in the detection of cancer by screening general populations or groups at high risk of developing cancer. Second, immunodiagnostic assays may assist in distinguishing between patients with cancer and those with benign disease, among patients coming to physicians with signs or symptoms consistent with, or suggestive of, cancer. In addition, immunologic procedures might be employed in patients with known cancer, to help in its localization, to determine prognosis and type of therapy, and to monitor patients for clinical recurrences or metastases.

A systematic evaluation of potentially useful immunodiagnostic procedures is underway at the National Cancer Institute (NCI), in which this author is involved. The most important point to resolve for a test thought to be applicable to human cancer is whether it can distinguish accurately between cancer patients and others with benign diseases or with no disease. In the evaluation of possible immunodiagnostic serum tests at the National Cancer Institute, a collection of specimens from patients with known diagnoses has proved most helpful. When a promising new test is recognized, an appropriate panel of sera from the NCI–Mayo Clinic Serum Bank is rapidly assembled and sent under code to the investigators.

For example, in a typical serum panel for the evaluation of gastrointestinal (GI) cancer, a sizeable number of specimens (at least 20) are collected from patients with GI cancer in various stages of disease, including localized lesions, and in the main before therapy. Control sera are taken from patients with benign diseases of the same organ systems, including particularly inflammatory diseases (e.g., ulcerative colitis and pancreatitis), and from age- and sex-matched normal individuals. Sera from patients with other types of cancer are also obtained in order to assess the specificity of the test.

Several problems associated with this type of evaluation may be described. The first concerns the fact that, while immunodiagnostic tests often successfully differentiate between cancer patients (especially those in advanced stages) and young, adult, normal controls, most of these tests are not sufficiently specific in distinguishing between cancer patients and those with benign diseases. For example, while the T-globulin test of Tal and Halperin (1970) initially appeared to be quite specific for cancer, a recent analysis of a large panel of coded sera showed many positive results with sera of patients with benign diseases (Tal et al., 1973), suggesting that the test in its present form is not sufficiently discriminatory to be practicable for the immunodiagnosis of cancer.

The second problem to be stressed is the influence of unconscious bias or subjectivity in the evaluation of test data. There is sometimes a tendency to interpret test results in light of available clinical information, rather than independently through use of a coded serum panel, with all clinical information withheld from the investigator until after data analysis has been completed.

A third problem relates to the fact that cutoff values for discriminating between cancer and control groups are often determined from the test data themselves. Such retrospectively set cutoffs provide an unwarranted optimistic appraisal of the data which, in fact, need to be validated by means of further prospective measurements.

It should also be emphasized that, while a single test may be inadequate, several tests applied together may provide highly discriminating information. When such results are obtained, it becomes important to evaluate the possible additive or synergistic effects of the several immunodiagnostic tests. The recent study of Ravry et al. (1974), demonstrating a significant increase in the detection rate of metastatic gastric carcinoma by the combined use of two markers, is a good example of this phenomenon.

Several types of immunologic approaches are potentially applicable in screening for cancer. Attempts to detect antigenic markers in tumor-bearing individuals have been frequently undertaken. Because tumor cells may contain antigens undetectable or present in much smaller amounts in normal cells, antibodies against these antigens, whether in the patients' sera or in the sera of animals immunized against them, are potentially useful for discriminating between tumor cells and normal cells.

To be of clinical significance in immunodiagnosis, the tumor antigens should be common to a variety of tumors, at least to those of the same histologic type. Studies in animal model systems have shown that tumors induced by chemical carcinogens as well as some spontaneous tumors contain distinct tumor-associated transplantation antigens that are absent in other types of tumors induced by the same agent (Prehn and Main, 1957). Such antigens would not be diagnostically useful, because antibodies prepared against one tumor would not be expected to react with other tumors.

Common antigens on tumors have been identified. In general, they fall into three categories: 1) virus-induced or associated antigens, 2) fetal or carcinoembryonic antigens, and 3) tissue antigens. Tumors induced by the same virus, even when they differ in morphologic appearance, share some tumor-associated antigens. While no human tumors have yet unequivocally been shown to be induced by viruses, several viruses and their antigens are clearly and closely associated with certain human tumors. For example, Epstein-Barr virus is associated with Burkitt's lymphoma and nasopharyngeal carcinoma (Henle et al., 1969; Henle et al., 1970), herpes simplex virus with cervical carcinoma (Aurelian and Strnad, 1976) and cancers of the head and neck (Hollinshead and Tarro, 1973), and mouse mammary tumor virus with breast cancer (Black et al., 1974). Even without a direct etiologic significance, such virus-associated antigens could be useful diagnostic markers.

Antigens present on normal fetal cells may also be present in a variety of tumor cells and may be applicable in cancer screening, regardless of their etiologic importance. Finally, normal tissue antigens may be expressed in large amounts in tumor cells, and some may be specific for the organ from which the tumor is derived. The converse situation, namely, the loss of some normal antigens, organ specific or not, from tumor cells may also be useful in immunodiagnosis. For example, loss of blood group antigens has been correlated with a tendency for metastasis (Davidsohn and Ni, 1969).

Depression in the immune competence of cancer patients may also be exploited for diagnostic purposes. Decreased immune surveillance has, in fact, been suggested as an important factor in tumor development (Burnet, 1957). Furthermore, tumor growth can also produce immunosuppression (Herberman, 1974a). In either case, the decreased immune competence relative to levels in normal individuals or in those with benign disease has diagnostic implications.

Many tumor-associated antigens can elicit an immune response in tumor-bearing individuals. Such antigens can often be recognized by the host even when present in very small amounts, suggesting that immunologic reactions could be detected while tumors were still small and localized. Humoral antibodies, cell-mediated immune responses, and serum factors blocking cellular immune reactions are all potential markers for cancer control efforts.

The use of immunologic tests for cancer screening is probably the most difficult of all the potential applications. If a test is shown to discriminate between cancer and control groups, it must then be evaluated for screening utility by means of an appropriately designed study. A number of factors can affect the feasibility of a particular test for screening purposes. These need to be carefully considered before any screening programs are initiated.

The assay system must be relatively simple and applicable to the testing of large numbers of specimens or individuals. The method must be sufficiently developed and standardized, so that reproducible results can be obtained over time and in multiple laboratories. Furthermore, the test, which presumably would be offered to large numbers of normal individuals, should pose little or no risk to the recipients.

A suitable population must be available for study. It is especially desirable to identify populations or family groups at high risk of developing cancer. Examples of such high risk groups currently being used to evaluate screening techniques are heavy smokers, industrial workers exposed to carcinogens, and families genetically predisposed to cancer. The population must be sufficiently accessible to permit retesting as necessary and to make it possible for test-positive screenees to undergo extensive clinical evaluation. Equally important, the initially disease-free individuals in the population must be available for clinical follow-up over a period of several years in order to identify and to characterize those who subsequently develop cancer.

Prospective studies are often expensive to perform and require long periods of time to complete. An alternative approach is to collect and store serologic or other specimens from individuals being screened for other purposes. Years later, when a promising diagnostic test is developed, it could be validated by applying it to specimens from individuals known to have developed cancer after the initial screening and from individuals known to have remained free of cancer. For example, serum specimens are now being collected from smokers undergoing screening for lung cancer and from elderly persons submitting to periodic health examinations. Such prospective studies done in retrospect may prove useful in assessing a test's potential for screening. An important qualification is that the serum constituents of interest may be affected by long-term storage, even at $-70°C$. Fortunately, most known antigens and antibodies are stable when the sera have been carefully collected, processed, and stored at sufficiently low temperatures.

A fundamental requirement is the specificity of the immunologic assay. The test must be able to detect a consistent difference between cancer and noncancer. The difference should preferably, but not necessarily, be qualitative. The presence of a marker in cancer patients and its absence in nonneoplastic disease states, or the loss of a normal component in cancer patients, would provide the basis for the development of a useful diagnostic test. However, quantitative differences in parameters between cancer patients and controls could also suffice. In this case, it would be necessary to determine the normal range of values and, as discussed above, the appropriate cutoff point. A valid diagnostic test should have a high degree of specificity, that is, very few false-positives should exist among screenees without cancer.

The screening test should be very sensitive, with relatively few false-negative results. In other words, it should detect cancer in a large proportion of cancer patients, including those with small, localized tumors as well as those with recurrent or metastatic deposits. To be useful for early detection the test should also be able to localize the tumor mass. This is especially important for the occult or clinically undetectable cancers. A rational approach to cancer control certainly requires more than the diagnosis of a "cancer, type, and site unknown." Accordingly, the developers of potential screening instruments should strive to achieve a specificity of the immunologic test for a particular organ site or histologic type of cancer.

It is difficult to make general statements about acceptable levels of specificity and sensitivity for screening tests. A major factor that must be considered is the prevalence and incidence of the type of cancer being screened in the population of interest. High specificity is particularly important in screening for cancers that occur with low frequency. For example, a test may yield a 2% rate of false-positives, which one might otherwise consider to be quite acceptable. However, if the incidence of the cancer in the population were 20 per 100,000 and if the test were 100% sensitive, 99 out of every 100 positive tests would be false- positives.

Another consideration of great practical importance is the ability of a test to detect cancer at a time prior to the development of clinical symptoms and, particularly, prior to metastatic spread. The longer the lead time (i.e., the interval between test positivity and clinical detection of disease), the more likely it is that the test will contribute to the screenee's survival and response to therapy. It should be noted that, in order to accurately determine the lead time for a particular assay, tests need to be performed repeatedly to establish the point in the disease at which the test first becomes positive.

The amount of lead time provided by a test and the clinical benefits conferred by early detection of disease are, to some extent, determined by the tumor's growth rate. Screening tests are more apt to be useful for slow growing tumors with long latent periods than for explosively growing tumors that metastasize early.

Another factor not to be ignored concerns the consequences of positive test results in a screened individual. False-positives often present a number of psychological, logistic, and economic problems. Such screenees must undergo additional diagnostic procedures in order to arrive at the proper diagnosis, but this must be done in such fashion as to avoid undue alarm.

The nature of the clinical procedures needed to establish or rule out the presence of the particular type of cancer has a substantial influence on the specificity required of a screening test. A test in which only 1% of the positives actually had cancer might be very useful if it detected most, or all, of the cancers and if it involved only a simple and low risk, noninvasive diagnostic procedure. By way of contrast, if an extensive surgical procedure were needed to establish the diagnosis, such a screening test would be considerably less acceptable.

CURRENT STATUS OF IMMUNODIAGNOSTIC TESTS FOR CANCER

Many human tumors have been found to contain common tumor-associated antigens. Antibodies against these antigens can be prepared to test tissue biopsies or exfoliated cells for neoplasms. At present, this potentially useful approach has not been fully exploited. Much of the emphasis has been on the detection of antigens released from tumor cells and present in the circulation. The development of a radioimmunoassay (Thomson et al., 1969) to the carcinoembryonic antigen (CEA) of Gold and Freedman (1965), which made it possible to screen large numbers of serum specimens, provided a major impetus to this area of research.

The original paper on the clinical application of CEA suggested high specificity and sensitivity. In addition, there were indications that the CEA values became elevated prior to the clinical manifestations of cancer. However, recent studies, using patients with benign GI disease and cancer patients with localized disease, reveal that a considerable number of false-positives are obtained and that many patients with localized GI cancer do not have increased levels of CEA at all (Zamcheck et al., 1972). In addition, many patients with a variety of non-GI cancers have elevated levels of CEA.

Although large numbers of specimens from cancer patients and from variously selected controls have already been tested, no prospective studies of CEA have been undertaken. However, there is one study in which adequate clinical follow-up was compiled for 4 years on Australian patients whose sera had been previously collected (Stevens, MacKay, and Cullen, 1975). The findings are summarized in Table 1. Overall, the false-positive rate was only 3.8%. Viewed in terms of its predictive value, however, the assay was false-positive among 81% of positive screenees. Even more disappointing was the failure of the CEA assay to detect cancer in three-quarters of those who subsequently developed carcinoma of the GI tract, lung, or breast, sites that had previously been associated with elevated CEA values. These data may provide an overly pessimistic view, however, because some of the tumors might have become manifest several years after the serum had been collected.

Table 1. Use of CEA in screening for cancer

| | CEA levels in 1969 | | | |
| | Elevated | | Normal | |
Health status in 1973	Number	Percent	Number	Percent
Cancer: GI, lung, and breast	6	14	18	2
Cancer: Other sites	2	4	34	4
Smokers	15	34	95	10
Benign diseases	2	4	44	5
Normal	19	43	721	79

Percentage of false-positive tests: 3.8
Percentage of false-negative tests:
    Total cancer   87
    GI, lung, and breast   75
    Other sites   94

Source: Stevens, MacKay, and Cullen, 1975.

The use of CEA as a diagnostic adjunct rather than as a primary screening instrument is only now being systematically evaluated. The potential use of CEA to indicate prognosis and to monitor therapy has been suggested by a number of investigators (Chu, Holyoke, and Murphy, 1974; Mach et al., 1974; Sorokin et al., 1974). However, all of the published reports involved small numbers of patients and rather short follow-up periods. About 5 years ago, a prospective study was initiated at the Roswell Park Memorial Institute in Buffalo, New York, to evaluate CEA in monitoring large numbers of patients with GI cancer (Herrara, Chu, and Holyoke, 1976). Although it is still in progress, the study has already provided some interesting data. More than 100 patients with colorectal cancer have been entered into the study at the time of surgery. Postoperatively, 23 patients have thus far developed recurrent disease. These patients were matched with 23 patients who have had no recurrences after a follow-up of at least 12 months. The preoperative CEA levels appear to have some prognostic value in this situation. Among patients with localized tumors at the time of surgery, elevated CEA levels were found significantly more often in those patients who subsequently had recurrent disease than in those who did not. All patients with recurrent or metastatic disease at the time of surgery had elevated CEA levels.

Thus, elevated CEA levels at the time of surgery seem to be correlated with a poor prognosis. However, this correlation is certainly not complete. Postoperative CEA levels tended to rise in many patients so that the test had no apparent clinical significance up to 3 months later. After 3 months, serial CEA determinations did correlate fairly well with clinical events. However, a single elevation in CEA had no predictive value. Only when three consecutive values obtained at monthly intervals were elevated did the immunologic data correlate well with the clinical course of disease. This type of data has been used to support the practice of "second look" surgery. It should be noted, however, that 4 of 23 patients with no disease recurrence in more than a year had elevated CEA levels. It remains to be seen whether such results represent false-positives or whether they are giving a very early indication of recurrent cancer.

As already noted, the occurrence of false-positive results with sera from patients with benign diseases and with other types of cancer has interfered with the use of CEA assays in screening in colorectal cancer. Recently, Edgington, Astarita, and Plow (1975) isolated a CEA fraction termed CEA-S, which seems to have a high degree of specificity in radioimmunoassay. A coded panel of sera was sent to them for testing. The CEA-S assay detected a higher proportion of patients with GI cancer and had a remarkably low incidence of false-positive results in noncancer patients when compared with conventional CEA assays as performed by Go (see Ravry et al., 1974). Although these results are encouraging, they must be interpreted with caution. More than one-half of the patients with GI cancer had CEA levels in the normal range; thus, the test may not be sufficiently sensitive for the detection of early disease. The CEA-S test also needs to be evaluated in respect to the various clinical parameters discussed above.

Alpha-fetoprotein (AFP), after its initial description by Abelev (1971), has been extensively studied as an immunodiagnostic marker for hepatomas, teratomas, and other tumors. A number of investigators have used AFP assays for large-scale screening in populations with a relatively high incidence of hepatoma. The data from two of these studies are summarized in Table 2. Leblanc, Tuyns, and Masseyeff (1973) screened almost 10,000 individuals in Senegal, where the incidence of primary hepatocarci-

Table 2.   Alpha-fetoprotein in screening for primary liver cancer

Item	Leblanc, Tuyns, and Masseyeff (1973)	Coordinating Group (1974)
Screening site	Senegal	China
Incidence of primary liver cancer	>45/100,000	?
Number screened	9,864	343,999
Number with elevated AFP	6	147
Elevated AFP rate	60/100,000	43/100,000
Number of apparent false-positives	0	18
Number of false-negatives/total evaluable	3/9,864	7/11,004
Number elevated AFP in asymptomatic/ total evaluable liver cancer	3/9	33/53

nomas exceeds 45 per 100,000. Only six screenees tested positive, but this is equivalent to a rate of 60 per 100,000, a figure only one-third larger than the overall incidence of the disease. The program failed to detect three cases of primary liver cancer, and, of those detected, only one-half were found prior to the appearance of clinical signs and symptoms. Apparently, there were no false-positives at all.

Investigators in China have mounted a large screening project that has already involved the testing of more than 300,000 people (Coordinating Group, 1974). They screened a similar proportion of positive cases, 43 per 100,000. Although their false-positive rate was very low (about 0.005%), these screenees accounted for more than 10% of all positive tests. Seven cases failed to be detected among 11,000 individuals, suggesting that the test may have detected fewer than one-half of the individuals with hepatic cancer. An encouraging aspect of this study is that more than one-half of the evaluable hepatoma patients were detected prior to the appearance of clinical evidence of disease. However, no information was available on the effect of this screening program on patient survival.

Both of the above studies employed relatively insensitive immunodiffusion assays for AFP. Purves (1973), using a more sensitive radioimmunoassay, failed to detect a single case of elevated AFP (defined by a cutoff of > 100 ng/ml) among 5,000 asymptomatic Bantu miners. This is surprising since the incidence of primary liver cancer among this population was 1 per 2,700 overall. The investigators attempted to explain this disappointing result on the basis of a very rapid doubling time (about 10 days) for this particular type of cancer.

Medullary carcinoma of the thyroid is a neoplasm for which an accepted and sensitive immunologic test exists, namely, the radioimmunoassay for thyrocalcitonin. Because this disease can be inherited within some families as an autosomal dominant trait, a high risk population is available for screening. Tashjian, Wolfe, and Voelkel (1974) screened 258 members of 5 kindreds and performed thyroidectomies on 38 asymptomatic individuals because their calcitonin assays were positive. Nearly 90% of these patients had medullary carcinomas of the thyroid. Particularly encouraging was the finding that 40% of these patients had localized disease, which has a much better prognosis than if the lesion had extended beyond the gland. Wells et al. (1975) screened 40 individuals, and 4 false-negatives with basal calcitonin and calcium infusion tested positive after pentagastrin.

Although these data are impressive, their significance is not yet completely established. For example, it is not yet known what the expected incidence of fatal thyroid cancer is among such families and whether all localized and asymptomatic cases necessarily progress to invasion. Furthermore, some of the positive screenees were found to have only C cell hyper-plasia without any signs of malignancy. Although C cell hyperplasia has been postulated as a preinvasive lesion (Wolfe et al., 1973), there is presently no direct evidence on its malignant potential.

Elevated calcitonin levels are not entirely pathognomonic for medullary carcinoma of the thyroid, because some patients with subacute thyroiditis also have high basal levels (Cervi-Skinner and Castleman, 1973). So, too, do some patients with oat cell carcinoma of the lung (Silva et al., 1974) and other cancers (Coombes et al., 1974). Tests for basal levels of calcitonin do not appear to be sufficiently sensitive for detecting patients with thyroid cancer. However, infusion of calcium and particularly of pentagastrin (Wells et al., 1975) has considerably improved the diagnostic accuracy of this test.

It remains to be seen whether these procedures can detect all (or nearly all) patients with medullary carcinoma of the thyroid and what the impact on survival will be. The very success of the calcitonin screening test has made it difficult to organize controlled studies of these questions.

One tumor-associated marker, found not in serum but in gastric juice, has provided the basis for a large screening study for gastric cancer (Table 3). Häkkinen (1974) observed that fetal sulfoglycoprotein antigen (FSA) was associated with gastric cancer. He screened 13,612 people in Finland, a country which has a relatively high incidence of this disease, approximating 30 per 100,000 in the age range screened. The results provide an example of the potential problems of screening. While the overall false-positive rate was

Table 3. Fetal sulfoglycoprotein (FSA) in screening for gastric cancer

Screening locale	industrial and rural Finland
Number screened	13,612
Number FSA positive	461
Industrial, % positive	3
Rural, % positive	6
Total, % positive	3.3

Diagnoses in FSA + screenees	Number	Percent
Gastric cancer or polyposis	5	1
Gastritis	61	13
Ulcer	10	2
Atrophy	23	5
Other benign	32	6
No detectable disease	330	71

Percent false-positive	3.3	Incidence of gastric cancer	~30/100,000
Percent false-negative	0	Incidence of total cancer	~37/100,000

Source: Häkkinen, 1974.

Table 4.   Three markers in sera from Framingham Study[a]

Marker	True-positives		False-positives	
	Number	Percent	Number	Percent
CEA	5	29	7	21
AFP	1	6	0	0
HCG	1	6	4	12

Source: Williams et al., 1977.
[a] Cases: 9 carcinomas of pancreas; 8 carcinomas of stomach.
Controls: 34 matching, without cancer.

only 3.3%, only 1.1% of those with a positive test actually had gastric cancer detectable by gastroscopy. Häkkinen has suggested that the screening successfully detected all gastric cancers in the population. If this is correct, the test may still prove useful for screening, because the confirmatory diagnostic procedures required for the positive screenees pose little risk to the patients.

In a recent study the use of multiple tumor markers was evaluated for screening purposes (Williams et al., 1977). The investigators made use of sera collected since 1948 as part of the Framingham Heart Study. Most of the study population has been followed for development of cancer as well as for other types of disease. It was possible to select cases in which sera were drawn prior to the development of pancreatic or gastric cancer. For every such individual, two control specimens were selected from individuals who did not develop cancer, and who matched the cancer cases in age, sex, smoking history, and other characteristics. The results of screening tests for AFP, CEA, and human chorionic gonadotropin (HCG) are summarized in Table 4. The radioimmunoassay for CEA proved to be the most sensitive test because it detected 29% of the cancers. However, its false-positive rate was almost as high. The dual problems of false-positives plus low sensitivity are similar to those seen in the other studies of CEA (Stevens, MacKay, and Cullen, 1975). AFP testing added very little, because of its low sensitivity. The results with HCG were particularly unsatisfactory, with only one cancer positive and four false-positive. Furthermore, the specimens with elevated AFP or HCG levels also had elevated CEA levels, so that the other two markers were not additive. However, the elevated marker levels did appear to increase the lead time by up to 12 months among those individuals who developed cancer (Table 5). This suggests that if the specificity and sensitivity of the CEA assays could be improved, the procedure might have some applicability in screening.

A large number of other human tumor-associated markers have been described, some of which might prove useful in cancer immunodiagnosis (Alpert, Coston, and Drysdale, 1973; Banwo, Versey, and Hobbs, 1974;

Table 5.   Framingham Cancer Study

| Diagnosis | Patient | Lead time (months) | Tumor markers in ng/ml | | |
			CEA	AFP	HCG
Pancreatic cancer	1	6	17.4		
	2	2	4.0		21
	3	12			
	4	2			
Gastric cancer	5	10	11.6		
	6	9	7.2		
	7	<1	4.8	84	
	8	11			

Source: Williams et al., 1977.

Benson et al., 1974; Braunstein et al., 1973; Buffe et al., 1972; Edynak et al., 1972; Gerwirtz and Yalom, 1974; Hendrick and Franchimont, 1974; Marcus and Zinburg, 1975; Roof et al., 1971; Rosen et al., 1975; Usategui-Gomez, Yeager, and Fernandez de Castro, 1973). These include markers based on the ectopic production of hormones and their detection by radioimmunoassay. The clinical applications and limitations of most of the other markers remain largely indeterminate at this time.

TESTS OF DIMINISHED IMMUNE COMPETENCE IN IMMUNODIAGNOSIS

The types of assays for decreased immunologic competence that might be useful in the study of cancer patients are summarized in Table 6. In accordance with immune surveillance theory, decreased immunologic reactivity

Table 6.   Assays for decreased immune competence as possible diagnostic procedures

1. Skin tests for delayed hypersensitivity
   a. Tests for previous natural sensitization with recall antigens
   b. Primary sensitization (e.g., dinitrochlorobenzene, hemocyanin)
2. Enumeration of circulating T and B lymphocytes
   a. Rosette assays
   b. Immunofluorescent and cytotoxic antibodies
3. Lymphocyte functions
   a. Proliferative response to mitogens, antigens
   b. Cytotoxicity, and generation of cytotoxic lymphocytes
   c. Production of lymphokines
4. Antibody production
5. Macrophage functions

might be found prior to development of clinical cancer or in the presence of early, localized disease (Herberman, 1974b). Theoretically, this might be useful in the prognosis and monitoring of cancers.

In most of the studies reported to date, impaired reactivity has been seen mainly in cancer patients with advanced rather than early disease. Skin tests for delayed hypersensitivity have been used most extensively. Many studies involved tests with recall antigens, to which many or most of the screenees had been naturally sensitized. So far, at least, the results have not proved diagnostically useful, because most patients, except those with widely disseminated disease, react to at least some of these antigens (Lamb et al., 1962; Miller, 1968; Soloway and Rapaport, 1965).

Tests for delayed hypersensitivity, involving sensitization to an antigen to which the individual has not been previously exposed, followed by a challenge, appear to be more sensitive indicators of immune depression. Failure of cancer patients to be sensitized to dinitrochlorobenzene (DNCB) has been found to be a useful prognostic indicator of unresectable disease or of early recurrence after surgery (Elber and Morton, 1970; Pinsky et al., 1971; Wells et al., 1973).

In vitro assays of cell-mediated immune reactivity have also been employed to look for decreased reactivity among cancer patients. Decreased proliferation of lymphocytes in response to mitogens has been extensively studied, but findings have largely been restricted to patients with advanced or inoperable disease (Han and Takita, 1972; Hersh and Oppenheim, 1965; Whittaker, Rees, and Clark, 1971). This approach needs to be tested for its prognostic or monitoring value in cancer patients. Other lymphocyte functions may also be depressed in cancer patients, including some with localized disease (Takasugi and Kinoshita, 1974). Alterations in macrophage function may also affect cancer patients, but little work has been done in this area.

In addition to functional assays, enumeration of the relative proportions and absolute numbers of T and B cells might prove useful in cancer immunodiagnosis. The most promising procedure is that of rosette formation of human T cells with sheep erythrocytes (E-rosettes). Many cancer patients have been found to have decreased percentages of E-rosette-forming cells before therapy. The best discrimination between cancer and control patients has been observed when the assays were performed under suboptimal conditions, so that only a proportion of the T cells formed rosettes (West et al., 1976; Wybran and Fudenberg, 1973). Most cancer patients, including those with localized disease, had decreased percentages of rosette-forming cells before treatment. Afterward, in the absence of evident disease, many of the patients returned to the normal range.

In contrast to the decreased cell-mediated immune competence seen in some cancer patients, most show no discernible evidence of decreased abililty to produce serum antibodies (Aizawa and Southam, 1960; Southam and Moore, 1954). However, the subject has not been intensively studied, and it is possible that with more sensitive and quantitative techniques, some immunologic deficits might be revealed.

None of these assays for immune competence has yet been adequately tested for potential use in clinical immunodiagnosis. Data are particularly scanty on the value of these tests for the detection or early diagnosis of particular neoplasms. Prospective studies of symptomatic patients and of population groups at increased cancer risk are needed.

A major impediment in evaluating immunodiagnostic approaches are the technical problems inherent in the assays. Test results, even among normal individuals, tend to fluctuate over a considerable range from day to day. To make these assays suitable for large-scale clinical application, it will be necessary to standardize them to reduce the variability of the procedures. This would allow a more careful determination of the normal range and might also narrow the range. The use of cryopreserved lymphocytes or sera as standard controls and ongoing quality control testing with specimens from normal individuals as well as from patients with benign diseases should help in this respect.

IMMUNE RESPONSES TO TUMOR-ASSOCIATED OR VIRUS-ASSOCIATED ANTIGENS

In addition to studies on the general immunologic competence of cancer patients, a number of investigators have evaluated immune responses to tumor-associated antigens. The types of techniques available for such studies are summarized in Table 7. Despite the immunodepression sometimes seen, many cancer patients have detectable immune responses to tumor-associated antigens.

Table 7.   Assays for immune response to tumor-associated antigens

1. Cell-mediated immunity
    a. Skin tests for delayed hypersensitivity, using extracts of tumor cells
    b. Cytotoxicity assays, against tumor cells of tumor-derived cells in culture
    c. Leukocyte migration inhibition by tumor antigens
    d. Proliferative response to tumor antigens
    e. Macrophage electrophoretic mobility test
    f. Leukocyte adherence inhibition
2. Humoral factors
    a. Antibodies against tumor antigens, measured by immunofluorescence, cytotoxicity, etc.
    b. Factors that block assays of cell-mediated immunity

There have been a number of studies on cell-mediated immunity to tumor antigens. Skin tests for delayed hypersensitivity to tumor extracts have been performed in a manner similar to that employed with recall antigens (Herberman, 1974a; Herberman et al., 1973). Reactions to antigens common to many tumors of similar histologic type have been observed in acute leukemia, intestinal cancer, breast cancer, malignant melanoma, and others. Since reactivity to leukemia-associated antigens seems to correlate with clinical state, skin tests with tumor extracts may prove useful for prognosis and monitoring response to therapy.

Skin tests also have potential application to screening and early diagnosis of cancer. However, a major difficulty lies in the possible hazards associated with inoculation of extracts from cancer tissues into cancer-free individuals. Although there is as yet no evidence of adverse effects from the large number of tests performed thus far, even a very small risk is unacceptable for the general population. However, among symptomatic patients it appears reasonable to administer such tests even in the presence of some risk, because benefits in improved cancer prognosis would probably outweigh any small exposure risks.

On this basis, skin tests with soluble and partially separated extracts of malignant melanoma have been evaluated for their utility in the differential diagnosis of ocular melanoma (Char et al., 1974). The results obtained thus far are promising; 26 of 27 patients with ocular melanoma gave positive reactions, whereas negative results were seen among none of 5 patients initially thought to have ocular melanoma who proved to have other nonmelanomatous ocular lesions.

Another possible approach to skin testing in cancer detection involved the use of extracts prepared from normal tissues. Because skin-reactive antigens in intestinal and lung cancer are also found in normal fetal cells (Hollinshead et al., 1970; Wells et al., 1973), fetal extracts should provide safe materials for such testing. Studies are now in progress to evaluate the use of fetal intestine and liver extracts in the detection of colorectal cancer in families with polyposis.

Cell-mediated cytotoxicity assays also have potential application to cancer immunodiagnosis. The Hellströms and others have reported that the lymphocytes of patients with various types of cancer can inhibit colony formation or can be cytotoxic against tissue culture cells derived from tumors of the same histologic type (Hellström et al., 1973). If only persons who developed tumors exhibited cell-mediated reactivity against histologic type-specific tumor antigens, a sensitive detection method might be available. However, this does not seem to be the case (Herberman and Oldham, 1975). A considerable number of normal individuals have been found to react significantly against cultured cells derived from tumors. In addition, cancer patients have reacted against cells derived from dissimilar types of cancer. At the moment, therefore, this assay does not appear to be suitable for practical clinical application.

Humoral factors, which can inhibit or facilitate cell-mediated cytotoxicity have also been described (Hellström et al., 1973). These may be correlated to some extent with clinical status. However, the findings to date are only tentative, and further standardization of the basic assay procedures will have to precede any final conclusions.

Reactivity to common tumor-associated antigens has also been detected by the leukocyte migration inhibition assay in patients with breast cancer (Cochran et al., 1972; McCoy et al., 1974), malignant melanoma (Cochran et al., 1972; McCoy et al., 1975), intestinal cancer (Bull et al., 1973), and lymphoma and leukemia (Braun et al., 1972). In most cases, the reactions have been against common antigens on tumors of the same histologic type, and normal reactivity has been infrequent. A major limitation to extensive use of this test is technical; the procedure is difficult to perform and requires large numbers of leukocytes. The leukocyte adherence inhibition assay (Maluish and Halliday, 1974) was developed as a possible simplified replacement for the migration inhibition assay, and preliminary results are encouraging.

Another assay resembling the leukocyte adherence inhibition assay is the macrophage electrophoretic mobility assay (Caspary and Field, 1971; Pritchard et al., 1973). The pattern of results with this test has differed from that seen with the cellular immunity assays described above. Most cancer patients give positive results with an antigen that appears to be common to a wide variety of tumors, while normal controls are negative. More patients with benign diseases need testing in order to evaluate the diagnostic potential of this assay.

Soluble extracts of autologous and allogeneic tumor cells, prepared with 3 M KCl, have recently been shown to stimulate and induce lymphocyte proliferation in cancer patients (Mavligit et al., 1973). It is postulated that these soluble antigens can stimulate only the lymphocytes of immune persons, in contrast with the ability of antigens on intact cells to elicit a primary proliferative response. Since extracts of some breast tumors and of normal leukocytes, prepared in the same fashion, were able to induce proliferation in a high proportion of lymphocytes from allogeneic normal donors (Dean et al., 1975), it is unlikely that the use of 3 M KCl tumor extracts will prove effective in early cancer detection. However, it is possible that the assay may be useful for disease monitoring in cancer patients for whom autologous tumor extracts are available.

Cercek, Cercek, and Franklin (1974) have used another technique to measure lymphocyte stimulation by "cancer basic protein," the same material used in the macrophage electrophoretic mobility test. Positive results were obtained in all patients with cancer and in very few normal individuals or patients with benign disease.

Detection of antibodies to tumor-associated antigens is a potentially sensitive and logistically simple procedure for cancer immunodiagnosis. Unfortunately, there have been relatively few advances in this area. Antibodies to common antigens on some tumors, for example, melanoma (Lewis et al., 1969; Morton et al., 1970) and osteosarcoma (Morton et al., 1970; Mukherji and Hirshaut, 1973), have been described. However, a considerable number of normal donors also gave positive reactions, and the specificity of the detected antigens has not been well documented. Morton et al. (1970) observed a good correlation between antibody titers and clinical status, and serial antibody determinations may prove useful for prognosis and for monitoring therapy.

Cancer immunodiagnosis based on immune reactivity to tumor-associated antigens appears to be a promising approach. One should be able to exploit the specific reactivity of tumor-associated antigens. However, progress has been impeded by the complexities of the antigens and of the immune response itself. One problem besetting almost all the assays is the lack of standardized, well-characterized sources of antigens or target cells. The number of tests has been small and the tumor specimens have been many and diverse. Efforts directed at cryopreservation of large numbers of tumor cells and at characterization of tissue culture lines derived from tumors may help to solve the problem.

Immune reactivity to viruses and to virus-associated antigens appears to be an important area for research related to cancer immunodiagnosis. Virtually 100% of patients with Burkitt's lymphoma and nasopharyngeal cancer have elevated titers of antibodies to Epstein-Barr virus (EBV)-associated antigens (Henle et al., 1969; Henle et al., 1970). This may prove helpful in distinguishing these tumors from histologically similar ones in which the frequency of positive titers or elevated levels is much lower. The level of the antibody titers is correlated to some extent with the stage of disease and its clinical course.

Similarly, antibodies to antigens associated with herpes simplex virus have been associated with cervical cancer (Aurelian, Davis, and Julian, 1973) and with squamous cell carcinomas of the head and neck (Hollinshead and Tarro, 1973). Mouse milk containing mammary tumor virus has been reported to give positive results in the leukocyte migration inhibition test of patients with breast cancer but not of normal controls (Black et al., 1974). This reactivity of breast cancer patients has correlated well with reactivity to tumor-associated antigens and also with the clinical stage of disease. Some other recent advances in cancer immunodiagnosis are discussed in the

Compendium of Assays for Immunodiagnosis of Human Cancer
(Herberman, 1979).

REFERENCES

Abelev, G. I. 1971. Alpha-fetoprotein in ontogenesis and its association with malignant tumors. Adv. Cancer Res. 14:295–358.

Aizawa, M., and Southam, C. M. 1960. Serum antibodies following homotransplantation of human cancer cells. Ann. N.Y. Acad. Sci. 87:293–298.

Alpert, E., Coston, R. L. and Drysdale, J. W. 1973. Carcino-fetal human liver ferritins. Nature 242:194–196.

Aurelian, L., Davis, H. J., and Julian, C. G. 1973. Herpesvirus Type 2-induced tumor specific antigen in cervical carcinoma. Am. J. Epidemiol. 98:1–9.

Aurelian, L., and Strnad, B. C. 1976. Herpesvirus Type 2-related antigens and their relevance to humoral and cell-mediated immunity in patients with cervical cancer. Cancer Res. 36:810–820.

Banwo, O., Versey, J., and Hobbs, J. R. 1974. New oncofetal antigen for human pancreas. Lancet 1:643–645.

Benson, R. C., Jr., Riggs, B. L., Pickard, B. M., and Arnaud, C. D. 1974. Radioimmunoassay of parathyroid hormone in hypercalcemic patients with malignant disease. Am. J. Med. 56:821–826.

Black, M. M., Moore, D. H., Shore, B., Zachran, R. E., and Leis, H. P., Jr. 1974. Effect of milk samples and human breast tissues on human leukocyte migration indices. Cancer Res. 34:1054–1060.

Braun, M., Sen, L., Backman, A. E., and Pavlovsky, A. 1972. Cell migration inhibition in human lymphomas using lymph node and cell line antigens. Blood 39:368–376.

Braunstein, G. D., Vaitukaitis, J. L. Carbone, P. P., and Ross, G. T. 1973. Ectopic production of human chorionic gonadotrophin by neoplasms. Ann. Intern. Med. 78:39–45.

Buffe, D., Rimbaut, C., Fuccaro, C., and Burtin, P. 1972. Isolation and characterization of α_2 ferroprotein: α_2H globulin. Ann. Inst. Pasteur Lille 123:29–42.

Bull, D. M., Leibach, J. R., Williams, M. A., and Helms, R. A. 1973. Immunity to colon cancer assessed by antigen-induced inhibition of mixed mononuclear cell migration. Science 181:957–959.

Burnet, M. 1957. Cancer—A biological approach. I. The processes of control. Br. Med. J. 1:779–786.

Caspary, E. A., and Field, E. J. 1971. Specific lymphocyte sensitization in cancer—Is there a common antigen in human malignant neoplasia? Br. Med. J. 2:613–615.

Cercek, L., Cercek, B., and Franklin, C. I. V. 1974. Biophysical differentiation between lymphocytes from healthy donors, patients with malignant diseases and other disorders. Br. J. Cancer 29:345–352.

Cervi-Skinner, S. J., and Castleman, B. 1973. Thyroid nodules in a man with a family history of thyroid carcinoma and pheochromocytoma. N. Engl. J. Med. 289:472–479.

Char, D. H., Hollinshead, A., Cogan, D. G., Ballantine, E., Hogan, M. J., and Herberman, R. B. 1974. Cutaneous delayed hypersensitivity reactions to soluble melanoma antigen in patients with ocular malignant melanoma. N. Engl. J. Med. 291:274–277.

Chu, T. M., Holyoke, E. D., and Murphy, G. P. 1974. Carcinoembryonic antigen. Current clinical status. NY State J. Med. 74:1388–1398.

Cochran, A. J., Spilg, W. G. S., Mackie, R. M., and Thomas, C. E. 1972. Postoperative depression of tumor-directed cell-mediated immunity in patients with malignant disease. Br. Med. J. 4:67–70.

Coombes, R. C., Hillyard, C., Greenberg, P. B., and MacIntyre, I. 1974. Plasma-immunoreactive-calcitonin in patients with non-thyroid tumors. Lancet 1:1080–1083.

Coordinating Group for the Research of Liver Cancer, China. 1974. Application of serum alpha feto-protein assay in mass survey of primary carcinoma of liver. In: C. Maltoni (ed.), Proceedings of the 2nd International Symposium on Cancer Detection and Prevention, pp. 655–658. Excerpta Medica, Amsterdam.

Davidsohn, I., and Ni, L. Y. 1969. Loss of isoantigens A, B, and H in carcinoma of the lung. Am. J. Pathol. 57:307–334.

Dean, J. H., Silva, J. S., McCoy, J. L., Leonard, C. M., Middleton, M., Cannon, G., and Herberman, R. B. 1975. Lymphocyte blastogenesis induced by 3 M KCl extracts of allogeneic breast carcinoma and lymphoid cells. J. Natl. Cancer Inst. 54:1295–1298.

Edgington, T. S., Astarita, R. W., and Plow, E. F. 1975. Association of an isomeric species of carcinoembryonic antigen (CEA-S) with neoplasia of the gastrointestinal tract. N. Engl. J. Med. 293:103–106.

Edynak, E. M., Old, L. J., Vrava, M., and Lardis, M. P. 1972. A fetal antigen associated with human neoplasia. N. Engl. J. Med. 286:1178–1183.

Eilber, F. R., and Morton, D. L. 1970. Impaired immunologic reactivity and recurrence following cancer surgery. Cancer 25:362–367.

Gerwirtz, G., and Yalom, R. S. 1974. Ectopic ACTH production in carcinoma of the lung. J. Clin. Invest. 53:1022–1032.

Gold, P., and Freedman, S. O. 1965. Specific carcinoembryonic antigen of the human digestive system. J. Exp. Med. 122:467–481.

Häkkinen, I. P. T. 1974. A population screening for fetal sulfoglycoprotein antigen in gastric juice. Cancer Res. 34:3069–3072.

Han, T., and Takita, H. 1972. Immunologic impairment in bronchogenic carcinoma: A study of lymphocyte response to phytohemagglutinin. Cancer 30:616–620.

Hellström, I., Hellström, K. E., Sjögren, H. O., and Warner, G. A. 1971. Demonstration of cell-mediated immunity to human neoplasia of various histological types. Intl. J. Cancer 7:1–16.

Hellström, I., Warner, G. A., Hellström, K. E., and Sjögren, H. O. 1973. Sequential studies on cell-mediated immunity and blocking serum activity in ten patients with malignant melanoma. Int. J. Cancer 11:280–292.

Hendrick, J. C., and Franchimont, P. 1974. Radioimmunoassay of casein in the serum of normal subjects and of patients with various malignancies. Eur. J. Cancer 10:725–730.

Henle, G., Henle, W., Clifford, P., Diehl, V., Kafuko, G. W., Kirya, B. G., Klein, G., Morrow, R. H., Munube, G. M. R., Pike, M., Turkei, P. M., and Ziegler, J. L. 1969. Antibodies to Epstein-Barr virus in Burkitt's lymphoma and control groups. J. Natl. Cancer Inst. 43:1147–1157.

Henle, W., Henle, G., Ho, H. C., Burtin, P., Cochen, Y., Clifford, P., de Schryner, P., de-The, G., Diehl, V., and Klein, G. 1970. Antibodies to Epstein-Barr virus in nasopharyngeal carcinoma, other head and neck neoplasms, and control groups. J. Natl. Cancer Inst. 44:225–231.

Herberman, R. B. 1974a. Cell-mediated immunity to tumor cells. Adv. Cancer Res. 19:207–263.

Herberman, R. B. 1974b. Delayed hypersensitivity skin reactions to antigens on human tumors. Cancer 34:1469–1473.

Herberman, R. B. (ed.). 1979. Compendium of Assays for Immunodiagnosis of Human Cancer. Elsevier-North Holland, New York.

Herberman, R. B., Hollinshead, A. C., Alford, T. C., McCoy, J. L., Halterman, R. H., and Leventhal, B. G. 1973. Delayed cutaneous hypersensitivity reactions to extracts of human tumors. Natl. Cancer Inst. Monogr. 37:189–195.

Herberman, R. B. and Oldham, R. K. 1975. Problems associated with study of cell-mediated immunity to human tumors by microcytotoxicity assays. J. Natl. Cancer Inst. 55:749–753.

Herrara, M. A., Chu, M. T., and Holyoke, E. D. 1976. Carcinoembryonic antigen (CEA) as a prognostic and monitoring test in clinically complete resection of colorectal carcinoma. Ann. Surg. 183:5–20.

Hersh, E. M. and Oppenheim, J. J. 1965. Impaired in vitro lymphocyte transformation in Hodgkin's disease. N. Engl. J. Med. 273:1006–1012.

Hollinshead, A., Glew, D., Bunnag, B., Gold P., and Herberman, R. B. 1970. Skin-reactive soluble antigen from intestinal cancer-cell membranes and relationship to carcinoembryonic antigens. Lancet 1:1191–1195.

Hollinshead, A. C., and Tarro, G. 1973. Soluble membrane antigens of lip and cervical carcinomas—Reactivity with antibody for herpesvirus nonvirion antigens. Science 179:698–700.

Lamb, D., Pilney, F., Kelly, W. D., and Good, R. A. 1962. A comparative study of the incidence of anergy in patients with carcinoma, leukemia, Hodgkin's disease and other lymphomas. J. Immunol. 89:555–558.

Leblanc, L., Tuyns, A. J., and Masseyeff, R. 1973. Screening for primary liver cancer. Digestion 8:8–14.

Lewis, M. G., Ikonopisov, R. L., Narin, R. C., Phillip, T. M., Hamilton-Fairley, G., Bodenham, D. C., and Alexander, P. 1969. Tumor-specific antibodies in human malignant melanoma and their relationship to the extent of the disease. Br. Med. J. 3:547–552.

McCoy, J. L., Jerome, L. F., Dean, J. H., Cannon, G. B., Alford, T. C., Doering, T., and Herberman, R. B. 1974. Inhibition of leukocyte migration by tumor-associated antigens in soluble extracts of human breast carcinoma. J. Natl. Cancer Inst. 53:11–17.

McCoy, J. L., Jerome, L. F., Dean, J. H., Perlin, E., Oldham, R. K., Char, D. H., Cohen, M. H., Felix, E. L., and Herberman, R. B. 1975. Inhibition of leukocyte migration by tumor-associated antigens in soluble extracts of malignant melanoma. J. Natl. Cancer Inst. 55:19–23.

Mach, J. P., Jaeger, P., Bertholet, M. M., Ruegsegger, C. H., Loosil, R. M., and Pattavel, J. 1974. Detection of occurrence of large-band carcinoma by radioimmunoassay of circulating carcinoembryonic antigen (CEA). Lancet 2:535–540.

Maluish, A., and Halliday, W. J. 1974. Cell-mediated immunity and specific serum factors in human cancer: the leukocyte adherence inhibition test. J. Natl. Cancer Inst. 52:1415–1420.

Marcus, D. M., and Zinburg, N. 1975. Measurement of serum ferritin by radioimmunoassay: Results in normal individuals and patients with breast cancer. J. Natl. Cancer Inst. 55:791–795.

Mavligit, G. M., Ambus, V., Gutterman, J. V., and Hersh, E. M. 1973. Antigen solubilized from human solid tumors: Lymphocyte stimulation and cutaneous delayed hypersensitivity. Nature (New Biology) 243:188–190.

Miller, D. G. 1968. The immunologic capability of patients with lymphoma. Cancer Res. 28:1441–1448.

Morton, D. L., Eilber, F. R., Joseph, W. L., Wood, W. C., Trahan, E., and Ketcham, A. S. 1970. Immunological factors in human sarcomas and melanomas: A rational basis for immunotherapy. Ann. Surg. 172:740–749.

Mukherji, B., and Hirshaut, Y. 1973. Evidence for fetal antigen in human sarcoma. Science 181:440–442.

Pinsky, C. M., Oettgen, H. F., El Domeiri, A., Old, L. J., Beattie, E. J., and Burchenal, L. H. 1971. Delayed hypersensitivity reactions in patients with cancer. Proc. Am. Assoc. Cancer Res. 12:100.

Prehn, R. T., and Main, J. M. 1957. Immunity to MCA induced sarcomas. J. Natl. Cancer Inst. 18:769–775.

Pritchard, J. A. V., Moore, J. L., Sutherland, W. H., and Joslin, C. A. F. 1973, Evaluation and development of the macrophage electrophoretic mobility (MEM) test for malignant disease. Br. J. Cancer 27:1–9.

Purves, L. R. 1973. Primary liver cancer in man as a possible short duration seasonal cancer. South African J. Sci. 69:173–178.

Ravry, M., McIntire, K. R., Moertel, C. G., Waldmann, T. A., Schutt, A. J., and Go, V. L. W. 1974. Brief communication: Carcinoembryonic antigen and alpha-fetoprotein in the diagnosis of gastric and colonic cancer: A comparative clinical evaluation. J. Natl. Cancer Inst. 52:1019–1021.

Roof, B. S., Carpenter, B., Fink, D. J., and Gordon, G. S. 1971. Some thoughts on the nature of ectopic parathyroid hormones. Am. J. Med. 50:686–694.

Rosen, S. W., Weintraub, B. D., Vaitukaitus, J. S., Sussman, H. H., Hershman, J. M., and Muggia, F. M. 1975. Placental proteins and their subunits as tumor markers. Ann. Intern. Med. 82:71–83.

Silva, O. L., Becker, K. L., Primack, A., Doppman, J., and Snider, R. H. 1974. Ectopic secretion of calcitonin by oat-cell carcinoma. N. Engl. J. Med. 290:1122–1124.

Soloway, A. C., and Rapaport, F. T. 1965. Immunologic responses in cancer patients. Surg. Gynecol. Obstet. 121:756–760.

Sorokin, J. J., Sugarbaker, P. H., Zamcheck, N., Piseck, M., Kupchik, H. Z., and Moore, F. D. 1974. Serial carcinoembryonic antigen assays: Use in detection of cancer recurrence. JAMA 228:49–53.

Southam, C. M., and Moore, A. E. 1954. Anti-virus antibody studies following induced infection of man with West Nile, Ilheus, and other viruses. J. Immunol. 72:446–452.

Stevens, D. P., MacKay, I. R., and Cullen, K. J. 1975. Carcinoembryonic antigen in an unselected elderly population: A four year follow-up. Br. J. Cancer 32:147–151.

Takasugi, M., and Kinoshita, K. 1974. Specific antibody activation of lymphocytes for cell-mediated cytotoxicity against cultured target cells. J. Natl. Cancer Inst. 53:1539–1544.

Tal, C., and Halperin, M. 1970. Presence of serologically distinct protein in serum of cancer patients and pregnant women. Israel J. Med. Sci. 6:708–716.

Tal, C., Raychaudhuri, A., Herberman, R. B., and Buncher, C. R., 1973. Simplified technique for the T-globulin cancer test. J. Natl. Cancer Inst. 51:33–43.

Tashjian, A. H., Jr., Wolfe, H. J., and Voelkel, E. F. 1974. Human calcitonin, immunologic assay, cytologic localization and studies on medullary thyroid carcinoma. Am. J. Med. 56:840–849.

Thomson, D. M. P., Krupey, J., Freedman, S. O., and Gold, P. 1969. The radioimmunoassay of circulating carcinoembryonic antigen of the human digestive system. Proc. Natl. Acad. Sci. (USA) 122:467–481.

Usategui-Gomez, M., Yeager, F. M., Fernandez de Castro, A. 1973. A sensitive immunochemical method for the determination of the Regan isoenzyme. Cancer Res. 33:1574–1577.

Wells, S. A., Jr., Burdick, J. F., Christiansen, C., Ketcham, A. S., and Adkins, P. C. 1973. Demonstration of tumor-associated delayed hypersensitivity reactions in patients with lung cancer and in patients with carcinoma of the cervix. Natl. Cancer. Inst. Monogr. 37:197–203.

Wells, S. A., Jr., Ontjes, D. A., Cooper, G. W., Hennessy, J. F., Ellis, G. J., McPherson, H. T., and Sabiston, D. C., Jr. 1975. The early diagnosis of medullary carcinoma of the thyroid gland in patients with multiple endocrine neoplasia type II. Ann. Surg. 182:362–368.

West, W. H., Sienknecht, C. W., Townes, A. S., and Herberman, R. B. 1976. Performance of a rosette assay between lymphocytes and sheep erythrocytes at 29°C to study patients with cancer and other diseases. Clin. Immunol. Immunopathol. 5:60–66.

Whittaker, M. G., Rees, K., and Clark, C. G. 1971. Reduced lymphocyte transformation in breast cancer. Lancet 1:892–893.

Williams, R. R., McIntire, K. R., Go, V. L. W., Feinleib, M., Waldmann, T. A., Kannel, W., Dawberg, T., Castelli, W., and McNamara, P. 1977. Tumor associated antigen levels (CEA, HCG, AFP) antedating the diagnosis of cancer in the Framingham study. J. Natl. Cancer Inst. 58:1547–1551.

Wolfe, H. J., Melvin, K. E. W., Cervi-Skinner, S. J., Al Saadi, A. A., Juliar, J. F., Jackson, C. E., and Tashjian, A. H. 1973. C cell hyperplasia preceding medullary thyroid carcinoma. N. Engl. J. Med. 289:437–441.

Wybran, J., and Fudenberg, H. H. 1973. Thymus-derived rosette-forming cells in various human disease states: Cancer, lymphoma, bacterial and viral diseases. J. Clin. Invest. 52:1026–1032.

Zamcheck, N., Moore, T. L., Dhar, P., and Kupchik, H. Z. 1972. Immunologic diagnosis of human digestive tract cancer: Carcinoembryonic antigens. N. Engl. J. Med. 286:83–86.

7

The Epidemiologic Significance of
Cytologic and Histologic Data

Leopold G. Koss

For those interested in problems relating to cancer epidemiology, some grasp of the significance, accomplishments, and pitfalls of cytopathology and histopathology in the diagnosis of cancer and precancerous states is essential. For example, some time ago in Atlanta, Georgia, a group of knowledgeable epidemiologists were attempting to evaluate the effects of the contraceptive pill on precancerous states of the uterine cervix epithelium. A set of data was collected with the help of a competent local pathologist. Two "experts" were invited to double check these data. By the time the experts had completed their review of the histologic diagnoses, they disagreed thoroughly not only with the local pathologist but also with each other. This ruined the paper, which was potentially an important contribution. One of the critical issues in cancer epidemiology is the evaluation of diagnostic data from a variety of laboratories. Interpretation of cancer morphology, whether by cytology or histology, is very subjective and variable, dependent not only on the training, skill, and experience of the pathologist, but also on his or her personal philosophy and biases.

Some of the basic principles, accomplishments, and pitfalls of the cytologic techniques in the evaluation of cancer and precancerous lesions are discussed below. This subject can be approached by giving some illustrative examples from particular organs. In many ways these examples can be expanded to include a number of other organs which for a variety of reasons, anatomic or other, have not been similarly investigated.

SEQUENCE OF EVENTS IN EPITHELIAL CARCINOGENESIS

To appreciate the biologic background of morphologically abnormal cells that are evaluated in the detection of precancerous states, it may be useful to consider the theory of the *fitter cell*, proposed by Cairns (1975). This contributes to our understanding of the origins of cancer, especially epithelial neoplasms, for example, those of the uterine cervix and the skin. This theory is based on the fact that normal epithelial renewal is the result of mitotic activity occurring exclusively at the level of a single layer of *basal* cells that are, therefore, *immortal*. These cells give rise, on the one hand, to other immortal cells that continue the proliferative process within the basal layer of the epithelium and, on the other hand, to cells that can no longer divide and whose destiny is to differentiate and mature along certain preexisting patterns (Figure 1). The latter may be termed *mortal cells*. In the epidermis or in the squamous epithelium of the cervix these mortal cells mature by becoming large, keratin-forming, squamous cells.

It is assumed that cancer originates with the appearance of a new immortal cell, in a location where such immortal cells should not be present. Instead of the normal situation in which immortal cells are confined to the basal layer, genetic errors—either spontaneous or induced by carcinogenic substances or viruses—result in one or more cells capable of reproduction within the epithelium. Such new immortal cells have a significant advantage over mortal cells and are, thus, *fitter* cells (Figure 2). A sequence of genetic errors may occur in subsequent generations, until a clone of cells emerges that has the capacity to produce invasive carcinoma. It is conceivable that a number of such transformations are required until the cell abnormality is finally visible at the level of the light microscope. This theory has immense appeal because it is biologically and intellectually satisfying and because it is applicable to nearly all the causative concepts of cancer that have been proposed.

CANCER CELLS VERSUS
NORMAL CELLS: MORPHOLOGIC DIFFERENCES

A brief review of some of the essential morphologic differences between fixed and stained human cancer cells and normal cells may be in order (Figure 3). Cancer cells may have an abnormal shape when compared with normal cells. The nucleus of the cancer cell is often enlarged and filled with dark, opaque granules of chromatin. The nucleolus may also be enlarged and irregular when compared with the nucleolus of a normal cell. In Figure 3, the cancer cell is drawn without any attachments, whereas the normal cell has a desmosomal attachment to an adjacent cell. This symbolizes the fact that normal cells adhere to each other by a variety of mechanisms. By way of contrast, cancerous cells, although usually forming cell attachments, do not adhere very well. This has an important and practical implication: it is relatively easy to remove cancer cells from their natural environment.

NORMAL SQUAMOUS EPITHELIUM

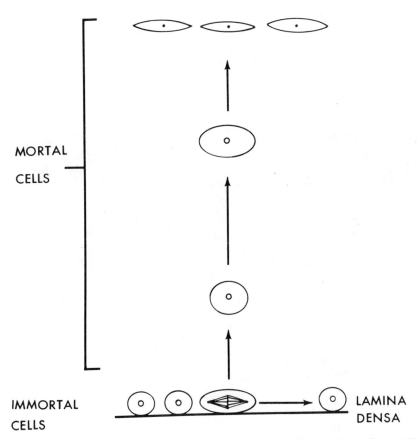

Figure 1.   Theory of fitter cells. Function of normal squamous epithelium. Source: Koss, 1979.

Furthermore, cancer cells will exfoliate from the surface of a tissue much more readily than normal cells.

CERVICAL CANCER DETECTION

In citing examples of carcinogenesis in man, it is useful to consider the epithelium of the uterine cervix, an organ from which a great deal of knowledge has already been acquired at the levels of cytopathology and his-

tology. The story of cervical cancer detection can be traced to a paper by
Schauenstein (1908), who suggested that, because of histologic similarity,
certain lesions found on the surface of the uterine cervix epithelium are
precursors of invasive carcinoma. Although he did not invent the term *carcinoma in situ*, Schauenstein showed that some cancers, especially those of

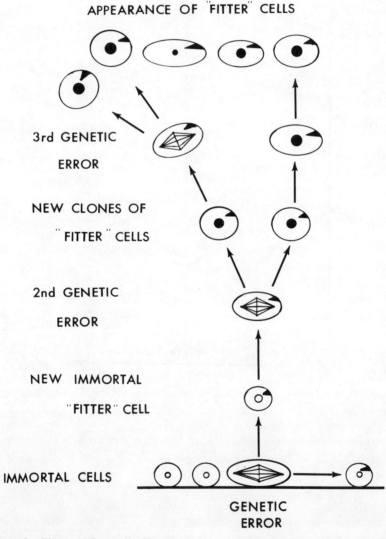

Figure 2. Theory of fitter cells. The origin of cancer. Abnormal fitter cells are identified by black triangles. Source: Koss, 1979.

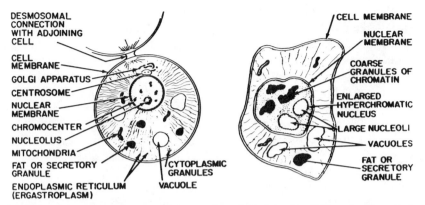

Figure 3.   Schematic differences between a hypothetical benign (left) and a hypothetical malignant cell (right). Source: Koss, 1979.

the epithelial tissues, are preceded by precursor lesions that are confined to the epithelium of origin.

Hence, the lesion known as *carcinoma in situ* can be defined as *a lesion confined to the epithelium of origin that histologically resembles invasive carcinoma of the same origin.* This is a common sense definition that has been modified by a number of committees, but these modifications do not appear to serve any useful purpose. Papanicolaou (1943) demonstrated that by a simple and painless procedure one can remove a sample of cells from the cervix or the vagina and determine whether or not there is microscopic evidence of a precancerous malignant process, such as carcinoma in situ. This procedure, now widely used as the *Pap test,* has contributed a great deal to our knowledge and understanding of the sequence of events in carcinogenesis of the uterine cervix epithelium.

Much has been learned in the last 25 years about carcinogenesis in the uterine cervix. This disease has been extensively studied from many points of view including cytologic samplings, histologic studies, colposcopic inspection under high magnification, and epidemiologic and biologic studies. It is known that the vast majority of uterine cervix cancers originate within a rather well-defined area of squamous epithelium abutting on the glandular endocervical epithelium. Within this epithelium the previously described events leading to the appearance of *fitter* cells occur. This area is often referred to as the *squamocolumnar junction* or, in the language of colposcopy, as the *transformation zone.* It is, in fact, a zone where there is more mitotic activity than anywhere else in the normal epithelial lining of uterine cervix. Because cells replicate here with considerable frequency, genetic errors are more likely to occur than in a quiescent epithelium.

Microscopic examinations of cells and tissues have shown that certain stages in the development of cervical cancer can be differentiated. The first change, presumably the initial manifestation of the *fitter* cell, occurs at the level of the cell nucleus, which becomes very much enlarged when compared with the nucleus of normal cells. The cells, however, are not otherwise significantly modified. Papanicolaou (1949) termed this phenomenon *dyskaryosis*, reflecting the fact that the first visible events involved the nucleus of the cells. Because these events may progress and expand, the tendency has been to attempt to classify the various intraepithelial lesions preceding invasive carcinoma according to the level of cytologic and histologic abnormality, namely, *dysplasia* and *carcinoma in situ*.

The precancerous events occur as a series of sequential morphologic changes. However, even very "early" and barely visible precancerous lesions are capable of producing invasive carcinoma. In other words, what is observed at the level of light microscopy is presumably not the first generation of *fitter* cells, as would have been expected, but rather one of the many succeeding generations. It is likely that morphologic changes perceptible at the light microscopic level represent clones of cells that are capable of producing clinical, invasive cancer.

Precancerous states or carcinoma in situ are generally not palpable, visible, or otherwise clinically identifiable as cancer. The search for such lesions must therefore be a deliberate one. It has often been noted that some of the less advanced morphologic changes, commonly referred to as borderline lesions or *dysplasia*, occur in younger women than does carcinoma in situ. The latter, in turn, occurs in younger women than does invasive carcinoma.

In view of the above, it has customarily been assumed that the early intraepithelial lesions occur 10 years or so before the more advanced intraepithelial lesions which, in turn, develop about 10 years before invasive carcinoma. This sequence would account for a total natural life history of approximately 20 years for human carcinoma of the cervix (Koss, 3rd ed., 1979; Koss, 1970). In reality, enormous variations exist between individual patients. One can sometimes observe the development of invasive cancer in a young woman within a time span of not more than 2, 3, or 4 years. On the other hand, one can also observe precancerous lesions that never develop into invasive cancer of the uterine cervix.

The natural history of the untreated precancerous lesions was investigated a number of years ago (Koss et al., 1963). The lesions were grouped into two categories: carcinoma in situ and lesser or borderline lesions (Table 1). A certain number of lesions in both categories disappeared after a diagnostic or minor therapeutic procedure. Some of the lesions persisted without

Table 1. Patterns of behavior of lesions of the cervical epithelium

Behavior	Carcinoma in situ		Borderline lesions		Total	
	Number	Percent	Number	Percent	Number	Percent
Disappeared	17	25.4	10	38.5	27	29
Persisted	41	61.2	4	15.4		
Progressed to carcinoma in situ	0		11	42.3		
Progressed to questionable invasion	5	7.5	0		66	71
Progressed to invasive carcinoma	4	5.9	1	3.8		
Total	67		26		93	

Source: Koss et al., 1963.

significant morphologic change, and others progressed to more significant changes. Some patients in both groups developed invasive carcinoma.

One of the most perplexing dilemmas in cancer biology today is not why cancer develops but why precancerous states disappear. It is possible that clones of fitter cells are developing in all of us, at all times, in many organs. Despite this, the events leading to clinical cancer apparently occur relatively infrequently. The explanations for these phenomena merit investigations by epidemiologists as well as immunologists.

Other studies have confirmed the fact that morphologically less impressive lesions of the cervix epithelium, often referred to as *dysplasia*, are important precancerous lesions. If one takes two groups of patients, with and without such lesions, the group with prior dysplasia will have a far greater possibility of developing carcinoma in situ, as demonstrated by Stern and Neely (1963).

Similarly, Richart and Barron (1969) followed a number of patients with the morphologically lesser abnormalities of the cervical epithelium without treatment. The study had to be interrupted when several of the patients developed invasive cervical cancer. Richart calculated that there was a 60% probability for lesions known as dysplasia to progress to carcinoma in situ after 10 years. The progression rate of lesions known as severe dysplasia was so marked as to obviate the need for any differentiation between them and the so-called carcinomas in situ. Richart suggested that all the precancerous states, regardless of the degree of morphologic abnormality, ought to be considered under a single term, *cervical intraepithelial neoplasia* (CIN), encompassing the entire spectrum of neoplastic disease in the uterine cervix from mild dysplasia to carcinoma in situ. While the probability of progression to invasive carcinoma varies with the degree of morphologic abnormality, progression may occur with any of these intraepithelial lesions.

It should also be recognized that there are enormous differences among individual observers in efficiency of detection and perception of the lesions. Sedlis et al. (1974) took two smears from the cervix, one immediately after another, from a large number of patients. Important precancerous lesions were missed, either on the first or on the second smear, for a combined total error rate of approximately 30%. The first smear did not prove to be necessarily more reliable than the second. It would appear that the failure rate in cytologic detection of precancerous stages of the uterine cervix by means of a single routine smear is about 25%. Repeated screenings of a given population would be required to achieve maximal efficacy by this method of detection.

Similar observations were reported by Nyirjesy (1972). He pointed out that follow-up of patients with a cytologic diagnosis of *atypia* may disclose invasive or preinvasive carcinomas of the uterine cervix. This suggests that there are significant differences in the individual perceptibility of pathologists and technologists in the evaluation of smears. These facts must be considered when attempts are made to establish valid incidence and prevalence rates for precancerous states of the uterine cervix.

Another interesting and practical point from the epidemiologic perspective is the unreliability of cytology as a follow-up tool. If a patient with an abnormal smear has a second smear performed, the chances of obtaining a negative smear in the presence of an important lesion is very high, presumably 40% (Koss, 1970). For example, 12 patients in Nyirjesy's group initially had a suspicious smear. The subsequent smear was negative in 9 patients and atypical in 3 of these patients, atlhough all 12 patients had either invasive carcinoma, carcinoma in situ, or dysplasia. It seems that the utility of cytologic screening for cancer of the cervix has to be carefully evaluated. Contrary to many assertions, the method is far from being 100% accurate.

The histologic examination, as well as the cytologic method, is inaccurate. Cocker, Fox, and Langley (1968) submitted 30 biopsies of the cervix to two pathologists. Significant differences were apparent in the interpretation of the slides. The same material was shown again to one of the pathologists 18 months later, and he significantly disagreed with himself. Similar findings are on record from other surveys (Committee on Reproducibility of Histopathologic Diagnosis, 1969; Siegler, 1956). These represent serious epidemiologic problems. When attempting to evaluate any set of laboratory data, a large number of variables related to educational background, perception, ability, training, experience, and personal bias of the observers must be taken into account.

The differential diagnosis between various levels of intraepithelial abnormality, whether mild, moderate, or severe dysplasia, or carcinoma in situ, is not reproducible among different observers. Hence, all the data based on subclassifications of these cervical lesions are of questionable validity. One man's dysplasia is another man's carcinoma in situ (Hulme and Eisenberg, 1968). While this may be disturbing to epidemiologists, it is fortunately not crucial to cervical cancer prevention. All patients, regardless of degree of cytologic or histologic abnormality, should have the benefit of a clinical examination, combined with colposcopic inspection of the uterine cervix. The latter serves to identify areas of epithelial abnormality not otherwise visible to the naked eye, permits the delineation of the size of the lesion, and facilitates removal of tissue samples for further study prior to treatment. The treatment may consist of local removal of the diseased tissue with full preservation of reproductive function.

URINARY BLADDER CANCER DETECTION

Another organ in which much investigative effort has been expended and in which cytopathology and histology of precancerous lesions play important roles is the urinary bladder. For many years, a large group of workers exposed to a potent bladder carcinogen, para-aminodiphenyl or xenylamine (Koss, Melamed, and Kelly, 1969), were carefully followed. Among 503 exposed workers, approximately 10% developed cancer of the bladder. There was no correlation between the degree of exposure and bladder cancer risk. Some of the men who developed cancer had maximal exposure, while others had only intermittent or slight exposure. Two of the latter were not even production workers; they were in charge of the upkeep of the gutters leading from the production room to the outside of the plant. Disease risk was also not correlated with time. Some of the subjects developed cancer within 2 or 3 years of exposure, while others developed cancer after 30 years. These differences have not yet been explained.

All of these workers were followed by cytologic examination of the urinary sediment as one of the tools for the detection of bladder cancer. In a rather large group of workers, cancer cells were found in the urinary sediment in the absence of clinical evidence of bladder cancer. It was concluded (Koss et al., 1965) and subsequently proven (Koss, Melamed, and Kelly, 1969) that the neoplasms of these men arose from nonpapillary urothelial carcinoma in situ.

Like cervical cancer, carcinoma in situ of the urinary bladder is neither visible nor palpable, although its biologic behavior is considerably different. Carcinoma in situ and related states of the uterine cervix have an unpredictable behavior. Some lesions may develop into an invasive cancer after many years; others may remain arrested, while still others may vanish. By way of contrast, carcinoma in situ of the bladder is a disease capable of progression to invasive cancer within a relatively short period of time. Of 95 cases of this disease observed until 1972, 57 progressed to invasive cancer within less than 5 years (Koss, 1975).

VARIABLES AFFECTING EPIDEMIOLOGIC STUDIES OF CANCER

Cytology is a useful tool for the detection of precancerous states in various organs. However, in the study of precancerous states, a number of important factors must be considered. The first is the availability of abnormal cells that are shed from a precancerous lesion. The rate at which this occurs is probably extremely variable, even for the uterine cervix.

A second factor is the interpretation of microscopic findings. Each interpreter will have his or her own way of looking at and assessing the lesions. If one works with more than one interpreter, the data are not necessarily comparable. Yet, the diagnosis of cancer should never become a matter of plebiscite.

The third, and perhaps most important factor, is that precancerous states appear to vary from organ to organ in their behavior pattern. There are the relatively innocuous lesions, such as carcinomas in situ of the uterine cervix or of the endometrium, and morphologically similar lesions that have a much more aggressive behavior. Examples of the latter include non-papillary carcinomas in situ of the urinary bladder, bronchogenic carcinomas in situ, and carcinomas in situ of the esophagus and stomach. These three factors represent major limitations to our understanding of human cancer and obstacles in our efforts in cancer control.

CONCLUSIONS

Epidemiologic studies on the early stages of human carcinogenesis must take into account a great many factors. Perhaps the most important of these concerns interpretative differences in microscopic findings with reference to cells and tissues. The light microscopic diagnosis of cancer and precancerous states carries with it a major observer bias that renders data from one laboratory not readily comparable with data from another. A second set of variables has to do with biologic factors responsible for the variability in the future behavior of a precancerous lesion which cannot be accurately predicted. The third set of variables relates to the differences in the behavior of morphologically similar lesions between one organ and another. For example, carcinoma in situ of the uterine cervix has a generally protracted course, whereas carcinoma in situ of the urinary bladder progresses rapidly to invasive carcinoma in most cases. Perhaps the most interesting biologic question deserving of further study is not why some precancerous epithelial lesions progress to cancer but why some disappear.

REFERENCES

Cairns, J. 1975. Mutation selection and the natural history of cancer. Nature 255:197–200.

Cocker, J., Fox, H., and Langley, F. A. 1968. Consistency in the histological diagnosis of epithelial abnormalities of the cervix uteri. J. Clin. Pathol. 21:67–70.

Committee on Reproducibility of Histopathologic Diagnosis. 1969. Joint position statement by the cancer control program. Acta Cytol. 13:309–310.

Hulme, G. W., and Eisenberg, H. S. 1968. Carcinoma in situ of the cervix in Connecticut. Am. J. Obstet. Gynecol. 102:415–425.

Koss, L. G. 1961. Diagnostic Cytology and Its Histopathologic Bases. J. B. Lippincott Company, Philadelphia. [3rd ed., 1979.]

Koss, L. G. 1970. Concept of genesis and development of carcinoma of the cervix. Obstet. Gynecol. Surv. 24:850–860.

Koss, L. G. 1975. Tumors of the urinary bladder. In: Atlas of Tumor Pathology, fascicle 11, 2nd series. Armed Forces Institute of Pathology, Washington, D.C.

Koss, L. G., Melamed, M. R., and Kelly, R. E. 1969. Further cytologic histologic studies of bladder lesions in workers exposed to para-aminodiphenyl: Progress report. J. Natl. Cancer Inst. 43:233–243.

Koss, L. G., Melamed, M. R., Ricci, A., Melick, W. F., and Kelly, R. E. 1965. Carcinogenesis in the human urinary bladder. Observations after exposure to para-aminodiphenyl. N. Engl. J. Med. 272:767–770.

Koss, L. G., Stewart, F. W., and Foote, F. W., Jordan, M. J., Bader, G. M., and Day, E. 1963. Some histological aspects of behavior of epidermoid carcinoma in situ and related lesions of the uterine cervix. Cancer 9:1160–1211.

Nyirjesy, I. 1972. Atypical or suspicious cervical smears: An aggressive diagnostic approach. JAMA 222:691–693.

Papanicolaou, G. N. 1949. Survey of actualities and potentialities of exfoliative cytology in cancer diagnosis. Ann. Int. Med. 31:661–674.

Papanicolaou, G. N., and Traut, H. F. 1943. Diagnosis of Uterine Cancer by the Vaginal Smear. Commonwealth Fund, New York.

Richart, R. M., and Barron, B. A. 1969. A follow-up study of patients with cervical dysplasia. Am. J. Obstet. Gynecol. 105:386–393.

Schauenstein, W. 1908. Histologische Untersuchungen uber atypisches Plattenepithel an der Portio und an der Innenflache der Cervix uteri. Arch. Gynäk. 85:576–616.

Sedlis, A., Walters, A. T., Balin, H., Hontz, A., and Lo Sciuto, L. 1974. Evaluation of two simultaneously obtained cervical cytological smears: A comparison study. Acta Cytol. 18:291–296.

Siegler, E. E. 1956. Microdiagnosis of carcinoma in situ of the uterine cervix: A comparative study of pathologists' diagnoses. Cancer 9:463–469.

Stern, E., and Neely, P. M. 1963. Carcinoma and dysplasia of the cervix: A comparison of rates for new and returning populations. Acta Cytol. 7:357–361.

8

The Implications of Chemotherapy for Cancer Control

C. Gordon Zubrod

Drugs are playing and will continue to play an important role in the treatment of cancer and, therefore, in the prospects for cancer control. This chapter begins with a review of what has been accomplished through cancer chemotherapy and then speculates on what this may mean for ultimate reduction in cancer morbidity and mortality.

HISTORICAL PERSPECTIVE

During the 1940s, before the recognition that drugs could affect the regression of clinical cancers, it was apparent that death rates were remaining constant in spite of extraordinary improvements in medicine, surgery, and radiation therapy. The increasing incidence of cancer and the growing size of the elderly population, coupled with the consequent increase in the number of deaths from cancer, made it seem as if we were losing ground.

The reason for the failure to reduce death rates was that the improvements in surgery and radiation therapy were directed at the control of local disease, that is, the primary tumor and its regional extension, whereas it was the distant or metastatic disease that was responsible for the deaths. In other words, local treatment cannot be expected to control nonlocalized cancer. Because metastases occur anywhere in the body, systemic therapy is required to kill those tumor cells that have wandered away from the local lesion.

Therefore, the primary scientific objective was to discover something to control metastatic disease. Before 1940, there were only faint suggestions that metastatic disease could be influenced by systemic therapy. For example, arsenic or urethane had some effect upon the chronic leukemias, and ovariectomy had been shown to influence metastatic breast cancer (Beatson, 1896), although this latter observation had not been exploited. Huggins and Hodges (1941) demonstrated that orchiectomy, or estrogen administration, brought about regression of metastases from prostatic cancer. A similar hormonal dependency of breast cancer was re-recognized.

The first nonhormonal drug to be discovered was nitrogen mustard (Gilman and Philips, 1946), and the first antimetabolite to be identified was aminopterin (an antifolate agent) (Farber et al., 1948). These observations led to an increased interest in the potential of cancer chemotherapy, to the discovery of a number of agents, and, in 1955, to a national program for drug development (Zubrod et al., 1966). At the present time, at least 44 drugs can cause regression of one or more forms of clinical cancer (Table 1).

Up to the mid-1950s, the available agents led only to partial and transient remissions. Conceptually, control of metastatic cancer by chemotherapy was opened up by the use of methotrexate to cure metastatic choriocarcinoma (a cancer of trophoblastic tissues) (Li, Hertz, and Spencer, 1956). This was followed by the observation of Burkitt, Hutt, and Wright (1965) that cyclophosphamide could be used in the cure of metastatic Burkitt's lymphoma. Although many other cancers, especially the hematologic malignancies, were sensitive to single agents, regressions were partial and transient.

In the early 1960s, combinations of drugs seemed to show promise in acute lymphocytic leukemia, and Freireich, Karon, and Frei (1964) demonstrated that a regimen of four antileukemia drugs yielded a high percentage of complete remissions. This led to extensive studies in the use of drugs in the treatment of acute lymphocytic leukemia and, later, in the treatment of advanced Hodgkin's disease; at the present time, cures for both diseases have been achieved (De Vita, Serpick, and Carbone, 1969; George

Table 1. Types of antitumor compounds

Compound	Total	Different structures	Used in curative regimens
Alkylating agents	9	4	3
Antimetabolites	6	5	2
Mitotic inhibitors	2	1	1
Antibiotics	6	5	2
Random synthetics	8	6	1
Hormones	12	5	1
Enzymes	1	1	0
Total	44	27	10

Table 2.   Cure rates in 11 drug responsive tumors

Tumor	Estimated percent cured before addition of chemotherapy	Estimated percent cured after chemotherapy
Wilms' tumor	50	90
Choriocarcinoma	20	80
Ewing's sarcoma	10	70
Burkitt's lymphoma	5	70
Retinoblastoma	20	55
Acute lymphocytic leukemia	0	50
Mycosis fungoides	5	50
Rhabdomyosarcoma	10	50
Advanced Hodgkin's disease	5	40
Histiocytic lymphoma	0	25
Metastatic embryonal carcinoma, testicular	0	10

et al., 1968). Using the outcome criterion of normal life expectancy of treated cancer patients as compared to demographically similar cohorts in the total population, it has been shown that drugs have been the critical factor in the cures of 11 different cancers (Table 2).

VARIATIONS IN DRUG SENSITIVITY OF CANCERS

The successful use of drugs to cure these uncommon cancers, and the failure to cure metastatic disease in common tumors such as breast and colon cancer, led to considerable investigation of the reasons for the susceptibility of cancer to drugs (Skipper, Schabel, and Wilcox, 1964). It was first noted that the growth rates of susceptible tumors were much more rapid than those of the nonsusceptible tumors. The rapid growth rate was due to the large growth fraction, that is, to the large percentage of cells whose DNA was replicating at any instant of measurement of uptake of tritiated thymidine (Malaise, Chavaudra, and Tubiana, 1973). Conversely, cancers that grew slowly had small growth fractions.

Because the antitumor drugs have their greatest killing power during DNA synthesis, or, in a few instances, during mitosis, their varying degrees of effectiveness can be explained on this basis. Cancers with 90% of cells synthesizing DNA will be easily destroyed by such agents, whereas slow growing tumors with small growth fractions will have, for example, less than 10% of cells killed by chemotherapy. It has also been recognized that the growth fraction of tumors is a function of their age, so that young tumors grow rapidly and have large growth fractions, while old tumors grow slowly and have small growth fractions (Schabel, 1969). We can conclude that drug-sensitive tumors are those that are discovered when they are young and consequently have large growth fractions and rapid growth rates. Tumors that remain unrecognized until they are old have by that time developed a small growth fraction, have slowed in their growth rate, and have become relatively insensitive to drugs.

ADJUVANT CHEMOTHERAPY

The latter situation is usually true for the common tumors, raising the question of how chemotherapy can be used to gain control over tumors such as lung and colon cancer that are discovered when they are biologically quite old. Several years ago, Simpson-Herren, Sanford, and Holmquist (1974) published an experimental observation that provided an important clue. These researchers measured the growth fraction in Lewis lung tumors of mice, both in the primary tumor and in the pulmonary metastases, at a number of points (in days) after primary tumor transplantation. At 20 days, for example, the growth fraction of the primary tumor was small, while that of the younger metastases was quite large. This suggested that the metastases (termed *micrometastases* because they were so small) would be susceptible to drugs, even though the primary tumor was not. Hypothetically, if the primary tumor could be removed by surgery, and the micrometastases killed by drugs given soon after surgery, then a permanent cure would result. Experiments in a number of animal models by Schabel (1976) showed that this indeed was the case.

In the clinical application of these data, it should be pointed out that such adjuvant chemotherapy following surgery and irradiation had been successful in a number of pediatric tumors such as Wilms', Ewing's, rhabdomyosarcoma, and retinoblastoma. However, these successes did not provide an adequate test of the hypothesis because these tumors were characterized by growth fractions that were larger than those of the common carcinomas.

Many studies of the common tumors are under way, but these are recent and the capacity of adjuvant chemotherapy to reduce mortality in the common tumors is still unknown. In premenopausal breast cancer, Fisher et al. (1975) have demonstrated that L-phenylalanine mustard given after radical mastectomy significantly reduces the relapse rate as compared to recurrences in women who have had radical mastectomy alone. Similarly, Bonadonna et al. (1976) have shown that a combination of drugs used adjuvantly significantly reduces the relapse rate in breast cancer. This may provide a clue to the reduction of mortality from the common cancers, but such reductions have yet to be proved, and there is much to be done in determining the appropriate drugs or drug combinations, the optional schedule, the duration of administration, and the relation to radiation therapy, as well as the requisite hormonal manipulation and immunotherapy. The choice of optimal regimen may well depend on the ability to relate completeness of cell kill to the proliferative state of the tumor.

The best clues to improving chemotherapy may come from direct measurement of growth fraction (as assessed from percentage of tumor cells labeled following tritiated thymidine) in clinical cancers and from correlation of the values with success and failure of drug treatment. Recently, Sulkes, Livingston, and Taylor (1976) have shown that only 3% of patients with breast cancer metastases with labeling indices of less than 8.1% responded to combination chemotherapy. When the labeling index was greater than 8.1%, 43% had tumor regression. This suggests that if the growth fraction could be increased in the metastases, then response rates could also be improved.

In experimental systems, Schenken and Hagemann (1976) have shown that after the suppression of proliferation by an initial course of combination chemotherapy in tumors with small growth fractions there is a substantial proliferative rebound. By timing the second course of chemotherapy to the peak of proliferative rebound, the investigators were able to achieve a 90% cure rate in animal tumors that were previously incurable. Application of such studies to man will be required to design highly effective dosage schedules for metastases with small growth fractions.

IMPLICATIONS FOR CANCER CONTROL

What are the implications of chemotherapy for cancer control? It must first be pointed out that the term *cancer*, like the term *infection*, collectively describes a hundred or more different diseases. Judgment on the efficacy of disease control must come from measurements of improvement made in the specific disease rather than in the whole wastebasket of diseases. Major reductions in mortality from specific cancers are obscured if one looks only at total mortality from all cancers. For example, mortality from Hodgkin's disease is falling rapidly, but if one looks only at total cancer deaths, this major improvement is hidden by the sharply rising incidence of (and total deaths from) a much more common tumor, lung cancer.

Cancer control, by which is meant the achievement of significant reductions in morbidity and mortality through universal application of known medical knowledge, is at hand for the cancers listed in Table 1. It seems that it is not sufficient for every physician to be merely aware of the potential for cure of these 11 cancers. It is time to plan the universal application of curative measures, even though the diseases on the list represent but 10% of total clinical cancer. Such application would be far more complex than, for example, implementing a vaccination plan for poliomyelitis, because it would involve screening and early diagnosis, organization or multidisciplinary management by a health team that is traditionally committed to monomodal approaches, the development of psychosocial rehabilitation resources, and many other coordinative maneuvers that cut across traditional modes.

It is difficult to imagine that such organization of control measures can be carried out as governmental programs either on a national or statewide level or, indeed, through medical societies or medical schools. Instead, cancer control directed at the unusual tumors could perhaps best be accomplished on a regional basis, through the natural networks that are developing around cancer centers. These centers are closely connected with the physicians and organizations in the community as well as with the universities, and are in an excellent position to help with the application of the new knowledge to the specific regional problems.

Depending upon the outcome of ongoing adjuvant studies and the results of new and innovative approaches, the control of the common cancers may still be in the distant future. In terms of such control, chemotherapy at the moment offers little compared to the benefits to be derived from the screening of high risk populations for early cancer, such as the Pap smear for carcinoma of the cervix, and from intensive educational programs for the early detection of breast and colon cancer. Even so, a great deal can be accomplished in reducing cancer morbidity and mortality by intensive regional efforts and by a coordinating of efforts of all interested parties in each region.

CONCLUSIONS

Over the past 35 years, considerable progress has been recorded in the development of drugs to cure cancer. The following conclusions may be drawn:

1. Metastatic forms of some types of cancer can presently be cured by the use of drugs.
2. Those cancers that are highly drug sensitive have a large percentage of their cells in an active proliferative phase.
3. Conversely, those tumors with a small percentage of their cells dividing are presently not curable by drugs; these are generally the common carcinomas.
4. Recent studies of the kinetics of cancer cell growth show that multidisciplinary management (e.g., local treatment, such as surgery, plus systemic therapy, such as chemotherapy) can cure otherwise incurable animal tumors.

5. Early results of the application of the above principle to patients show a reduction in morbidity from breast cancer, but it is as yet premature to judge the effect on mortality.
6. There is an opportunity to control the uncommon drug-sensitive tumors by application of present knowledge on a regional scale, perhaps through cancer centers.
7. Control of some of the common cancers by means of drugs may be partially attainable if the promises of ongoing research are borne out.

REFERENCES

Beatson, G. T. 1896. On the treatment of inoperable cases of carcinoma of the mamma: Suggestions for a new method of treatment, with illustrative cases. Lancet 2:104–107, 162–165.

Bonadonna, G., Brusamolina, E., Valagussa, P., Rossi, A., Brugnatelli, L., Brambilla, C., De Lena, M., Tancini, G., Bajetta, E., Musumeci, R., and Veronesi, U. 1976. Combination chemotherapy as an adjuvant treatment in operable breast cancer. N. Engl. J. Med. 294:405–410.

Borsa, J., and Whitmore, G. F. 1969. Cell killing studies on the mode of action of methotrexate on L-cells. Cancer Res. 29:737–744.

Burkitt, E., Hutt, M. S. R., and Wright, D. H. 1965. The African lymphoma. Preliminary observations on response to therapy. Cancer 18:399–410.

DeVita, V. T., Jr., Serpick, A., and Carbone, P. P. 1969. Combination chemotherapy of advanced Hodgkin's disease: The NCI program, a progress report. Proc. Am. Assoc. Cancer Res. 10:19.

Ensminger, W., Frei, E., III, Pitman, S., Wick, M., and Raso, V. 1976. Prevention of methotrexate toxicity by thymidine in man. Proc. Am. Assoc. Cancer Res. 17:282.

Farber, S., Diamond, L. K., Mercer, R. D., Sylvester, R. F., Jr., and Wolff, J. A. 1948. Temporary remissions in acute leukemia in children produced by folic-acid antagonist, 4-amino-pteroylglutamic acid (aminopterin). N. Engl. J. Med. 238:787–793.

Fisher, B., Carbone, P., Economou, S. G., Frelick, R., Glass, A., Lerner, H., Redmond, C., Zelen, M., Band, P., Katrych, D. L., Wolmark, N., and Fisher, E. R. (and other cooperating investigators). 1975. L-phenylalanine mustard (L-PAM) in the management of primary breast cancer. N. Engl. J. Med. 292:117–122.

Freireich, E. J., Bodey, G. P., de Jongh, D. S., Curtis, J. E., and Hersh, E. M. 1970. Supportive therapeutic measures for patients under treatment for leukemia-lymphoma. In: Leukemia-Lymphoma, pp. 275–284. Proceedings of the 14th Annual Clinical Conference on Cancer Sponsored by the University of Texas M. D. Anderson Hospital and Tumor Institute at Houston. Yearbook Medical Publishers Inc., Chicago.

Freireich, E. J., Karon, M., and Frei, E., III. 1964. Quadruple combination therapy (VAMP) for acute lymphocytic leukemia of childhood. Proc. Am. Assoc. Cancer Res. 5:20.

George, P., Hernandez, K., Hustu, O., Borella, L., Holton, C., and Pinkel, D. 1968. A study of "total therapy" of acute lymphocytic leukemia in children. J. Pediatr. 72:399–408.

162   Zubrod

Gilman, A., and Philips, F. S. 1946. The biological actions and therapeutic applications of the β-chloro-ethyl amines and sulphides. Science 103:409–415.
Henderson, E. S., and Samaha, R. J. 1969. Evidence that drugs in multiple combinations have materially advanced the treatment of human malignancies. Cancer Res. 29:2272–2280.
Huggins, C., and Hodges, C. V. 1941. Studies on prostatic cancer I. The effect of castration, of estrogen and of androgen injection on serum phosphatases in metastatic carcinoma of the prostate. Cancer Res. 1:293–297.
Jaffe, N., Frei, E., III, Traggis, D., and Bishop, Y. 1974. Adjuvant methotrexate and citrovorum-factor treatment and osteogenic sarcoma. N. Engl. J. Med. 291:994–997.
Li, M. C., Hertz, R., and Spencer, D. G. 1956. Effect of methotrexate therapy upon choriocarcinoma and chorioadenoma. Proc. Soc. Exp. Biol. Med. 93:361–366.
Malaise, E. P., Chavaudra, N., and Tubiana, M. 1973. The relationships between growth rate, labelling index and histological type of human solid tumors. Eur. J. Cancer 9:305–312.
Mitchell, M. S., Wawro, N. W., DeConti, R. C., Kaplan, S. R., Papac, R., and Bertino, J. R. 1968. Effectiveness of high dose infusions of methotrexate followed by leucovorin in carcinoma of the head and neck. Cancer Res. 28:1088–1094.
Schabel, F. M., Jr. 1969. The use of tumor growth kinetics in planning "curative" chemotherapy of advanced solid tumors. Cancer Res. 29:2384–2389.
Schabel, F. M., Jr. 1976. Concepts for treatment of micrometastases developed in murine systems. Am. J. Roentgenol. Radium Ther. Nuclear Med. 126:500–511.
Schenken, L. L., and Hagemann, R. F. 1976. Recruitment oncotherapy schedules for enhanced efficacy of cycle active agents. Proc. Am. Assoc. Cancer Res. 17:88.
Simpson-Herren, L., Sanford, A. H., and Holmquist, J. P. 1974. Cell population kinetics of transplanted and metastatic Lewis lung carcinoma. Cell Tissue Kinet. 7:349–361.
Skipper, H. E., Schabel, F. M., Jr., and Wilcox, W. S. 1964. Experimental evalua-(subhuman and human) relationships. Cancer 21:600–610.
Skipper, H. E., Schabel, F. M. Jr., and Wilcox, W. S. 1964. Experimental evaluation of potential anticancer agents. XIII. On the criteria and kinetics associated with the "curability" of experimental leukemia. Cancer Chemother. Rep. 35:3–111.
Sulkes, A., Livingston, R., and Taylor, G. 1976. Pretreatment labelling index (LI%) in breast carcinoma patients as a predictor of response to combination chemotherapy (CC). Proc. Am. Assoc. Cancer Res. 17:59.
Ziegler, J. L., Bluming, A. Z., Morrow, R. H., Fass, L., and Carbone, P. 1970. Central nervous system involvement in Burkitt's lymphoma. Blood 36:718–728.
Zubrod, C. G. 1971. Historical perspective of curative chemotherapy. In: R. L. Clark, R. W. Cumley, J. E. McCoy, and M. Copeland (eds.), Oncology, 1970, pp. 337–343. The Proceedings of the 10th International Cancer Congress, Year Book Medical Publishers, Inc., Chicago.
Zubrod, C. G., Schepartz, S., Leiter, J., Endicott, K. M., Carrese, L. M., and Baker, C. G. 1966. The chemotherapy program of the National Cancer Institute: History, analysis and plans. Cancer Chemother. Rep. 50:349–540.

Part IV
Advances in the Detection of Breast Cancer and Other Cancers

9
Breast Fluid Analysis in Breast Cancer Detection

Nicholas L. Petrakis

At the present time, early detection offers the greatest hope for cure of breast cancer. Although regular breast examination by self or physician, needle biopsy, and other techniques are immensely valuable in the early diagnosis of palpable tumors, they have almost no potential for the detection of nonpalpable intraductile or lobular carcinomas *in situ.* Mammography, demonstrated to be of value in the detection of minimal breast cancer, has recently had its safety in mass screening programs brought into question. New approaches to the early detection and diagnosis of breast cancer to supplement or even replace current methods are needed.

Some promising aspects of the author's research involving nipple aspiration of breast fluid, a technique that may have value in the cytologic and biochemical detection of breast cancer, are dealt with here. In addition, a model hypothesis for studies in breast cancer epidemiology that evolved from the author's investigations on the physiology of breast secretion is proposed.

The work from which this hypothesis has evolved is based on the long-known but seemingly overlooked fact that mature nonlactating breast alveoli secrete and reabsorb fluid. Epithelial cells lining the ducts and the alveoli are desquamated into this fluid and are eventually digested. Their products and the secreted fluid itself are continuously reabsorbed by the ductal epithelium. The secreted fluid passes down the ductules into the main ducts and ampullae at the base of the nipple from which, in the healthy

This work was supported by Public Health Service Grant CA-13556 and Contract CB-33882 from the National Cancer Institute and by a gift from Mrs. Viola K. Schroeder. We would also like to thank the Marin Mastectomy Services in Marin County, California, for their help.

breast, it is prevented from escaping by the smooth muscle around the ampullae and by keratin plugs in the nipple openings.

Breast secretions obtained from nipples aspirated for the early detection of cancer cells have been studied by a number of investigators in the past, including Ringrose (1966) and Masukawa, Lewison, and Frost (1966). The approach has not been widely utilized, primarily because the methods used for obtaining adequate amounts of breast fluid were unsatisfactory. Recently, however, a breast aspiration pump for cytologic and physiologic studies that has been found to be successful in obtaining ductal fluid from a relatively high proportion of women tested has been developed by Sartorius, (1973). By means of this breast pump—a small cup connected to a 10-cc syringe with a plastic tube—it is possible to aspirate ductal secretions from the nipple (Petrakis et al., 1975). When applied to the nipple, each cubic centimeter on the syringe generates about 30 mm of negative pressure. Fluid can be obtained from most Caucasian women with the syringe drawn to the 5- or 6-cc mark. The procedure causes a mild pinching sensation, but is quite acceptable to most women.

If the aspiration is successful, the fluid that appears at the nipple orifices can be collected in capillary tubes and sent to a laboratory for cytologic and biochemical studies. Ordinarily, from 50 to 300 ml of fluid can be obtained from each breast.

BIOLOGIC ASPECTS OF BREAST SECRETION

The frequency of breast secretors in various races is shown in Table 1. Fluid was successfully obtained from 158 of 225 (i.e., 70%) Caucasian women. The lowest proportion of secretors was among Chinese women (57 of 236, or 24%). Other groups fell somewhere in between. Fluid yield was related to age, menopausal status, and earwax type (Petrakis et al., 1975).

The frequency of breast fluid secretors by age and menopausal status is presented in Tables 2 and 3. A decrease in the frequency occurred after age 50 in all groups studied, although this was most marked among the Chinese.

Table 1. Breast fluid aspiration from women of various racial groups

Group	Number examined	Number of secretors	Percent of secretors
Caucasian	225	158	70.2
Filipino	10	7	70.0
Negro	37	23	62.2
Mexican-American	71	37	52.1
Japanese	27	8	29.9
Chinese	236	57	24.1

Table 2.   Age and frequency of successful breast fluid aspirations from women of various racial groups

Age group (years)	Number of secretors/Number of women examined (percent)			
	Caucasian	Negro	Mexican-American	Chinese
≤20	4/6 (66.6)	3/6 (50.0)	2/2 (100.0)	0/0
21–30	36/48 (75.0)	11/19 (57.9)	10/17 (58.8)	9/37 (24.3)
31–40	44/57 (77.2)	5/8 (62.5)	8/14 (57.1)	20/66 (30.3)
41–50	37/47 (78.7)	4/4 (100.0)	11/22 (50.0)	18/52 (34.6)
51–60	21/35 (60.0)	0/0	4/10 (40.0)	5/33 (15.2)
≥61	16/32 (50.0)	0/0	2/6 (33.3)	5/48 (10.4)
Total	158/225 (70.2)	23/37 (62.2)	37/71 (52.1)	57/236 (24.1)

Approximately 80% of premenopausal and 60% of postmenopausal Caucasian women yielded fluid. In contrast, there was a much lower overall yield of fluid in premenopausal Chinese women (30%) and virtually no fluid (3.8%) in most postmenopausal Chinese women tested.

Both the ceruminous (earwax) glands and the breast are modified apocrine glands. The group of Chinese women with genetic wet-type earwax was more likely to have secretions of fluid than the group who had dry-type cerumen. This suggests that an apocrine-related genetic factor may affect the secretory activity of the breast (Table 4). It was also found that the frequency of secretors among Chinese women of all ages was lower in those with dry cerumen than in those with the wet type. A marked drop in the proportion of secretors occurred after age 50, suggesting that little secretion was occurring in the Oriental women studied.

BREAST FLUID CYTOLOGY

Epithelial abnormalities of the breast ducts such as hyperplasia, atypical hyperplasia, dysplasia, and carcinoma in situ have previously been identified

Table 3.   Menopausal status and frequency of successful breast fluid aspirations from Caucasian and Chinese women

Group	Number examined	Number of secretors	Percent of secretors[a]
Caucasian			
Premenopausal	138	112	81.2
Postmenopausal	77	46	59.7
Chinese			
Premenopausal	156	47	30.1
Postmenopausal	80	3	3.8

[a] $p < 0.001$.

Table 4.   Cerumen type and frequency of successful breast fluid
aspirations from Chinese women

Type	Number examined	Number of secretors	Percent of secretors[a]
Wet	110	38	34.5
Dry	126	19	15.1
Total	236	57	24.2

[a] $\chi^2 = 12.1, p < 0.001$.

in association with carcinoma of the breast (Gallager and Martin, 1969; Kern and Brooks, 1969; Wellings, Jensen, and Marcum, 1975), and these may reflect a sequence of cytologic events resulting in frank cancer. Papanicolaou et al. (1958) suggested that exfoliative cytology might play a role in the diagnosis of early and preclinical breast cancer.

Cytologic findings of nipple secretions obtained by breast aspiration were analyzed to determine total cellularity and differential cell distribution, to identify abnormal and malignant cells, and to compare the cytologic with the histologic findings and the clinical status of the breast (King, Barrett, and Petrakis, 1975). Methods for preparing cells for microscopic examination as well as earlier findings have been reported previously (King et al., 1975; King, Barrett, and Petrakis, 1975).

Aspirations were attempted in more than 4,000 women with various physiologic and pathologic conditions of the breast. The present report is based upon the cytologic evaluation of nipple aspirates from 2,636 breasts. Aspirates from 503 of these were unsatisfactory because of absence of both duct epithelial cells and foam cells. Aspirates from an additional 354 breasts were excluded because they were from pregnant or lactating patients. Of the remaining specimens from 1,779 breasts, abnormal cells were found in aspirates from 197, of which tissue was available for 42—14 from patients with breast cancer and 28 from patients with lesions in the spectrum of so-called mammary dysplasia. Among the remaining 1,582 breasts with benign cytology, tissue was available for comparison from 80, of which 9 were from patients with breast cancer and 71 from patients with benign breast lesions in the mammary dysplasia complex.

Each microscopic field was examined for the presence of abnormal cells. These were differentiated from normal duct epithelial cells by their larger size (ranging from one and a half to three times the size of normal duct cells), by their increased nuclear-cytoplastic ratio, and by the presence of hyperchromatic nuclei with accentuated parachromatin. Abnormal cells classified as hyperplasia, atypical hyperplasia, dysplasia, and carcinoma were easily distinguished from normal cells. However, subtle gradations

Table 5. Comparison of cytologic and histologic findings in 1,779 breasts

| Cytology | Pathology | | | Total |
	Malignant	Benign	None	
Abnormal	14	28	155	197
Benign	9	71	1,502	1,582
Total	23	99	1,657	1,779

were also found among the various abnormal categories, ranging in severity from hyperplastic to clearly malignant cells.

The tissue was initially examined without reference to the cytologic findings. The principal lesions and accompanying pathologic changes were listed and duct epithelial abnormalities were recorded according to type and extent, using a system similar to the one reported by Black and Chabon (1969). The tabulated data from the cytologic and histologic evaluations were then directly compared in order to relate the cellular findings to specific histologic lesions.

Abnormal cells were found in 197 of the 1,779 breasts from which fluid was obtained. Correlation of these changes with tissue histology was possible in 122 breasts. Abnormal cells were observed in 14 of 23 women with a subsequent histologic diagnosis of breast cancer, and in 28 of 99 women with benign breast pathology (Tables 5 and 6). Tissue from patients with breast cancer revealed a tenfold greater frequency of epithelial abnormalities in the large ducts when abnormal cells were found in nipple secretions as compared to specimens lacking significant cellular abnormalities.

Attention has been directed by a number of investigators to the transformation of duct epithelium from normal to premalignant to carcinoma in situ. These changes appear to be significant in respect to the cytologic findings in those 42 cases in which tissue was available for comparison. However, the potential role of cytology in breast cancer control

Table 6. Breast fluid cytopathology in relation to histology

| Cytology | Pathology | |
	Malignant	Benign
Carcinoma	2	0
Carcinoma in situ	3	1
Dysplasia	7	4
Atypical hyperplasia	2	17
Hyperplasia	0	6
Total	14	28

Table 7.   Breast fluid cytology and clinical status
(no tissue)

Cytology	Clinical status	
	Lump	Normal
Abnormal	64	87
Benign	241	319
Total	305	406

will eventually be revealed by following clinical developments in women who have cellular abnormalities without clinical evidence of disease. Among the first 2,636 breasts examined, 87 were in this category (Table 7). Such women deserve especially close attention at follow-up examination over adequate intervals of time to characterize the biologic behavior of their lesions and the role of cytology in the recognition of incipient breast neoplasia.

BIOCHEMICAL AND IMMUNOLOGIC STUDIES OF BREAST FLUIDS

Certain biochemical aspects of the composition of breast fluid that may be of value in clinical diagnosis have been investigated. Breast fluid contains many of the components of colostrum and milk, including immunoglobulin, IgA, IgG, IgM, albumin, α-lactalbumin, lactose, cholesterol, fatty acids, and various enzymes (glucose-6-phosphate dehydrogenase, lactic dehydrogenase, etc.) (Petrakis et al., 1975).

In view of the presence of immunoglobulins in breast fluids and of the immune disturbances reportedly associated with human breast cancer (Edynak, Lardis, and Vrana, 1971; Priori et al., 1971; Roberts, Bathgate, and Stevenson, 1975; Springer, Desai, and Scanlon, 1976), immunoglobulin levels were measured in breast fluid and serum from women with breast cancer and benign breast disease as well as women with normal breasts (Petrakis et al., 1977). Laurell Rocket electrophoresis was performed on agarose gel slides containing monospecific IgA, IgG, and IgM antisera of goat or rabbit origin.[1]

The subjects included: 1) 55 women with normal breasts, 2) 95 with benign breast disease, and 3) 29 with breast cancer (of whom 9 had newly diagnosed primary breast cancer and 20 had a prior mastectomy, but without clinical evidence of recurrence). Diagnoses of normal breasts and breasts with benign disease were made by palpation and mammography. In some women, the diagnosis of benign breast disease was established by biopsy. All new diagnoses of breast cancer were based on histologic examination at operation.

---

[1] Obtained from Millipore, Biomedica, 15 Craig Road, Acton, Massachusetts.

Mean immunoglobulin levels in fluids from normal breasts and in those with benign disease resembled those reported for colostrum (Table 8 and Figures 1, 2, and 3). Mean IgA levels in breast fluids were elevated markedly above plasma IgA levels, whereas the reverse was true for IgG and IgM, where mean plasma levels were higher than mean breast fluid levels.

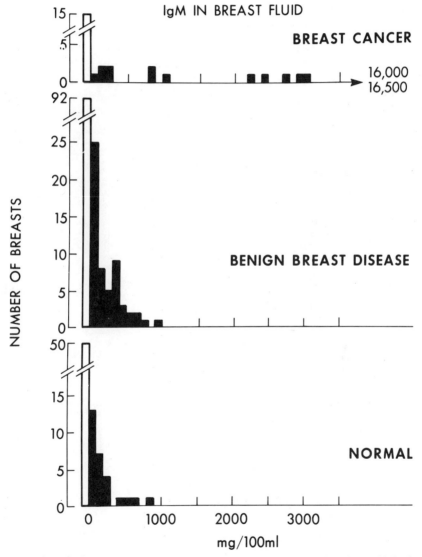

Figure 1. IgM levels (mg/100 ml) in breast fluid of normal women and of those with benign and malignant breast disease.

Table 8. Immunoglobulin levels in breast fluid and plasma

Condition of breasts	IgA			IgG			IgM		
	Number	Mean	SE[a]	Number	Mean	SE	Number	Mean	SE
Normal									
Breast fluid	86	1709	± 168	84	249	± 61	85	66	± 16
Plasma	55	247	± 23	55	1063	± 60	52	194	± 15
Benign disease									
Breast fluid	160	1784	± 132	157	214	± 31	155	84	± 14
Plasma	95	279	± 81	93	1116	± 52	89	189	± 12
Cancer									
Breast fluid	12	1620	± 593	11	258	± 104	11	1629	± 580
Plasma	9	114	± 14	9	1059	± 181	9	189	± 40
Prior mastectomy									
Breast fluid	20	1968	± 567	20	254	± 85	20	2150	± 1115
Plasma	20	168	± 26	20	861	± 78	20	152	± 20

[a] Standard error of the mean.

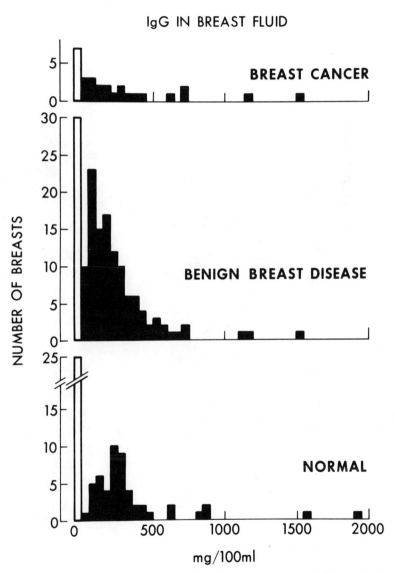

Figure 2.   IgG levels (mg/100 ml) in breast fluid of normal women and of those with benign and malignant breast disease.

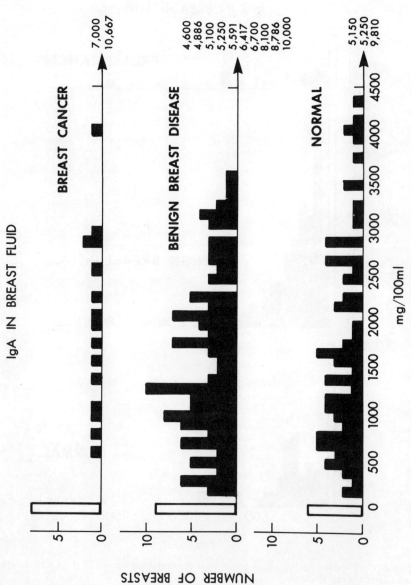

Figure 3. IgA levels (mg/100 ml) in breast fluid of normal women and of those with benign and malignant breast disease.

In women with breast cancer, the IgA level in breast fluids was elevated above plasma levels in all age groups. The reverse was observed for IgG, in which the highest mean levels occurred in plasma rather than breast fluids.

Mean levels of IgM in breast fluids from normal and benign disease breasts were similar and lower than those in plasma in all groups. A striking elevation of the mean IgM level compared with corresponding plasma IgM levels was found in breast fluids from cancerous breasts and from those later removed by mastectomy. In Figure 1 the distribution of IgM values for breast fluid from the three groups is presented. Of the individual IgM values from normal and benign-disease breasts, 95% were under 400 mg/100 ml, with most being under 100 mg/100 ml. A few were as high as 900 mg/100 ml. Six of 9 patients with newly diagnosed breast cancer and 5 of 15 with a prior mastectomy had significantly increased levels of IgM ranging from 800 mg/100 ml to 16,000 mg/100 ml.

In many samples of breast fluid, IgA, IgG, and IgM could not be detected. Ten of 30 cancerous breasts (33%) lacked IgA, compared with 5 of 81 (6.1%) normal breasts ($p < 0.001$), and 9 of 160 (5.6%) benign-disease breasts ($p = 0.001$). Nine of 31 (29%) cancerous breast fluids and 33 of 84 (39%) normal fluids lacked IgG, a difference that is not significant. However, breasts with benign disease lacked IgG in only 32 of 156 (21%) samples, a significant difference from normal breasts ($p < 0.001$). IgM was absent in 56 of 85 (66%) normal breasts, in 93 of 154 (60%) benign-disease breasts, and in 15 of 30 (50%) cancerous breasts.

These studies suggest that the concentration of IgM increases significantly in the breast fluids of many women with breast cancer or prior mastectomy. A large number of these women also lack IgA in their breast fluids. At present we can only speculate about the significance of these findings. In studies pertinent to these data, Roberts, Bathgate, and Stevenson (1975) found that one-third of cancerous breast tissue extracts contained higher concentrations of IgM, whereas IgG levels were reduced in such extracts.

Recently, Lentino (1975) reported that serum IgM levels were elevated in breast cancer patients with sinus histiocytosis in regional lymph nodes. In addition, serum IgG values were increased in breast cancer patients with axillary metastases.

The function of immunoglobulins in the breast fluid secretions of non-pregnant women is unknown. In addition to their presence in serum, immunoglobulins exist in other sites (Tomasi and Bienenstock, 1968). IgA is found in saliva, tears, milk, and the secretions of the gastrointestinal and respiratory tracts and other mucous membranes. Serum IgA is probably derived from lymphocytes in the Peyer's patches of the intestinal tract. Lesser concentrations of IgG and IgM are also present in these secretions.

IgA is transferred from the blood into glandular secretions, probably by the production of secretory piece by the epithelial cells, which may protect IgA from enzymatic degradation. Absence of IgA in breast fluid but not in plasma may represent a local deficiency of qualitative alteration of secretory piece produced by breast alveolar cells. As yet, breast fluid for secretory piece has not been studied.

Recurrent infections have been reported in subjects with IgA deficiency, which may indicate that IgA plays a role in immunity to bacterial and viral infections (Petrakis et al., 1975). IgA deficiency has also been associated with a variety of other diseases including malignancies (Wellings, Jensen, and Marcum, 1975). As noted in the study reported here, 33% of fluids from cancerous breasts lacked IgA compared to 5% for normal and benign-disease breasts. The significance of the absence of IgA in breast fluids and its role, if any, in the pathogenesis of breast cancer is unknown.

Why IgM concentrations are elevated in the breast fluids of cancer patients is also unknown. Moderate to high elevations in serum IgM may occur in association with bacterial infections; however, there was no evidence of breast infection in the patients studied. Marked elevations of serum IgM, comparable to the breast fluid findings, have been found in children with immune-deficiency diseases, and in the jejunal secretions of adults with coeliac disease (Hobbs et al., 1969; Rosen et al., 1961). It has been conjectured that these high levels of IgM might be a compensatory response to a quantitative decrease in IgA or to a qualitative impairment of IgA and IgG production or function.

The elevations of breast fluid IgM and the absence of IgA seen here may represent a locally aberrant immune response of mononuclear cells to tumor-specific antigens secreted into the breast fluids of many women with breast cancer. The ability of the secreted substances to provoke local immunologic responses in the breast is under investigation.

Study of the diagnostic and prognostic implications of these findings will be continued. It may be significant that 33% of women with prior mastectomy and 5% of those with benign-disease and normal breasts had elevated levels of IgM. Prospective studies of women at breast screening centers may provide information on the clinical significance of the observed variations in immunoglobulin content of human breast secretions.

BREAST SECRETORY ACTIVITY AND
THE EPIDEMIOLOGY OF BREAST CANCER

It is well known from studies of lactating mothers that drugs, chemicals, and food substances are rapidly secreted into breast milk (Knowles, 1965). Based on such reports, the secretion of extrinsically derived substances into breast fluids has been studied. The findings suggest that many exogenously derived substances are rapidly secreted into the fluid of the nonlactating breast. The dynamic rate of secretion is indicated by the observation that intravenously administered radioactive technetium (^{99m}Tc) was detectable in breast fluids within 5 minutes, reaching a plateau at 3 to 4 hours and disappearing by 24 hours (Figure 4).

By means of gas-liquid chromatography–mass spectrometry the secretion of such substances as phenobarbital, tannic acids, nicotine, nornicotine, and cotenine into breast fluids has been measured. Findings indicate that almost all ingested, inhaled, or intravenously administered chemical substances are taken up and secreted by the breast epithelium, suggesting that the secretory activity of the nonlactating breast may result in the exposure of breast epithelia to environmental carcinogens. These considerations have lead to the formulation of a working hypothesis relating secretory activity and carcinogenesis (Figure 5).

It is proposed here that the turnover rate of secreted substances and their rates of reabsorption are primary determinants of the extent and duration of exposure of the breast epithelium to environmental and endogenous carcinogens. The endocrine-dependent secretory activity of the nonlactating breast can provide a mechanism that permits potential initiating mutagens and cocarcinogenic factors to reach the breast epithelium, leading over time to the accumulation of mutant cells. Many histologic studies of the human breast have demonstrated striking increases in the frequency of alveolar atypia and metaplasia in the breasts of women over 30 years of age.

This model may help to explain the differential risk of breast cancer between Caucasian and Oriental women and the significantly lower rates in the latter group. The lower risk may be due to the overall decrease in secretory activity in Oriental women, especially marked in those with genetically dry-type apocrine systems. A low or absent epithelial secretory activity may minimize the contact of the breast with exogenous carcinogens with a concomitant reduction of mutant cells.

Utilizing the results of published studies on breast development and function as well as the findings on secretory activity reported in this chapter the epidemiologic features of breast cancer can be reinterpreted from the viewpoint of the hypothesis described above. During the growth period between 9 and 12 years of age, the breast is activated into development. This process is probably an uneven one, with some alveoli developing or functioning later than others. Secreted initiating and promoting substances would, at this time, begin to have the opportunity to act on the developing breast and to induce nonrandom somatic mutations that could eventually lead to the formation of latent cancer cells in the breast alveolar tissue of nulliparous women.

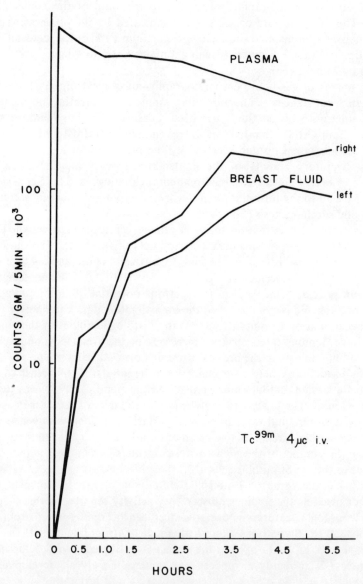

Figure 4.   Uptake of radioactive technetium (99mTc) in right and left breast fluids and plasma.

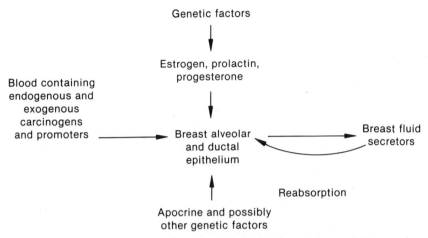

Figure 5.   Working hypothesis to relate secretory activity and cancer of the breast.

Early and late first pregnancies would have different effects on the breast and, therefore, different influences on the risk of breast cancer. In young primipara, the diffuse duct and alveolar cell death associated with the relatively severe engorgement and milk stasis regression would lead to a random loss of many of these latent cells, thereby reducing the number of latent tumor cells in the postpartum breast. Simultaneously, the secretion of colostrum and milk would remove the relatively static and potentially harmful secretions that have accumulated in the ducts since the onset of puberty. In the nulliparous woman, atypical, abnormal, and latent cells would accumulate in the duct and gland system with advancing age, resulting in a cancer risk higher than that in the young primipara.

The significantly increased risk of breast cancer observed in older primiparas may be due to the accumulation of mutant cell clones resulting from exposure to secreted environmental carcinogens (similar to the situation in nulliparous women) *plus* the endocrine stress of pregnancy acting on initiated but latent cancer cells. In older primipara, the process of milk stasis engorgement is known to involute less efficiently and, in addition, due to the stimulatory effect of hormones operating during pregnancy, might result in a marked increase in abnormal cells. It seems likely that such cells would be relatively autonomous with respect to hormone regulation. Following regression, these breasts would contain a much greater proportion of latent cancer cells than the breasts of nulliparous or early primiparous women, leading to a greater risk of breast cancer in older primipara.

Many avenues for physiological, genetic, clinical, and epidemiologic research are suggested by these studies. It is hoped that these may lead to new advances in the etiology, diagnosis, and prevention of breast cancer.

REFERENCES

Black, M. M., and Chabon, A. B. 1969. In situ carcinoma of the breast. Pathol. Annu. 4:185–210.

Edynak, E. M., Lardis, M. P., and Vrana, M. 1971. Autogenic changes in human breast neoplasia. Cancer 28:1457–1461.

Gallager, H. S., and Martin, J. E. 1969. Early phases in the development of breast cancer. Cancer 24:1170–1178.

Hobbs, J. R., Hepner, F. W., Douglas, A. P., Crabbé, P. A., and Johansson, S. G. O. 1969. Immunological mystery of coeliac disease. Lancet 2:649–650.

Kern, W. H., and Brooks, R. N. 1969. Atypical epithelial hyperplasia associated with breast cancer and fibrocystic disease. Cancer 24:668–675.

King, E. B., Barrett, D., King, M.-C., and Petrakis, N. L. 1975. Cellular composition of the nipple aspirate specimen of breast fluid. I. The benign cells. Am. J. Clin. Pathol. 64:728–738.

King, E. B., Barrett, D., and Petrakis, N. L. 1975. Cellular composition of the nipple aspirate specimen of breast fluid. II. Abnormal findings. Am. J. Clin. Pathol. 64:739–748.

Knowles, J. A. 1965. Excretion of drugs in milk—A review. J. Pediatr. 66:1068–1082.

Lentino, J. A. 1975. Immunological studies in breast cancer. Allergologia et Immunopathologia 3:279–288.

Masukawa, T., Lewison, E. F., and Frost, J. K. 1966. The cytologic examination of breast secretions. Acta Cytol. 10:261–265.

Papanicolaou, G. N., Holmquist, D. G., Bader, G. M.,and Falk, E. A. 1958. Exfoliative cytology of the human mammary gland and its value in the diagnosis of cancer and other diseases of the breast. Cancer 11:377–409.

Petrakis, N. L., Doherty, M., Lee, R., Mason, L., Pawson, S., Hunt, T., and Schweitzer, R. 1977. Immunoglobulin levels in fluids of women with breast cancer. Clin. Immunol. Immunopathol. 7:386–393.

Petrakis, N. L., Mason, L., Lee, R., Sugimoto, B., Pawson, S., and Catchpool, F. 1975. Association of race, age, menopausal status, and cerumen type with breast fluid secretion in nonlactating women, as determined by nipple aspiration. J. Natl. Cancer Inst. 54:829–834.

Priori, E. S., Seman, G., Dmochowski, L., Gallager, H. S., and Anderson, D. E. 1971. Immunofluorescence studies on sera of patients with breast carcinoma. Cancer 28:1462–1471.

Ringrose, C. A. D. 1966. The role of cytology in the early detection of breast disease. Acta Cytol. 10:373–375.

Roberts, M. M., Bass, E. M., Wallace I. W. J., and Stevenson, A. 1973. Local immunoglobulin production in breast cancer. Br. J. Cancer 27:269–275.

Roberts, M. M., Bathgate, E. M., and Stevenson, A. 1975. Serum immunoglobulin levels in patients with breast cancer. Cancer 36:221–224.

Rosen, F. S., Kevy, S. V., Merler, E., Janeway, C. A., and Gitlin, D. 1961. Recurrent bacterial infections and dysgamma-globulinemia: Deficiency of 7S gamma-globulins in the presence of elevated 19S gamma-globulins. Pediatrics 28:182–195.

Sartorius, O. 1973. Breast fluid cells help in early cancer detection. JAMA 224:823–827.

Springer, G. F., Desai, P. R., and Scanlon, E. F. 1976. Blood group MN precursors as human breast carcinoma-associated antigens and "naturally" occurring human cytotoxins against them. Cancer 37:169–176.

Tomasi, T. B., Jr., and Bienenstock, J. 1968. Secretory immunoglobulins. Adv. Immunol. 9:1–96.

Wellings, S. R, Jensen, H. M., and Marcum, R. G. 1975. An atlas of subgross pathology of the human breast with special reference to possible precancerous lesions. J. Natl. Cancer Inst. 55:231–273.

10
Considerations in Breast Cancer Screening

Sam Shapiro

There are few chronic conditions with as much favorable evidence on the efficacy of screening as breast cancer. Nevertheless, significant issues, a number of which are likely to remain unresolved in the immediate future, arise in considering the balance between benefits and risks in breast cancer screening. On the benefit side of the equation are such matters as the ages to be covered, the periodicity of screening, the relative value of available detection modalities, and the long-term versus short-term benefits of screening. The risk side of the equation is influenced by such potentially measureable factors as the radiogenic effect of x-ray procedures and the increased biopsy rates, both of which are also related to many of the benefit issues.

Superimposed on these considerations are cost, efficiency, and quality questions that are critically important when decisions are being made on the extension of screening to large segments of the population. Breast cancer detection demonstration projects now underway in the United States should provide a diversity of information to evaluate these and other related issues. This chapter focuses on what might be viewed as the underlying rationale for our concern with implementation, that is, the risks versus benefits of screening. Three questions form the framework for the discussion that follows:

1. What basis is there for determining the age range of interest for breast cancer screening?
2. What is the evidence on benefits from breast cancer screening, and what more needs to be determined?
3. What should be included as risks associated with screening, and what do we now know about these risks?

Supported in part by contracts PH 43-63-49 and NIH 69-88 from the National Institutes of Health to the Health Insurance Plan of Greater New York.

THE AGE FACTOR

The significance of age in breast cancer can be examined from several standpoints. By directing our attention to aggregations of data on breast cancer, we can heighten appreciation of the importance of the relatively young age groups. Figure 1 shows three cumulative distributions related to breast cancer for the age range between 20–24 years and 75–79 years. Older age groups are excluded because of the very high death rates from all causes to which such women are subject.

The lowest curve cumulates the proportion of total breast cancer deaths at each age, using as the denominator the total number of breast cancer deaths occurring between the ages of 20 and 79 years (Vital Statistics of the United States, 1971). The contour of the curve is affected not only by the age-specific death rates but also by the age distribution of women in the population. The fact that there is a substantially larger number of women in the younger age groups than in the older age groups results in one-fifth of all breast cancer deaths occurring between the ages of 35 and 49, despite low rates at these ages.

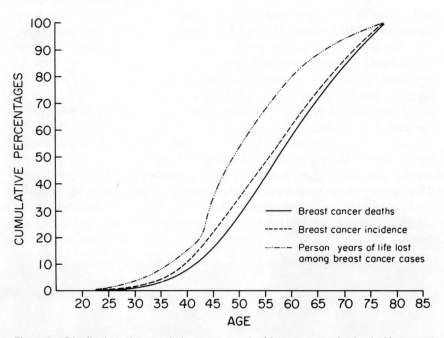

Figure 1.   Distributions (by cumulative percentages) of breast cancer deaths, incidence, and person years of life lost.

When incident cases are considered (the next higher curve in Figure 1) this proportion increases moderately (Third National Cancer Survey, 1975). However, when attention is directed to the cumulative number of years of life lost due to breast cancer (the top curve), the ages under 50 assume a new importance (End Results in Cancer, 1972). About two-fifths (41%) of the years of life lost from breast cancer detected in patients under 80 years of age are associated with the cases diagnosed at ages 34–49, one-third (34%) with cases diagnosed at ages 40–49, and a similar proportion (38%) with cases diagnosed at ages 50–64 years.

Accordingly, breast cancer among women 35–49 years old (especially 40–49) must command even greater attention than indicated by mortality or incidence rates. Unfortunately, no hard evidence is yet available that screening for breast cancer at these ages results in benefit, as measured by reduction in mortality from breast cancer.

EVIDENCE ON EFFICACY OF SCREENING

The only data available on the effect of screening on breast cancer mortality in which a control group was drawn from the same population as the group offered screening come from the Breast Cancer Screening Project, conducted by the Health Insurance Plan (HIP) of Greater New York (Shapiro et al., 1972). This study took the form of a randomized trial in which women between the ages of 40 and 64 years were assigned to either a study or a control group, each numbering about 31,000. A high degree of comparability between the two groups was demonstrated for a wide range of demographic and other characteristics as well as for general mortality other than from breast cancer (Fink, Shapiro, and Roeser, 1972).

Study group women were offered screening examinations; the 65% who appeared for an initial examination were offered three additional examinations at annual intervals, unless earlier follow-up or biopsy was indicated. All but a small proportion (12%) of these women underwent at least one additional annual examination. The screening consisted of a clinical examination, usually conducted by a surgeon, plus mammography. Independence between the two screening modalities was strictly maintained so that it could be determined which was responsible for the chain of events leading to biopsy. Control women were not screened, but they continued to receive their usual medical care.

Over a 7-year period of follow-up, the number of deaths due to breast cancer in the total study group (i.e., the combined experience of women screened and those who refused screening) was 70, or approximately one-third less than in the control group (108) (Table 1). The screenees'

186   Shapiro

Table 1.   Breast cancer deaths by time interval from date of entry

Completed years from date of entry	Cumulative number of deaths with breast cancer as underlying cause[a]	
	Study[b]	Control
2	11	8
3	17	20
4	25	38
5	40	63
6	56	88
7	70	108

[a] Follow-up through December 31, 1974. Data exclude breast cancer deaths among women first diagnosed as having breast cancer more than 5 years after entry.

[b] Includes women screened and women who refused screening.

advantage was restricted entirely to women in the age groups 50–59 and 60–69 years, whether age at death, age at diagnosis, or age at entry is employed as an independent variable (Table 2). No advantage was apparent among women screened at ages 40–49 years.

Cumulative case fatality rates for 5 and 6 years after diagnosis reveal a similar advantage to screenees over control subjects, after taking into account an estimated 1 year's artifactual lead time in breast cancer detection, which is attributable to the screening program (Table 3). Nearly all of the survival advantage by the end of years 5 and 6 was gained by screenees in the age group 50–59 years (Table 4). Above this age, screenees also

Table 2.   Breast cancer deaths by age: 7 years of follow-up from date of entry

	Number of deaths	
	Study[a]	Control
Total deaths	70	108
Age at death		
40–49 years	17	16
50–59 years	32	59
60–69 years	21	33
Age at entry		
40–49 years	33	39
50–59 years	30	54
60–69 years	7	15
Age at diagnosis		
40–49 years	27	21
50–59 years	31	60
60–69 years	12	27

[a] Includes women screened and women who refused screening.

Table 3. Cumulative case fatality rates (per 100) among confirmed breast cancer cases[a]

| | Number of cases | Years after diagnosis | | |
		1	5	6[b]
Total study	299	6.4	25.6	29.5 (2.7)
Study group				
Detected through screening	132	2.3	12.9	18.3 (3.4)
Interval cases	93	6.5	38.1	41.0 (5.2)
Refused screening	74	13.5	32.5	34.3 (5.6)
Control group	285	7.7	41.3	43.5 (3.0)
Total study (adjusted)[c]	299	8.0	28.0	30.5 (2.7)

[a] Cases detected within 5 years after entry; follow-up through December 31, 1974.

[b] Numbers in parentheses give standard error of case fatality rate.

[c] Lead time of 1 year included for cases detected through screening.

gained a survival advantage but to a lesser degree; at ages 40–49 years, there was almost no difference in mortality rates between the study and control groups.

Additional comparisons have been made utilizing data from the National Cancer Institute end results study of cancer experience in various regions of the country (End Results in Cancer, 1972). Applying estimated 5-year age-specific case fatality rates to the corresponding numbers of breast cancers in the HIP study's control group yields an overall expected rate of 41.3 per 100, which is identical to the rate observed in the control group. The rates estimated from the end results report are: 37 per 100 at ages under 50, 41 per 100 at ages 50–59 years, and 47 per 100 at ages 60–69 years. Introducing these rates does not affect the conclusion that the screening program did not reduce breast cancer mortality at ages 40–49 years. Our confidence in the existence of an advantageous effect at ages 50–59

Table 4. Cumulative case fatality rates (per 100)[a] by age at diagnosis

| | Year 5 | | Year 6 | |
Age at diagnosis	Total study[b]	Control	Total study[b]	Control
40–49 years	32.4	33.4	32.4	35.1
50–59 years	25.7	49.2[c]	28.5	51.1[c]
60 and over	27.4	35.3	32.6	38.3

[a] Cases detected within 5 years after entry; follow-up through December 31, 1974.

[b] Lead time of 1 year included for cases detected through screening.

[c] Differences between total study and control groups statistically significant ($p < 0.01$).

years is strengthened, and we also move closer to accepting the evidence, based on breast cancer mortality data, that screening has a salutary effect at ages 60–69 years as well.

The absence of a difference between study and control groups under age 50 in the HIP study cannot be taken as conclusive evidence that screening does not have value for women in this age group. It can be shown statistically that a 20% or 30% differential could easily be missed in a study of the size that was conducted. Furthermore, the results of the HIP study must be interpreted in reference to the specific screening procedures employed. Mammography proved relatively ineffective in detecting breast cancers among the younger women. Approximately 19% of these cases were positive only on mammography, as compared with 42% and 31% at ages 50–59 and 60–69 years, respectively. The significance of this derives from the very low case fatality rates among cases in which the initial basis for biopsy recommendation was mammography. If mammography today is a more effective modality than it was a decade ago, a new set of circumstances may exist.

Current screening programs may also differ in the types of personnel used for the physical examination. In the HIP study, primary dependence was on highly qualified surgeons, a situation that may not be feasible in most screening programs today. Follow-up is, of course, crucial, and this is not likely to be significantly improved in comparison with the HIP experience. Virtually every woman with a positive finding on screening was seen by a surgeon for a more definitive diagnostic work-up. In approximately 80% of the cases, the recommendation was confirmed, and four out of five such women underwent surgery.

ISSUES RELATED TO BENEFIT

The conclusion arrived at, then, is that the benefits of screening for breast cancer are limited to women 50 years of age and over. Below this age, the benefit, if any, has not been established. Thus, in estimating benefits from screening based on the available data, a benefit of zero would be assigned to women under 50, and benefits of about 45% and 35% to women of ages 50–59 and 60–69 years, respectively, over a 7-year follow-up period.

New studies are needed to test whether the HIP finding for the under 50 age group can be confirmed. That such data will not be easy to come by is suggested by other findings in the HIP study. The single most widely used indicator of breast cancer prognosis has been the presence or absence of axillary nodal involvement. In the HIP study, 68% of the cases detected through screening under 50 years of age had no axillary nodal involvement, an encouraging observation. However, in the total study group (screened plus unscreened), at these ages the figure was 53% compared to 49% for the control group. This suggests the importance of probing the possibility that patient selectivity may have played some role in the findings reported in this chapter. The same confounding factor must, of course, also be minimized in any new studies undertaken.

Another critical question to answer in relation to the benefits of screening concerns the incremental value of mammography. While an unequivocally precise statement on the subject will probably never be possible, useful approximations can be based on the available data. Two findings relevant to the possible effect of excluding mammography can be reported in this regard. In the HIP study, about one-third of the breast cancers detected through screening would have been missed without mammography and, as seen in Table 5, cases credited to mammography had an exceedingly low 7-year case fatality rate. It is not certain at what stage of disease the cases detected through mammography would otherwise have been diagnosed. However, the effect of excluding mammography can be speculated about under the assumption that cases credited to mammography in the HIP study would be detected at the same rate and with the same prognosis as all other cases in the screened population.

Two other issues of importance in assessing benefit should be mentioned. One concerns the periodicity of screening. Statistical models used in the HIP study indicate that the detection of breast cancer is advanced by an average of about 1 year through screening (Shapiro, Goldberg, and Hutchison, 1974). Other models (Zelen and Feinleib, 1969) suggest a longer

Table 5. Cumulative case[a] fatality rates (per 100) of cases detected through screening, by modality

Modality[b]	Number of cases	Years after diagnosis		
		5	6	7[c]
Total	132	12.9	18.4	21.1 (3.6)
Mammography only	44	4.5	7.0	9.7 (4.7)
Clinical only	59	11.9	19.0	19.0 (5.2)
Mammography and clinical	29	27.6	34.7	43.2 (9.6)
Cases positive on both modalities plus:				
Mammography only	73	13.7	18.0	22.9 (5.1)
Clinical only	88	17.1	24.1	26.8 (4.8)

[a] Cases detected within 5 years after entry; follow-up through December 31, 1974.

[b] Initial biopsy recommendation made independently on the basis of two modalities.

[c] Numbers in parentheses give standard error of case fatality rate.

time interval, but the important point is that estimates of average lead time are likely to have a lower bound close to 1 year and an upper bound of 2 years.

The absence of distributional data limits average lead time estimates as a basis for fixing the periodicity of screening. Limited as they may be, however, these averages suggest that, unless screening techniques have improved substantially since the HIP study, reasonable options for screening periodicity for breast cancer probably fall within a relatively narrow time range. Nevertheless, this does make a substantial difference from a cost and risk standpoint, if screening is annual or biannual. A decrease in benefit can be expected with longer screening intervals, but the magnitude of the decrease is critically important. While simulation models may be useful in approaching the question, given what is at stake, there seems to be a clear need for new randomized trials to settle the issue.

In all of this discussion, it should be borne in mind that estimates of benefit relate to follow-up periods of 5–7 years. To project benefits starting at age 50 and following women prospectively over their remaining life span, it would be necessary to make broad assumptions concerning the persistence of the benefits observed. The possibility that, in time, there will be some convergence in breast cancer mortality between study and control groups in the HIP study cannot be dismissed. Accordingly, while the benefit above age 50 appears to be substantial over the period of 5–7 years, results from longer term follow-up of the women are essential if we are to derive more secure estimates of the effect of screening over the total life span. Provisions have been made for such a follow-up of the HIP population.

ISSUES RELATED TO RISK

On the risk side of the equation, many factors must be taken into account. Only two are considered here: the radiogenic effects of mammography, and the possible increase in biopsies resulting from screening.

With respect to the hazards of radiation in inducing breast cancer, various conclusions are reached depending on the estimate of radiation dosage, the dose response model used, and whether comparisons are based on changes in incidence of breast cancer, mortality, or person years of life (Bailar, 1976). If a linear dose response model (Advisory Committee on the Biological Effects of Ionizing Radiation, 1972) is used to derive estimates of risk in an annual screening program with mammography and clinical examination, and if benefits are extrapolated on the basis of the HIP findings and a skin dose of 5 rads per examination is assumed, the result is a net benefit in person years of life for women 50 years of age and over (Chiacchierini,

Lundin, and Scheidt, 1976). The increment in risk associated with mammography performed at ages 35–49 years, although small, is not offset by benefits from screening.

The other risk factor to be considered concerns the biopsy rate. Here we are dealing with a morbidity effect with cost implications. The issue arises from the possibility of substantial increases in biopsies due to screening. This would occur only if the false-positive rate under screening conditions was appreciably different from the rate that is usually experienced, due to lack of specificity or to increased biopsies for highly equivocal screened cases that formerly would have been followed clinically. The reason for the emphasis on the false-positive rate is that screening does not, in the long run, substantially increase the number of breast cancers detected; its principal effect is to advance the date of diagnosis.

Only fragmentary bits of information are presently available on biopsy results. In the HIP study, among cases where screening led to the biopsy, about 1 in 5 (or 21%) of the biopsies were positive. This proportion was heavily influenced by the experience with women under age 50. Excluding this group in which confirmation of breast cancer occurred in only 1 out of 10 biopsies, the confirmation ratio was 1 out of 4 for cases over age 50. The latter may not be substantially different from what many hospitals are presently experiencing. Whether this situation has changed in recent years and how much variation in fact exists among screening programs certainly merits attention. To address this, an appropriate starting point could be the National Cancer Institute–American Cancer Society demonstration projects.

CONCLUSIONS

Based on the HIP study experience, the major risk issue in breast cancer screening is the effect of radiation exposure. Increased biopsy rates with large false-positive ratios were not a serious problem, but they could represent an issue in other screening programs and need to be considered. The balance between risks and benefits for women under age 50, regardless of how small the radiogenic risk may be, is not established as favorable and will remain so until new evidence on the issue becomes available. A great deal of attention is clearly warranted on the question of benefit in this age group.

Over age 50, a precise statement on the ratio of benefits and risks requires careful prospective analyses, some of which are underway. At this stage in our knowledge, there appears to be a definite gain in years of life saved through the inclusion of mammography in screening at these ages. This conclusion will be reexamined in the course of a long-term follow-up of the HIP study. Another important and unresolved question concerns the optional periodicity of screening, an issue which has implications for both cost and radiation exposure.

REFERENCES

Advisory Committee on the Biological Effects of Ionizing Radiation. 1972. Report on the Effects on Populations of Exposure to Low Levels of Ionizing Radiation. National Academy of Sciences–National Research Council, Washington, D.C.

Bailar, J. C., III. 1976. Mammography—contrary view. Ann. Intern. Med. 84:77–84.

Chiacchierini, R. P., and Lundin, F. E. 1977. Benefit risk ratio of mammography. In: W. Logan (ed.), Breast Carcinoma: The Radiologist's Expanded Role, pp. 15–28. John Wiley & Sons, New York.

End Results in Cancer. 1972. Report No. 4, National Institutes of Health, U.S. Department of Health, Education, and Welfare, Washington, D.C.

Fink, R., Shapiro, S., and Roeser, R. 1972. Impact of efforts to increase participation in repetitive screenings for early breast cancer detection. Am. J. Public Health 62:328–336.

Shapiro, S., Goldberg, J., and Hutchison, G. 1974. Lead time in breast cancer detection and implications for periodicity of screening. Am. J. Epidemiol. 100:357–365.

Shapiro, S., Strax, P., Venet, L., and Venet, W. 1972. Changes in 5-year breast cancer mortality in breast cancer screening program. Proceedings of the 7th National Cancer Conference, American Cancer Society, Inc., and National Cancer Institute, Los Angeles, pp. 663–678. J. B. Lippincott Company, Philadelphia.

Third National Cancer Survey. 1975. Incidence Data. National Cancer Institute Monograph 41. U.S. Department of Health, Education, and Welfare Publication No. (NIH) 75-787, Washington, D.C.

Vital Statistics of the United States. 1971. Life Table. 1970. Cause of Death. National Center for Health Statistics, U.S. Department of Health, Education, and Welfare, Washington, D.C.

Zelen, M., and Feinleib, M. 1969. On the theory of screening for chronic disease. Biometrika 56:601–614.

11
Cancers of the Lung, Pancreas, and Brain: Problems and Progress in Early Detection

Charles Ralph Buncher

In this chapter, three cancer studies for which the Division of Epidemiology and Biostatistics of the University of Cincinnati serves as the Central Statistical Group are discussed. Each of these studies, involving neoplasms of the lung, pancreas, and brain, represents an interesting effort to learn more about cancer screening, diagnosis, and treatment. Each study is described and some utilitarian conclusions are then drawn from the preliminary findings.

The descriptions of the three rather complicated studies are somewhat capsular because emphasis has been placed on methodological comparisons between them. The lung cancer study involves the clinical evaluation of a new diagnostic test to screen persons at high risk for lung cancer. The pancreatic cancer study involves no specific new developments but rather an empirical trial of a multiplicity of existing and imprecise diagnostic tests to ascertain whether any particular combination improves the earlier detection of this disease. The brain cancer study concerns a spectacular new technological development, computerized tomography, which has revolutionized certain aspects of clinical diagnosis and, in doing so, has become an example of how difficult it is to carry out controlled evaluations of widely accepted diagnostic instruments. On the clinical level, the three studies are completely independent of each other. Only the role of the Cincinnati Central Statistical Group is common to them. Administratively, all are funded by the Division of Cancer Biology and Diagnosis of the National

Supported by contract number NO1-CB-43868 from the National Cancer Institute of the U.S. Department of Health, Education, and Welfare.

This chapter is dedicated to the memory of William Pomerance, M.D., a superb administrator, teacher, and friend.

Cancer Institute and their project officer and guiding light was the late
William Pomerance.

LUNG CANCER

The lung is the most common site of cancer among Americans. More than
110,000 new cases occurred in 1979. The 5-year survival rate is a dismal 8%
in males and 12% in females (Anonymous, 1976). These figures increase to
9% for males and 13% for females with regional metastases alone, and to
29% and 48%, respectively, by sex, for those with localized disease. Only
about one case in six is detected while still in a localized stage. The most
depressing aspect is, of course, that most lung cancer could be prevented
by the simple expedient of eliminating cigarette smoking. For various reasons, sociocultural as well as economic, such an expedient has proved most
elusive.

It should also be remembered that even if everyone were to cease
smoking cigarettes, lung cancers would persist for some time. In addition,
there are certain respiratory tract neoplasms that bear no apparent relationship to cigarette smoking. For these reasons (among others), the question is
whether lung cancers can be diagnosed at a stage sufficiently early to allow
improvement of the prognosis. While most lay persons and even many
biomedical professionals believe that screening for lung cancer with x-ray
equipment saves lives, no more than perhaps one or two studies have been
able to document this belief. On the other hand, several studies have failed
to demonstrate that x-ray screening offers any advantage in the earlier diagnosis of lung cancer. X-ray screening has certainly detected early stage lung
cancers in specific individuals who have been cured of their disease.
However, such observations are by no means comparable to well-designed
epidemiologic studies that can demonstrate the effectiveness of a screening
modality in a population.

The question being tested in the present study is whether the addition of
sputum cytology in a screening program increases the survival of persons
diagnosed as having lung cancer. One can obtain a sputum sample containing
cells from the tracheobronchial tree, which can then be examined by a trained
cytopathologist and/or cytotechnician for evidence of cancer. This approach
is certainly not a new one; in fact, the development of sputum cytology preceded that of uterine cervical cytology in medical history. One might ask why
this technique was not adopted for lung cancer screening many years ago.
The underlying reason is that, unlike cervical cytology, a positive sputum
cytology does not sufficiently localize the tumor to permit surgery. In
contrast with radiographic techniques, for example, the detection of

abnormal sputum cells scarcely narrows the possibilities for the diagnostician.

The shortcomings of sputum cytology are exemplified by the cooperative study of the American Cancer Society and the Veterans Administration (Lilienfeld et al., 1966). Over a 3-year period of time, efforts were made to assess the value of sputum cytology and x-ray screening in an asymptomatic population of United States veterans. In an anecdotal report concerning this study, a positive sputum cytology was obtained for a subject, but nothing could be done until the tumor later became positive on an x-ray image. In another study (Delarue et al., 1971), the authors found it "disturbing that 25 of the 46 patients with positive [sputum] samplings have not yet otherwise declared the presence of the disease after an interval of 26 months." This problem of early diagnosis through screening encumbered by an inability to treat lung cancer early has posed a serious problem to all concerned. The frustration is compounded because the clinical utility of sputum cytology is compromised because of the need to delay treatment until the probability of metastases is high, so that there is no possibility of controlling lung cancer in this fashion.

The technological advance that made the present study possible is the advent of fiberoptic bronchoscopy, flexible tubes capable of carrying light (and vision) to a level several segments deep into the bronchial tree (Figure 1). With the rigid bronchoscope, one could only explore the upper segments of the trachea and major bronchi. With fiberoptic bronchoscopy, one can use either the oral or nasal route and probe the bronchial tree to the level of subsegmental bronchi. This medical breakthrough theoretically should permit the detection and localization of a neoplasm just days or weeks after the first positive sputum cytology. Accordingly, the time was ripe to test whether lung cancer can be controlled by means of sputum cytology screening coupled with fiberoptic bronchoscopy localization.

The study is designed to detect early lung cancer in asymptomatic persons who are at a relatively high risk of this disease. The three clinical centers involved in this work (and their principal investigators) are: the Mayo Clinic, Rochester, Minnesota (Dr. Robert S. Fontana); the Johns Hopkins Hospital, Baltimore, Maryland (Dr. John K. Frost); and Memorial Sloan–Kettering Cancer Center, New York, New York (Dr. Myron R. Melamed).

Study subjects in the three clinical centers must satisfy a number of eligibility criteria that put them at high risk of lung cancer. These include: 1) age of at least 45 years, 2) smoking of at least one pack of cigarettes per day until 1 year before enrollment, and 3) male sex. All subjects are advised to give up smoking as a means of reducing their risk of lung cancer and other diseases. However, as has been the experience of others, recommenda-

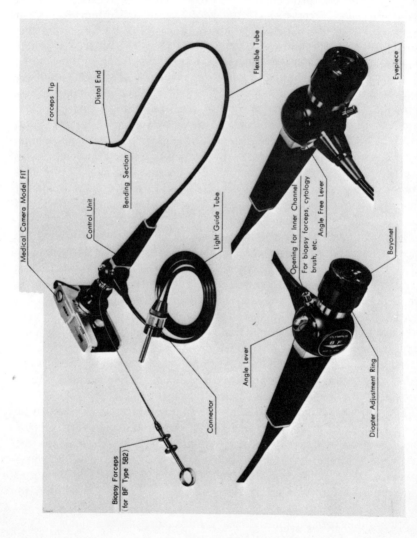

Figure 1.   Fiberoptic bronchoscope. (Courtesy of Olympus Corporation of America 2 Nevada Drive, New Hyde Park, New York 11040).

tions of this sort lead only a very small proportion to change their smoking habits.

Although one study is spoken of here, there are actually two study protocols. In the first protocol, at the Johns Hopkins Hospital and the Sloan-Kettering Cancer Center, the subjects are asymptomatic walk-in volunteers who are not patients at the institutions. At first examination, they are randomly divided into two groups. While all receive a chest x-ray examination (posterior-anterior and lateral), members of one of the groups receive a two-sample sputum cytology examination. The first of these is an induced sample that serves to break mucus loose from the subject's bronchial tree. After returning home, the subject is instructed to place sputum collected in the morning in a bottle for 3 consecutive days. This is mailed to the study center for cytologic evaluation. At 4 months and again at 8 months, sample containers are mailed to all participants with a request for additional sputum samples for examination. At the 1-year anniversary, the cycle begins again with the subject returning for x-ray examination and sputum sample collection, followed again by mailed sputum samples at 12, 16, and 20 months. The cycle recurs for 5 annual periods.

The comparison group receives an x-ray examination annually for 5 years. All subjects in both groups also fill out questionnaires on symptomatology, changes in cigarette smoking, health data, and other pertinent information. Since the two groups are alike in all respects except for the sputum samples obtained, any differences in outcome should help to answer the question of whether adding sputum cytology to a program of x-ray screening and symptom reporting will have any effect on lung cancer detection and survival.

The second protocol, the Mayo Clinic study, is somewhat different. The subjects are persons already attending the clinic and undergoing complete physical examination. If their characteristics fit the study design, they are invited to participate in the lung cancer screening program. All persons receive both chest x-ray and sputum cytology at their first examination, regardless of the group to which they were randomly assigned (Taylor and Fontana, 1972).

Although patients visiting the Mayo Clinic make their own choices concerning medical care, the clinic is currently recommending that persons at high risk of lung cancer should have both chest x-ray and sputum cytology examinations every year. In distinction to the other two studies, each subject in the highly screened group receives both a sputum cytology and a chest x-ray at 4-month intervals for the duration of the study. The x-ray examinations may be conducted at the Mayo Clinic, or, if performed elsewhere, provision is made for the films to be mailed, as are the sputum specimen containers.

The less highly screened group is not requested to undergo further chest x-ray or sputum cytology examinations, although those requesting will obviously receive them at the clinic or elsewhere. Thus, during the 5-year study period, the second group is contacted primarily through the annual questionnaire.

Clearly, the Mayo Clinic study can be expected to produce the largest possible screening difference between the two screenee groups in light of current medical standards and knowledge. At initial examination, the two groups are treated exactly alike, but one group is then persuaded to undergo 4-monthly sputum cytology and chest x-ray examinations, while the other is not.

Preliminary study results from the three clinical centers have been reported by Fontana et al. (1972), Marsh et al. (1976), Melamed et al. (1977), and Sanderson et al. (1974).

PANCREATIC CANCER

The incidence of pancreatic cancer has increased, and it is now the fourth leading cancer cause of death in the United States. About 23,000 new cases and 20,000 deaths from pancreatic cancer were projected for 1979. Five-year survival is 1% to 2%; even localized cases have a mere 3% to 4% 5-year survival rate (Anonymous, 1979).

The epidemiology of pancreatic cancer is quite confusing. There is good evidence that pancreatic cancer is associated with smoking cigarettes (relative risk of two or three). Viewed objectively, however, there is a dearth of solid epidemiologic information on pancreatic cancer. There are as yet no reasonable explanations as to why the disease is increasing. Those who are at high risk cannot be clearly delineated. How, then, can a study group be assembled that would make possible a prospective study of risk factors in, or early detection tests for, pancreatic cancer?

Two contrasting arguments have been made concerning the rationale of studying pancreatic cancer. One view holds that, because so little is known about this disease and because etiologic and diagnostic leads are so sparse, spending substantial sums of money on pancreatic cancer research is not justified. There is much to be said for this attitude. In the lung and brain cancer studies described elsewhere in this chapter, likely technological breakthroughs of sorts appeared to justify the expenditure of research dollars to evaluate or exploit the diagnostic advances. With pancreatic cancer, however, dollars saved could well be spent in other, more promising cancer research areas.

A second view holds that, despite the absence of breakthroughs, pancreatic cancer is an important disease. Accordingly, allocation of funds to advance knowledge and perhaps to generate a breakthrough would be justified. The study described here has been funded, suggesting that this second view prevails, at least for the moment.

The objective of the present study is to detect pancreatic cancers while still in a curable stage and thus prolong survival. The three participating clinics (and their principal investigators) are: the Mayo Clinic, Rochester, Minnesota (Dr. V. L. W. Go); Memorial Sloan-Kettering Cancer Center, New York (Dr. Patrick Fitzgerald); and the University of Chicago (Dr. A. R. Moossa). An important strength of this study is that the principal investigators represent different disciplines: surgery, pathology, and gastroenterology. To this may be added the Cincinnati Central Statistical Group's background in epidemiology and biostatistics and the late William Pomerance's expertise in obstetrics and gynecology. The fact that so many biomedical disciplines are represented is important in this particular study, which is designed to generate hypotheses, identify diagnostic instruments, and provide other insights that might subsequently be subjected to investigation by the more typical clinical or epidemiologic methods.

The study is designed to investigate individuals who are clinically, rather than epidemiologically, at high risk of pancreatic cancer. Some patients have relatively vague symptoms not clearly caused by other diseases; many of them will eventually be examined by laparotomy. The goal of the study is to examine persons undergoing laparotomy whom the clinicians think may have pancreatic cancer and who, following laparotomy, are definitively diagnosed as either having or not having the disease.

A major diagnostic complication here is that an individual may have a pancreatic disease other than cancer. Pancreatitis, for example, is sometimes difficult to differentiate from pancreatic cancer and other diseases of the abdomen. Alternatively, a subject may be suffering from cancer of a different organ in the anatomic neighborhood of the pancreas, rather than pancreatic cancer. Finally, there is the possibility of an entirely different disease, neither of the pancreas nor a neoplasm.

In view of the above, the patients have been classified into five diagnostic categories: pancreatic cancer, pancreatic disease other than cancer, cancer other than pancreatic, nonneoplastic disease of an organ other than the pancreas, and no discernible disease. Some of the diagnostic techniques utilized are relatively effective in distinguishing a diseased from a healthy pancreas. Others are useful in separating neoplastic from other diseases but without organ specificity. It is hoped that a particular combination of techniques to best diagnose pancreatic cancer can soon be identified.

Persons undergoing laparotomy are already symptomatic individuals and, therefore, cannot represent early disease. There are also patients who, on the basis of other tests and procedures, are not considered to be reasonable candidates for laparotomy. One might guess that a small proportion of these might later prove to have pancreatic cancer. These individuals may provide clues to characteristics that may be predictive of the early development of pancreatic cancer. Therefore, it would be extremely important to differentiate between the relatively early cases of pancreatic cancer and the otherwise comparable patients who do not have this disease.

The most appropriate patients to compare with the pancreatic cancer patients are persons undergoing laparotomy and careful diagnostic examination who are proved to be free of pancreatic cancer or other pancreatic diseases. However, some cases may fail to disclose a subsequently clinically apparent pancreatic neoplasm. Therefore, adequate follow-up procedures are an essential element in this study.

The diagnostic techniques used include ultrasound, angiography, endoscopy with retrograde pancreatoduodenography, radiography, computerized tomography, and a variety of laboratory tests. This wide variety of approaches is required because the pancreas is not easily accessible through either end of the alimentary tract nor is it near to a body surface. Its shape and position are not well-defined, and one must always contend with vagaries of its anatomic localization.

One valuable feature of the study is that at least one of the three study centers is a leader in each of the various diagnostic modalities utilized. Thus, personnel at the other centers can be helped to improve their own techniques.

Ideally, it might be suggested that a given diagnostic technique should not be used until it has been demonstrated that all three study centers can perform it equally well. In the case of lung cancer screening, this is exactly what has been attempted and actually accomplished. In this fashion, the diversity and talents of the centers are exploited and use of the diagnostic modalities by standardization is improved. However, this approach is not suitable for validating techniques already suspected to be highly useful.

Anecdotally, at the moment, it is probably fair to say that the ability to diagnose pancreatic cancer has increased in each of the participating screening centers. Whether this will ultimately be reflected in earlier diagnosis of pancreatic cancer and/or an improved survival rate remains to be seen.

Detailed information concerning preliminary results of this study may be found in Cubilla and Fitzgerald (1976), Fitzgerald (1976), Wood et al. (1976a), and Wood et al. (1976b).

BRAIN CANCER

The study of brain cancer, like that of the lung, is based on a medical breakthrough, namely, computerized tomography. Radiologists and information specialists have long recognized that more information could be produced by mathematically combining rays from different angles to generate a computed image. This concept reached fruition in England with the work of Godfrey Hounsfield, who produced a computer algorithm to reconstruct 160 separate and simultaneous transmission factors at 180 1° intervals (potentially 28,800 values) around a semicircle into an 80 by 80 matrix of density data (Gordon, Herman, and Johnson, 1975). The technique was first applied to the diagnosis of diseases of the head.

The National Cancer Institute initiated a collaborative clinical trial to compare the clinical performance of computerized tomography with radionuclide scanning, angiography, and pneumoencephalography, which were the accepted methods of the time. What makes this particular study interesting is that the collaborators undertook an extensive clinical trial of several years' duration to assess the efficacy of a truly revolutionary diagnostic technique. Two somewhat conflicting factors were operative here. First, there was the obvious need for a clinical trial if only to inform potential users of such equipment, costing more than one-third of a million dollars, whether the enormous expenditures are justified for use in hospitals or even office practices. Second, if the device is of scientific merit, this is likely to stimulate competition in our free enterprise system, with resulting improvements in the device and in its applications. Therefore, the technique being investigated would not, in fact, be precisely the technique in general use.

The five collaborating clinical centers (and their principal investigators) were: Columbia University, New York (Dr. Sadek K. Hilal); New York Hospital–Cornell University, New York (Dr. D. Gordon Potts); George Washington University, Washington, D.C. (Dr. David O. Davis); Massachusetts General Hospital, Boston (Dr. Paul F. J. New); and the Mayo Clinic, Rochester, Minnesota (Dr. H. L. Baker, Jr.).

The extraordinary rapidity with which the field of computerized tomography has been developing may be appreciated by considering the first such installation in the United States. This took place in June 1973, at the Mayo Clinic. The first publication on the subject, presenting results on the first 500 patients, appeared only 7 months later (Baker et al., 1974). This clearly reflects the great interest of all concerned with this new device.

The revolutionary nature of computerized tomography in clinical diagnosis continues to generate interest as well as rapid technological modifications. For example, the original technique was based on an 80 by 80 scanner, and a rather slow mathematical algorithm. By the time the study collaborators had conferred a few times, it was decided that the standard would be a 160 by 160 matrix machine and a fast Fourier series algorithm. This produces some 25,600 points of usable data, which is close to the 28,800 potentially available; any further improvements would therefore have to involve a complete redesign of the apparatus. Although the study was scheduled to start in June 1974, the date had to be postponed for 3 months until the company could retrofit the existing installations for the new design.

One advantage cited for computerized tomography is that it is a *noninvasive* technique. Previous diagnostic approaches involved injecting air into the spinal cavity for imaging by pneumoencephalography or injecting radiopaque material for angiography or radiopharmaceuticals for radionuclide imaging. While these have been made as safe as possible, an alternative noninvasive technique that could serve the same diagnostic and cancer control purposes would certainly be welcomed.

However, the current usage of the term *noninvasive* is somewhat vexing. As soon as the procedure was widely accepted, attempts to improve on it by injecting contrast-enhancing media were advocated. Thus, a truly noninvasive technique became invasive. Addition of the contrast medium transforms the procedure from an essentially hazard-free one to one that has a small but finite risk of fatality. The hazard-free characterization of computerized tomography is also somewhat less than accurate because, however small the dose, radiation is clearly a potential health hazard.

The term *noninvasive* can sometimes be misleading. The term *noninjection technique*, to indicate procedures such as radiography that do not require the injection of another material, may be preferable. Even this term might have to be expanded to include noningestion techniques. On the other hand, any technique that shoots beams of x-rays, an ionizing radiation that has been clearly shown to be carcinogenic in the right combination of doses and tissues, is clearly not as safe as a procedure such as thermography in which one merely measures, exterior to the body, the characteristic emissions of the body. We should distinguish between the truly noninvasive techniques of simple observation, the less invasive techniques measuring responses to external stimuli, and the more invasive techniques involving injection, ingestion, catheterization, and so forth.

Additional information on the clinical applications of computerized tomography for the diagnosis of neoplasms can be found in Baker (1975), Baker et al. (1975), Goodenough, Weaver, and Davis (1975), New and Scott (1975), and New et al. (1975). A useful discussion of image reconstruction from projections is that of Gordon, Herman, and Johnson (1975).

CONCLUSIONS

Three ongoing studies encompassing screening, diagnosis, and treatment of cancer have been discussed. Each has been initiated for different reasons. The lung cancer study came about because of the technical breakthrough of fiberoptic bronchoscopy, which permits the localization of lesions yielding a positive sputum cytology. This makes it possible to use sputum cytology to detect lung cancer either by itself or in conjunction with chest x-rays at such an early clinical stage that substantially more cases will be treatable or even curable by existing therapeutic methods. The success of this trial would be manifested by improved survival or decreased mortality from this disease. To prove the utility of the method at a statistically significant level has been estimated to require 5,000 men in each of the two comparison groups at each of the three study centers. With such numbers and an anticipated 50% reduction in the death rate, each center would have more than 9 chances in 10 of detecting a statistically significant difference if it existed. It should also be noted that this collaborative effort to determine the value of sputum cytology in lung cancer screening will cost millions of dollars.

The brain cancer study was designed around an enormous break-through in clinical medicine, computerized tomography. In this instance, the field is developing so rapidly that it has been difficult to design a specific study and carry it out according to protocol over periods of more than 6 months at a time. Experience has proved that, whenever decisions are made on the use of a particular apparatus for clinical study, major improvements or modifications are introduced within a matter of months. Even the use of angiography as a confirmatory test is precluded by changes in clinical practice that occurred less than a year after the introduction of com-puterized tomography into clinical practice. An additional complication is that this initially noninvasive technique has been changed into an invasive one involving the injection or infusion of contrast media into the patient.

These two studies are contrasted with the investigation of pancreatic cancer. The approach in this study, involving as it does no particular hypothesis, would in earlier times have been called "a fishing expedition." More recently, we have become sophisticated and termed such efforts "hypothesis-generating" studies. Pancreatic cancer exemplifies a situation such that, if studies are not initiated, nothing is going to be learned but, if they are, the probability of adding to our sorely deficient body of knowledge is increased. Unfortunately at the present, we must study patients primarily with advanced disease, even though our long-range goal is to develop methods for detecting and treating pancreatic cancer earlier and more effec-tively. This situation is exemplified by the fact that such crude clinical indi-cators of disease as a loss of more than 10% of body weight or jaundice are used, although these are most likely symptoms of late disease, especially of lesions involving the head of the pancreas. An important challenge in this field is for epidemiologists to identify groups at increased risk of pancreatic cancer.

204   Buncher

REFERENCES

Anonymous. 1976. Ca—A Cancer Journal for Clinicians 26:28–29.
Anonymous. 1979. Ca—A Cancer Journal for Clinicians 29:14–15.
Baker, H. L., Jr. 1975. The impact of computed tomography on neuroradiologic practice. Radiology 116:637–640.
Baker, H. L., Jr., Campbell, J. K., Houser, D. W., Reese, D. F., Sheedy, P. F., and Holman, C. B. 1974. Computer assisted tomography of the head: An early evaluation. Mayo Clin. Proc. 49:17–27.
Baker, H. L., Jr., Houser, O. W., Campbell, J. K., Reese, D. F., and Holman, C. B. 1975. Computerized tomography of the head. JAMA 233:1304–1308.
Cubilla, A. L., and Fitzgerald, P. J. 1976. Morphological lesions associated with human primary invasive nonendocrine pancreas cancer. Cancer Res. 36: 2690–2698.
Delarue, N. C., Pearson, F. G., Thompson, D. W., and Van Boxel, P. 1971. Sputum cytology screening for lung cancer. Geriatrics 26:130–143.
Fitzgerald, P. J. 1976. Pancreatic Cancer: The dismal disease. Arch. Pathol. Lab. Med. 100:513–515.
Fontana, R. S., Sanderson, D. R., Miller, W. E., Woolner, L. B., Taylor, W. F., and Uhlenhopp, M. A. 1972. The Mayo lung project: Preliminary report of "early cancer detection" phase. Cancer 30:1373–1382.
Goodenough, D. J., Weaver, K. E., and Davis, D. O. 1975. Potential artifacts associated with the scanning pattern of the EMI scanner. Radiology 117:615–620.
Gordon, R., Herman, G. T., and Johnson, S. A. 1975. Image reconstruction from projections. Sci. Am. 233:56–68.
Lilienfeld, A., Archer, P. G., Burnett, C. H., Chamberlain, E. W., Chazin, B. J., Davies, D., Davis, R. L., Haber, P. A., Hodges, F. J., Koprowska, I., Kordan, B., Lane, J. R., Lawton, A. H., Lee, L., Jr., MacCallum, D. B., McDonald, J. R., Milder, J. W., Naylor, B., Papanicolaou, G. N., Slutzker, B., Smith, R. T., Swepston, E. R., and Umker, W. O. 1966. An evaluation of radiologic and cytologic screening for the early detection of lung cancer: A cooperative pilot study of the American Cancer Society and the Veterans Administration. Cancer Res. 26:2083–2121.
Marsh, B. R., Frost, J. K., Erozan, Y. S., and Carter, D. 1976. New horizons in lung cancer diagnosis. Cancer 37(suppl.):437–439.
Melamed, M. R., Flehinger, B., Miller, D., Osborne, R., Zaman, M., McGinnis, C., and Martini, N. 1977. Preliminary report of the lung cancer detection program in New York. Cancer 39:369–382.
New, P. F. J., and Scott, W. R. 1975. Computed Tomography of the Brain and Orbit (EMI Scanning). Williams & Wilkins Company, Baltimore.
New, P. F. J., Scott, W. R., Schnur, J. A., Davis, K. R., Taveras, J. M., and Hochberg, F. H. 1975. Computed tomography with the EMI scanner in the diagnosis of primary and metastatic intracranial neoplasms. Radiology 114:75–87.
Sanderson, D. R., Fontana, R. S., Woolner, L. B., Bernatz, P. E., and Payne, W. S. 1974. Bronchoscopic localization of radiographically occult lung cancer. Chest 65:608–612.
Taylor, W. F., and Fontana, R. S. 1972. Biometric design of the Mayo Lung Project for early detection and localization of bronchogenic carcinoma. Cancer 30:1344–1347.

Wood, R. A. B., Hall, A. W., Moossa, A. R., Levin, B., and Skinner, D. B. 1976a. Pancreatic cancer diagnosis: Preliminary evaluation of a prospective study. J. Surg. Res. 21:113–115.

Wood, R. A. B., Moossa, A. R., Blackstone, M. O., Bowie, J., Collins, P., and Lu, C. T. 1976b. Comparative value of four methods of investigating the pancreas. Surgery 80:518–522.

Part V
The Delaney Clause: A Colloquy

12
Evolution of the Delaney Clause

Gilbert S. Goldhammer

The so-called Delaney Clause is a widely discussed and highly controversial subject. Its discussion is often charged with emotion and heat. A study of the evolution of the Delaney Clause is useful in comprehending its legislative rationale. Understanding its historical development in the context of congressional intent and changing concepts is helpful, if not essential, for a clear understanding of the subject.

What is the Delaney Clause? It is part of the 1958 Food Additives Amendment to the Federal Food, Drug, and Cosmetic Act, which requires that food additives be adequately tested for safety before marketing, and that the evidence of safety be submitted to the Food and Drug Administration (FDA). Marketing is permitted only after the FDA is satisfied from the scientific evidence presented that the safety of the additives for their intended uses has been established.

The Delaney Clause prohibits the FDA from approving a food additive if it has induced cancer in man or in animal when ingested. The prohibition is embodied in the following wording of the Delaney Clause: "Provided, that no additive shall be deemed to be safe if it is found to induce cancer when ingested by man or animal, or if it is found, after tests which are appropriate for the evaluation of the safety of food additives, to induce cancer in man or animal. . . ."

In 1959, Congress enacted the Color Additives Amendment and included a Delaney Clause provision applicable specifically to color additives.

In 1962, Congress modified the Delaney Clause to permit the use in animal feeds of drugs, such as diethylstilbestrol (DES), which had been found to induce cancer in animals, provided their use did not result in detectable drug residues in any edible animal tissue. This provision was subsequently carried over to the Animal Drug Amendments of 1968.

Fundamentally, the effect of the Delaney Clause is to deprive the FDA of any latitude or discretion in determining the safety of carcinogenic additives. Such additives are by statute deemed to be inherently unsafe. To the extent that the Delaney Clause reflects a deep concern about the effects of food additives on public health, its concept is not new. The fears that grip the public today are not very different from those that were manifested a century ago. For instance, during the late 1870s, Harvey W. Wiley, Chief of the United States Department of Agriculture's Bureau of Chemistry (FDA's predecessor agency), began a study of the quality and safety of marketed foods, which included the use of certain food additives, particularly chemical preservatives and artificial colors. Congress encouraged this endeavor by appropriating funds for similar studies in the ensuing years.

Wiley's work, as well as his crusade for a federal food and drugs law, stimulated public support and congressional interest that finally resulted in the enactment in 1906 of the Federal Food and Drugs Act. It is significant that between June 20, 1879 and June 30, 1906, no fewer than 190 proposals, designed in some way to protect the consumer of foods and drugs, were presented to Congress. Few of these ever got out of congressional committees, but the crusades of Wiley and others for food and drug legislation finally bore fruit in 1906. Wiley was destined to become the first administrator of the 1906 Federal Food and Drugs Act.

As one would anticipate, the 1906 law dealt with harmful food additives, and the applicable statutory provision reveals the intent of Congress to ban food additives that might adversely affect the public health. This purpose was to be achieved by a provision that defined a food as adulterated and, therefore, illegal for interstate commerce, ". . . if it contains any *added* poisonous or other *added* deleterious ingredient which *may* render such article injurious to health" (italics added). The law was silent as to the status of poisons found naturally in food.

In interpreting the statutory phrase "which may render the food injurious to health," the courts consistently held that the agency did not have to establish that the food containing the toxic substance was in fact injurious to health. It was enough to prove that it was poisonous and deleterious and that there was a reasonable possibility of injury to some segment of the consuming population.

That provision was law for 32 years, between 1906 and 1938. Because of the many deficiencies of the statute that became apparent during the 32 years of FDA experience with the law, Congress replaced it with the 1938 Federal Food, Drug, and Cosmetic Act. The new law addressed itself to natural as well as to added poisonous or deleterious substances in foods. It defined a food containing a *natural* poison as adulterated only if the poison was present in an amount that actually rendered the food injurious to health. The 1938 law also ruled out any *added* poisonous and deleterious substances regardless of amount if they were not necessary in the production of the foods, or could be avoided by good manufacturing practices. The law authorized the enforcing agency to establish safe limits, or tolerances, for poisonous additives that were necessary for the manufacture of the food or could not be avoided.

It is obvious that, in the 1906 and 1938 enactments, Congress sought to prevent the addition of even the smallest amounts of toxic substances to foods on the theory that, while not dangerous in any one food, in the aggregate they could become dangerous if used in many other widely consumed foodstuffs. Under both the 1906 and 1938 laws, the FDA regarded carcinogenic food additives as poisonous and deleterious substances and, therefore, not suitable for use in food. This accounts for the FDA's prompt action against foods containing carcinogenic additives even before the enactment of the Delaney Clause.

Prior to the 1958 Food Additives Amendment, the burden of proof for the illegality of foods containing added poisonous or deleterious substances under both the 1906 and the 1938 statutes was on the Food and Drug Administration. Before the FDA could ban such foods, it had to await conclusive evidence that the added ingredient was indeed poisonous or deleterious. The result of this was that often, for a period of time, foods containing such additives would be on the market unmolested by the enforcing agency until convincing evidence of toxicity had been established by animal experimentation.

Because of this serious weakness and the growing use of new chemical substances in food products and food technology, the House of Representatives created a select committee in 1950, chaired by Representative James J. Delaney (Democrat from New York) to investigate the chemical food additives problem. The Delaney committee filed its report on June 30, 1952, and urged amending the law so that chemicals employed in or on foods would be subjected substantially to the same safety requirements as existed in the law for new drugs. The Delaney report was followed by extended congressional efforts to implement the committee's work, which culminated in the passage of the 1958 Food Additives Amendment. The most important provision of this amendment was to shift the burden of establishing safety of additives from FDA to industry; industry would be required to conduct the tests necessary to establish safety of additives before marketing.

The bill, as originally introduced and passed by the House Interstate and Foreign Commerce Committee, did not contain a Delaney Clause. It was assumed that carcinogens would be ruled out simply on the proposition that they could not be established to be safe. Thus, the committee's report to the House of Representatives to accompany the bill made no reference to a cancer clause. However, after the Food Additives bill had been approved by the committee, Congressman Delaney pressed for inclusion of his now well-known clause, and the House of Representatives obliged by enacting it.

Unlike the House Committee report, the report to accompany the bill of the Senate Commerce Committee does discuss the Delaney Clause. The Senate Committee stated that it did not feel that the clause was necessary since the general preclearance provisions of the Food Additives Amendment would automatically result in nonapproval of additives that produced cancer in animal studies. The Food and Drug Administration also felt that the clause was not necessary, but influential scientists within the National Cancer Institute held a different view, namely, that because of the inability to establish a safe dose or period of exposure for a carcinogen it would be prudent to deny the enforcing agency any latitude to determine whether or not a carcinogen might be safe under certain conditions. This view prevailed with both the Secretary of Health, Education, and Welfare and with the House of Representatives. The Senate agreed with this view and enacted the Delaney Clause despite its Commerce Committee's advice that the clause was unnecessary.

One fact appears to be evident from the legislative history: Congress wanted to err on the side of caution. Cancer mortality rates were rising steadily, inexorably, and inexplicably, and Congress had little choice but to "play it safe."

Efforts have been made in Congress in the last 4 or 5 years to change the Delaney Clause to permit wider latitude on the part of the regulatory agency, but Congress has exhibited little disposition to change the Delaney Clause for the present. The FDA, while ambiguous on the subject, does not appear to be disposed at the present time to promote a change in the Delaney Clause.

No one knows whether any carcinogenic food additive in the amount present in food has ever caused any human cancer. That may, in fact, never be known. What is known is that some chemical agents have the potential to produce cancer in animals and, indeed, in man. But, aside from that, we are still groping in the dark. We know little concerning the mechanics of the transformation of normal cells into malignant cells, or how much exposure to the carcinogen is necessary for such transformation. That chemicals are in some way responsible for at least some of such transformations can no longer be doubted.

So the basic question facing Congress, the FDA, and the public remains: What is the best policy to pursue until the necessary facts are developed? If the trend of cancer mortality rates were declining, perhaps Congress and the public might be receptive to a change in the Delaney Clause. But, for decades, cancer mortality rates have been increasing. Can anyone be smug under such circumstances, especially when there are definite signs that the rate of increase may now be accelerating? That, in essence, is the central issue, and the controversy revolves about it. Should we continue the "play it safe" policy of the Delaney Clause or, by revising it, gamble that we are acting in the best public interest by permitting added carcinogens in food for possible economic or other gains?

13
A Healthy Law for Consumers

Anita Johnson

The U.S. Food and Drug Administration (FDA) is charged by law with eliminating foods that "may be injurious to health." For naturally occurring poisons, the FDA bears the legal burden of proving that the food is or may be unsafe. In the case of food additives, however, the food manufacturer bears the burden of proving safety.

A manufacturer wishing to add a chemical to food must generate test data and file a food additive petition at the FDA. The data are reviewed and the additive is cleared for marketing if the FDA deems "safety" to be adequately demonstrated. The law has a special proviso, namely,

> Provided, that no additive shall be deemed to be safe if it is found to induce cancer when ingested by man or animal, or if it is found, after tests which are appropriate for the evaluation of the safety of food additives, to induce cancer in man or animal . . . (U. S. Code, 1958).

This is the so-called Delaney Clause, enacted in 1958. It is unique in regulatory law in directing an agency to take action in the face of specific evidence. Most regulatory law merely directs an agency to act if the risks outweigh the benefits of a product, leaving it up to the agency to decide how to achieve this balance. The Delaney Clause does not allow a weighing of benefits and risks, once the agency determines that cancer is produced by an additive. An additive may not be used in any amount if it has been demonstrated to cause cancer to any degree in man or in animal studies.

The Delaney Clause does not operate at all until the FDA determines that the chemical causes cancer. If the FDA determines that cancer is caused by ingestion in animal tests, the chemical must be banned. If the study is poorly designed or poorly conducted, the FDA would not conclude that the chemical caused cancer. If tests other than ingestion tests demonstrate carcinogenesis, the FDA decides whether the tests are pertinent to food additive exposure. For example, if an additive caused cancer after being injected into animals, the FDA would use that test to trigger a Delaney Clause ban only if scientists deemed it relevant to the question.

Technically, the Delaney Clause applies only to approval of food additive petitions. The FDA has invoked it only three times, twice for chemicals in food packaging adhesives and once to ban diethylstilbestrol. In the 1969 cyclamate ban, the Delaney Clause was not applied because cyclamate was a so-called "generally recognized as safe" additive by virtue of the fact that it was on the market prior to passage of the law without noted adverse effect, rather than by virtue of an approved food additive petition. The only issue in the cyclamate case was whether, given three positive cancer studies (all flawed), the chemical could continue to be deemed "generally recognized as safe." The FDA said no, and required the filing of a food additive petition documenting well-designed chronic animal studies with negative results. Since such studies were not available, cyclamate went off the market. The FDA never officially determined that cyclamate was a proven carcinogen.

The Red Dye No. 2 case is similar. This dye had been granted "provisional" marketing status because it was on the market when the law was passed. It had never been cleared for safety. The FDA revoked the "provisional" status of the dye in January 1976 on the basis of studies that raised serious questions to the effect that the dye may cause cancer in man. The studies are flawed and do not prove that the dye causes cancer. Nevertheless, the dye is off the market because, given the doubts, no studies prove that it is safe. A similar situation exists with respect to the FDA's attempt to ban saccharin in 1977.

PRINCIPLE OF ZERO TOLERANCE

Although the Delaney Clause itself is relatively narrow, the Delaney principle of zero tolerance for carcinogens has been used to remove other chemicals from the food supply. In 1960, the FDA refused to authorize the use of safrole (oil of sassafras) under the transitional provision of the new Food Additives Amendment on the basis of its cancer-causing properties. Safrole was used as a flavoring agent in root beer. Oil of calamus, a flavoring agent in vermouth, was stripped of its "generally recognized as safe" status in 1968. Diethylprocarbonate (DEPC), used in soft drinks and believed to form urethan, a proven carcinogen, in combination with other ingredients, was stripped of its approved food additives petition under the general safety provisions of the law. An additive from rubber gaskets in contact with food was withdrawn because of its ability to form a carcinogen. In 1973, the interim status of Violet No. 1 was removed because of two rat studies showing it to be a carcinogen (United States Congress, 1974).

There has been opposition to the Delaney Clause from industry on the grounds that it arbitrarily prohibits food additives of economic value that are safe in small amounts (Oser, 1973). Speaking for the cattle-raising industry, which adds sex hormones to feed on the theory that this saves money by stimulating growth, then Secretary of Agriculture Earl Butz advocated changing the Delaney Clause because "it leaves no area for judgment" (Butz, 1976).

The industry opponents state that a "safe" amount of a carcinogen for man can be found by extrapolating from the "no-effect" level in those animal studies in which cancer is produced at high doses but not at low doses. In the words of Paul Hopper (1973), "What we are saying, in essence, is that for every substance in our environment, both natural and man-made, there is a dose-response curve. Too much water, too much salt, too much orange juice, too much sugar, too much anything can all cause severe effects in man. This should not be construed to mean that such substances should therefore be banned."

A large number of chemicals produce cancer at very low doses indeed, and a "no-effect" level in animal studies cannot be established. For example, diethylstilbestrol (DES), a sex hormone that appears as residues in beef because it is added to animal feed, produces cancer in rats at the lowest dose used, namely, 6.25 parts per billion (Gass, 1964).

Other chemicals induce cancer at high doses but seem inactive in animals at the lower doses that are more compatible with food exposure levels. Experimental evidence so far indicates that these "no-effect" levels are artificial, since repetition of the same tests with large numbers of animals results in cancer induction at that lower dose. For example, a chemical that induced cancer in one in 100 animals at dose x might appear to induce no cancer at that dose if only 50 test animals were used. Yet, at that rate, it might induce 2 million cases of human cancer if 200 million people were exposed (Epstein, 1974). The risk of contracting cancer clearly decreases as dose decreases. However, there is as yet no support for the theory that there is a dose that produces no cases of cancer. This is a matter of consensus among many cancer scientists (Ad Hoc Committee, 1970; Saffiotti, 1973).

How carcinogens cause the pertinent cell changes is still unknown, but they apparently have the ability to interact with the DNA or RNA of cells in minute amounts and do not need continued exposure to be toxic. The impact on the cell is thought to be permanent and cumulative; the cell apparently does not recover from nonfatal assaults as it does with other kinds of toxicants (Miller, 1970; Saffiotti, 1973).

Even if a no-effect level in an animal study were established, this would not establish the same in man even with the 100-fold safety margin used by the FDA for other types of injury. This is because man is probably more sensitive to chemicals than are laboratory animals. Humans may be exposed for longer periods of time to the same dose, because the metabolic rate of rodents is faster than that of humans. Furthermore, the human life span is much longer, presenting many more cell divisions within which neoplastic changes can appear, and increasing the extent of chronic accumulation. For example, β-naphthylamine is a highly potent carcinogen in man, but a weak carcinogen in mice, rats, and guinea pigs (Heuper, 1969).

Humans live in a chemical environment that is much more varied than the animal laboratory, and many other chemicals therein may potentiate the activity of the carcinogen. For example, N-dodecane, found in petroleum waxes, increases the incidence of skin cancer in mice 1,000 times more than exposure to a carcinogen alone (Weisburger and Weisburger, 1968). Moreover, carcinogens are thought to have a synergistic effect on each other (Ryser, 1971).

Humans are not genetically homogeneous as are laboratory animals, and subgroups may have sensitivities not seen in the animal strains chosen for study. Moreover, humans vary in their state of health, while laboratory animals tend to be vigorous and healthy at the time of study.

In summary, high dose animal studies are valuable for identifying carcinogens in a comparatively small number of animals. Currently, no methodology exists that can identify safe levels of carcinogens because the effects of small doses cannot be deduced from animal studies, because there are unknown species differences in sensitivity, and because there is enormous human variation in responses to carcinogens, whether attributable to inborn traits or varying chemical environments. There may be a safe dose. However, at the present time, there is no experimental basis for finding it (United States Congress, 1974).

WHY THE REGULATION ON ADDITIVES SHOULD BE STRICT

The Delany Clause is a *policy* judgment by Congress that no food additive is worth any risk of cancer. In the case of food additives, this judgment is comparatively easy to make. No additives with important or irreplaceable functions have yet appeared. The vast majority are cosmetics, designed to improve the appearance or taste of food that has suffered from extensive processing or adulteration. Additives permit manufacturers to sell simulated food products that are almost invariably less nutritious than the natural ones.

An absolute prohibition on carcinogenic food additives is much easier to make than, for example, one on workplace exposures or air pollution, where serious costs may sometimes be involved in achieving zero exposure. Nevertheless, the mandated judgment is a significant safeguard for consumers since it prevents the FDA from bending to what former FDA

Commissioner Alexander Schmidt has termed the "pressure cooker" situation created by manufacturers. Consumer groups do not and cannot provide lobbying input on behalf of safety that is equal to the lobbying of the well-funded trade associations and law firms of industry.

For food additives, moreover, there is no adequate mechanism for generating data on alleged benefits and for weighing these against the risks of cancer. The drug law requires drug manufacturers to prove that their products are effective by well-controlled scientific investigations. For food additives, no such proof is required, and industry has consistently opposed any formal requirement for proving benefit. Instead, the law merely requires proof that the additive performs its intended function. This means that a dye manufacturer must, for example, show that a chemical does in fact turn food red. This is a far cry from proving that red dye benefits anyone, and to what extent.

For this reason, discussions about the benefits of food additives are vague and speculative. At a 1975 National Academy of Sciences forum, a prominent scientist suggested that the benefit of saccharin to consumers could be shown by sales figures (Crampton, 1975). A book by economist Rita Campbell states that food dyes should be valued for their "psychic benefits"—presumably these are intuitively perceived. The villain DES has been used to decrease costs to cattle farmers. Yet the evidence that DES use in fact benefits the farmers is very weak. A House of Representatives Government Operations Subcommittee examined the evidence and found that beef-raising costs are greater, not less, with DES (United States Congress, 1973). Yet the public has tended to believe in the benefits claimed by the manufacturers to the point of accepting an unusually well-documented cancer risk.

Even if there were strong evidence of benefits, there is at present no scientific body that has the confidence of consumer groups in weighing the benefits and risks. Some bodies that have been suggested are quite alarming. The then Director of the FDA Bureau of Animal Drugs has suggested that industries, through their trade associations, weigh the risks and benefits. The National Academy of Sciences Food Protection Committee, which has been suggested as an appropriate body, has a long history of indifference to chronic environmental insults, documented in part by Boffey (1975). If a particular food additive whose benefits are important and irreplaceable appears, the matter should go to Congress for a decision on the specific substance.

Protection from carcinogenic additives would be enhanced if the FDA required well-designed chronic studies for many food additives. For example, a number of coal-tar dyes have been granted permanent approval without proper chronic safety studies. The same is true for additives that enter food from packaging or processing equipment. These chemicals are being ignored for purposes of testing requirements because they are present in "negligible" amounts. Sometimes present at levels as high as 1 to 5 parts per million (ppm), these chemicals may not be "negligible" to human health. Proper testing of food additives is and must remain a priority in cancer prevention.

The Delaney Clause does not protect consumers from all exposures to carcinogens in food. It does not apply to environmental contaminants of food such as DDT and natural carcinogens such as aflatoxin, which are produced by mold on peanuts, corn, etc. These substances have been regulated under a section of the Food, Drug, and Cosmetic Act that permits the FDA to set tolerances for so-called unavoidable dangers in foods (United States Code, 1976) and by action levels, which are informal promises by the FDA not to seize contaminated products if the contamination does not exceed a certain degree. The FDA's regulation of these carcinogens has been unsatisfactory. It permits aflatoxin in foodstuffs at a level that induces a 100% incidence of cancer in animals (Wogan and Newberne, 1967). The FDA also permits DDT at levels of 5 ppm in fish and 7 ppm in apples despite the fact that it has induced cancer in animals at 2 ppm in the diet (Saffiotti, 1973). Admittedly, these situations are not as simple as those relating to food additives. DDT residues pervade the environment due to decades of profligate use by farmers, and zero tolerance would jeopardize a major source of protein.

Food additives are chemicals of relatively small benefit. Once added to food, they are widely distributed, making their long-range effects on health impossible to trace, and of enormous potential danger. Exposures are easily prevented. Prohibition of carcinogenic food additives is, in view of present knowledge, a sane, manageable approach to the preservation of our health (Health Research Group).

REFERENCES

Ad Hoc Committee on the Evaluation of Low Levels of Environmental Carcinogens. 1970. Evaluation of Environmental Carcinogens. National Cancer Institute, Bethesda, Md.

Boffey, P. 1975. The Brain Bank of America. McGraw-Hill Book Company, New York.

Butz, E. 1976. Make calls on food scientists to take stand on issues. Food Chem. News 18:5.

Campbell, R. 1974. Food Safety Regulation. American Enterprise Institute, Washington, D.C.

Crampton, R. 1975. The question of benefits and risk. In: Sweeteners: Issues and Uncertainties, p. 128. National Academy of Sciences, Washington, D.C.

Epstein, S. 1974. Environmental determinants of human cancer. Cancer Res. 34:2425.

Gass, G. H., Coats, D., and Graham, N. 1964. Carcinogenic dose-response curve to oral diethylstilbestrol. J. Natl. Cancer Inst. 33:971–977.

Health Research Group. Cancer Prevention and the Delaney Clause. Public Citizen's Health Research Group, 2000 P Street, N.W., Washington, D.C. 20036.

Heuper, W. 1969. Occupational and Environmental Cancer of the Urinary Tract. Yale University Press, New Haven, Ct.

Hopper, P. 1973. The Delaney Clause. Prev. Med. 2:159.

Miller, J. A. 1970. Carcinogenesis by chemicals: An overview. Cancer Res. 30:559–576.

Oser, B. L. 1973. An emotionally charged law. Chem. Eng. News Aug. 13, p. 3.

Ryser, H. J. P. 1971. Chemical carcinogenesis. N. Engl. J. Med. 285:721–734.

Saffiotti, U. 1973. Comments on the scientific basis for the Delaney Clause. Prev. Med. 2.

United States Code. 1958. 21 U.S.C. 348 (c) (3) (A).

United States Code. 1976. 21 U.S.C. 346.

United States Congress, Government Operations Committee. 1973. Regulation of Diethylstilbestrol (DES) and Other Drugs Used in Food Producing Animals. Exhibit 10: Report to the House of Representatives, 93rd Congress, 1st Session, Washington, D.C.

United States Congress, House of Representatives. Subcommittee of the Committee on Appropriations Hearings. 1974. Agricultural, Environmental, and Consumer Protection Appropriations of 1975, pp. 215–220. Part 8, 93rd Congress, 2nd Session, GPO. Washington, D.C.

Weisburger, J. H., and Weisburger, E. K. 1968. Additives and chemical carcinogens: on the concept of zero tolerance. Food Cosmet. Toxicol. 6:235–242.

Wogan, G. N., and Newberne, P. M. 1967. Dose response characteristics of aflatoxin β_1 carcinogenesis in the rat. Cancer Res. 27:2370–2376.

14
The Delaney Clause and Food Safety

Robert W. Harkins

CANCER IN THE UNITED STATES AND IN THE WORLD

Cancer—a dreaded disease—strikes fear into the heart of every man. The fear is directly proportional to our inability to explain its origin, and our still feeble efforts at preventing its debilitating effects. When cancer occurs, it is meaningless to talk of statistical probabilities, for these are of no significance to the cancer victim. Despite the fears of the cancer patient and his or her family and friends, one must maintain a reasonable perspective on this galaxy of diseases. While the singular term *cancer* is employed here, the plural *cancers* should in fact be used because these diseases apparently have a multitude of causes and entail perhaps an even greater number of elements in their prevention.

It has been suggested that 80% of cancers in man are attributable to an environmental cause of one sort or another. Whatever the correct proportion may be, there is no doubt that environmental insults are positively correlated with some neoplasms. Some of these insults—exposure to asbestos, exhaust fumes from coke ovens, cigarette smoke, and the like—are in good measure preventable. Others, which may originate in sunlight, food, water, or air, are more difficult to identify and therefore much less readily avoidable. To the extent that noxious agents can be identified, reduced, or eliminated at a realistic economic and social price, all is well. Those agents that cannot presently be entirely avoided (e.g., sunlight) must be endured as risk factors of uncertain magnitude in an uncertain environment.

The results of carcinogenic environmental insults to humans are suggested by the histograms in Figure 1 which present the incidence of cancer in the United States by site among men and women. The most frequent cancer in men, that of the lung and bronchus, can largely be prevented by avoidance of cigarette smoking. Two of the three major sites of cancer in

223

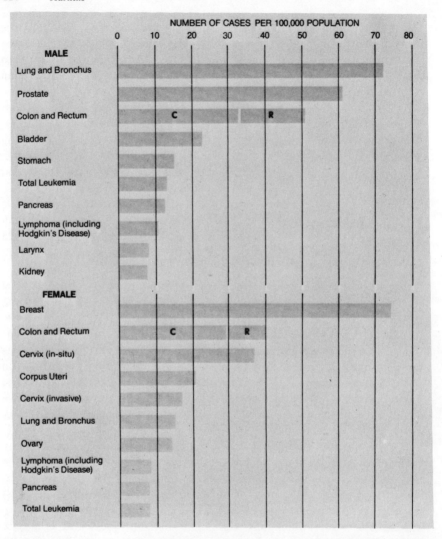

Figure 1.   Cancer incidence by site and sex: United States, 1969–1971 (age-adjusted to 1970 U.S. population).

women, breast and cervix, lend themselves to effective early detection and medical intervention. Clearly, personal decisions and life-style can make a difference in cancer risk.

Although absolute cancer incidence rates are important, it is also informative to examine changes in the relative frequencies of cancer by considering specific target organs. Time trends in cancer mortality for the leading sites among U.S. males and females are shown in Figure 2. The most dramatic change is apparent for lung cancer, which has increased almost twentyfold among men during the last 40 years. Women have been dying from lung cancer at a lower absolute rate, but this has recently begun to increase significantly.

Cancer of the stomach has been declining in both sexes, perhaps because of improved nutrition and better food sanitation practices, including refrigeration. No marked trends are apparent for cancers of the colon and rectum, prostate, or pancreas, or for leukemia. Over a 40-year period, we seem to be doing no better, despite increased public awareness and substantially expanded therapeutic and patient support programs.

How does the United States compare with other countries with respect to cancer incidence? Are Americans dying of cancer more frequently than are people of other countries? Data on cancer incidence among males of 23 developed countries are presented in Table 1. The rates were calculated on the basis of a variety of available sources.

Cancer incidence rates in the United States may be seen to be close to the average for the countries surveyed. However, in light of existing knowledge, for Americans prepared to undertake appropriate prophylactic steps, the incidence of lung cancer, the leading cause of cancer mortality, could be significantly reduced.

Table 1. Annual age-standardized[a] cancer incidence rates for all sites combined per 100,000 males

Country	Rate	Country	Rate
South Africa[b]	371.2	Puerto Rico	205.0
Rhodesia	304.9	Yugoslavia	204.1
Canada	264.5	Sweden	199.4
Finland	259.7	Japan	192.7
United Kingdom	246.9	Israel[e]	180.6
Colombia	245.9	Romania	176.9
German Federal Republic	244.4	Norway	174.8
New Zealand[c]	242.1	Poland	167.8
United States[d]	239.5	Hungary	164.0
Denmark	221.1	India	139.5
Jamaica	212.3	Nigeria	76.7
German Democratic Republic	211.7		

Source: Doll, Muir, and Waterhouse, 1970.

[a] Standard = estimated age distribution of males in 24 developed countries, primarily European and American.

[b] Whites only.

[c] European only.

[d] Including Hawaii.

[e] All Jews.

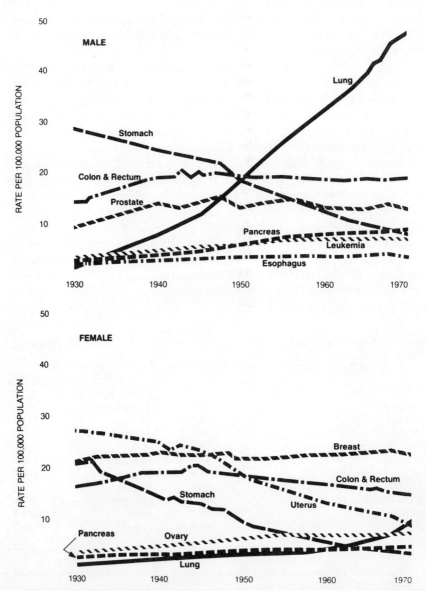

Figure 2.   Time trends in cancer mortality rates, by site and sex: United States, 1930–1970 (age-adjusted to 1940 U.S. population).

Does the American diet have unusual carcinogenic potential? To seek an answer to this question, the U.S. population was compared with five others, each with different genetic and geographic characteristics, but all from highly developed countries. The cancer incidence rates for six target sites in these populations are presented in Table 2. Stomach cancer incidence is lower in the United States than in any of the other nations, whereas colon cancer incidence is relatively higher, although substantially below that in New Zealand and close to the levels in Sweden and the United Kingdom. If the American diet were a major contributing factor to cancer, one would expect that the stomach and the colon would bear a proportionate share of the total cancer incidence burden. That these cancer rates are in fact intermediate or low suggests that the U.S. diet is similarly intermediate or low in carcinogenic potential.

Cancer rates in the United States for the two organs that are responsible for detoxification and excretion of metabolites, namely, the liver and the bladder, are somewhat higher than in the other countries. However, if the cancer incidence rates for these two organs plus those for the stomach and the colon are summed, the rates are seen to be similar in the United States, the United Kingdom, Hungary, Sweden, and New Zealand. Only in Japan is the total clearly different, being about twice as high as in the five other countries, primarily because of the extremely high stomach cancer incidence in that country.

Dietary Changes

The American diet is constantly evolving. While no value judgment can be applied to these changes, they are important insofar as changes in disease

Table 2.   Annual age-standardized[a] cancer incidence rates per 100,000 males, by site

Country	Stomach	Colon	Bladder	Liver	Total[b]	Bronchus, trachea	Melanoma, skin
United States[c]	15	18	14	4	51	35	3
United Kingdom	25	16	12	1	54	69	1
Japan	95	4	5	1	105	16	<1
Hungary	37	5	3	2	47	22	2
Sweden	25	15	10	3	53	19	3
New Zealand[d]	19	25	12	2	58	45	6

Source: Doll, Muir, and Waterhouse, 1970.

[a] Standard = estimated age distribution of males in 24 developed countries, primarily European and American.

[b] Sum of stomach, colon, bladder, and liver cancer incidence rates.

[c] Excluding Hawaii.

[d] European only, excluding Maori.

incidence and morbidity have been attributed to them. Gortner (1975) has recently compiled yearly statistics on the major nutrients contributing food energy to Americans for the period 1909–1974. Table 3, reproduced from his article, reveals the following:

1. The available supply of calories has changed minimally within a range of 3,110–3,530.
2. Dietary protein has remained nearly constant, varying only from 88 to 104 g/capita/day, during the 65-year period. However, the long-term trend is in the direction of an increased consumption of protein from

Table 3. Nutrients contributing food energy available for consumption/day, 1909–1974[a]

Year	Food energy (calories)	Carbo-hydrate (g)	Total (g)	Animal (g)	Vegetable (g)	Fat (g)
			Protein			
1909	3530	497	104	54	50	127
1910	3490	495	102	52	50	124
1911	3470	488	101	52	48	126
1912	3470	490	102	53	49	124
1913	3460	489	100	52	48	125
1914	3440	483	98	51	47	127
1915	3430	481	97	50	47	126
1916	3380	470	96	50	46	126
1917	3330	469	96	50	46	122
1918	3380	464	97	52	45	129
1919	3440	478	97	52	45	130
1920	3290	457	93	51	43	123
1921	3200	441	91	50	41	122
1922	3430	480	94	51	42	129
1923	3440	466	96	53	43	135
1924	3460	474	96	53	43	135
1925	3450	474	95	52	43	134
1926	3460	478	94	52	43	133
1927	3470	477	95	52	43	134
1928	3490	482	94	51	43	135
1929	3460	471	94	51	43	137
1930	3440	474	93	51	42	134
1931	3390	460	92	50	42	135
1932	3320	448	91	50	41	133
1933	3280	436	90	51	39	133
1934	3260	429	91	52	39	134
1935	3200	436	88	48	39	127
1936	3290	438	91	51	40	133
1937	3260	433	90	51	39	133

continued

Table 3.—*continued*

Year	Food energy (calories)	Carbo-hydrate (g)	Protein Total (g)	Protein Animal (g)	Protein Vegetable (g)	Fat (g)
1938	3260	433	90	51	40	133
1939	3340	439	92	53	39	139
1940	3350	429	93	54	39	143
1941	3410	443	94	55	39	144
1942	3320	425	97	56	41	140
1943	3360	428	100	59	41	142
1944	3350	426	99	60	39	142
1945	3300	418	102	62	40	138
1946	3320	412	102	63	39	143
1947	3290	412	97	62	35	143
1948	3200	397	94	60	34	140
1949	3200	399	94	60	34	140
1950	3260	402	94	60	34	145
1951	3160	391	93	59	34	139
1952	3190	389	94	61	33	143
1953	3170	386	95	62	32	142
1954	3150	380	94	63	32	142
1955	3180	378	95	64	32	146
1956	3180	378	96	65	31	146
1957	3110	372	95	64	31	141
1958	3120	375	94	63	31	142
1959	3170	376	95	64	31	147
1960	3140	375	95	64	31	143
1961	3120	374	95	64	31	142
1962	3120	373	94	64	31	142
1963	3140	371	96	65	31	145
1964	3180	374	97	66	31	147
1965	3140	371	96	65	30	145
1966	3170	371	97	67	30	147
1967	3210	373	98	68	31	150
1968	3260	378	99	69	31	154
1969	3280	381	100	69	31	154
1970	3300	380	100	70	30	157
1971	3320	380	101	71	30	158
1972	3320	381	101	71	30	158
1973	3300	385		68	31	155
1974[b]	3350	388		70	31	158

Source: Gortner, 1975; reprinted by permission.

[a] Quantities of nutrients computed by USDA, Agricultural Research Service, Consumer and Food Economics Institute, on the basis of estimates of per capita food consumption (retail weight), including estimates of produce of home gardens, prepared by the Economic Research Service. No deduction made in nutrient estimates for loss or waste of food in the home, use for pet food, or for destruction or loss of nutrients during the preparation of food. Civilian per capita only, 1941 to date.

[b] Preliminary.

animal sources at the expense of vegetable protein. This trend appears to be stabilizing at about 70 g of animal protein and 30 g of vegetable protein per day.
3. The daily carbohydrate intake has gradually decreased from an annual high level of nearly 500 g/day in 1909 to approximately 390 g/day at present.
4. Dietary fat intakes have risen gradually from about 125 g to more than 155 g/capita/day.

From these data it is apparent that adequate nutrients are available, but does this mean that Americans are well fed? Measured in terms of the availability of a diversity of foods in abundance, as seen in any super-market, the answer appears to be yes. Furthermore, if measured in terms of the availability of foods to meet nutritional needs, the answer clearly remains yes.

However measured, the U.S. diet meets or substantially exceeds the Recommended Daily Dietary Allowances established by the Food and Nutrition Board of the National Academy of Sciences–National Research Council (NAS–NRC). This is evident from an examination of the data in Table 4, which lists the percentages of U.S. Recommended Daily Allowances (U.S. RDA) for a number of important nutrients available for daily consumption. This analysis is based on U.S. RDA values derived by the Food and Drug Administration from the NAS–NRC guidelines, and on nutrients available for consumption per day (Code of Federal Regulations, 1975; Gortner, 1975).

Table 4. Percentage of U.S. recommended daily allowance (RDA) of nutrients available for consumption

Nutrient	U.S. RDA[a]	Nutrients available for consumption/day[b]	Percentage of U.S. RDA available for consumption/day
Vitamin A (I.U.)	5,000	8,200	164
Vitamin C (mg)	60	119	198
Thiamine (mg)	1.5	1.94	129
Riboflavin (mg)	1.7	2.33	137
Niacin (mg)	20	23.4	117
Calcium (g)	1.0	0.95	95
Iron (mg)	18	18.3	102
Vitamin B_6 (mg)	2.0	2.28	114
Vitamin B_{12} (mcg)	6	9.7	162
Phosphorus (g)	1.0	1.54	154
Magnesium (mg)	400	348	87

[a] Source: Code of Federal Regulations, 1975, 21 CFR 1.17.

[b] Source: Gortner, 1975.

Table 5.   Average life expectancy in years for white males

Year	At birth	Age 20	Age 40	Age 65
United States				
1900–1902	48.2	42.2	27.7	11.5
1909–1911	50.2	42.7	27.4	11.3
1919–1921	56.3	45.6	29.9	12.2
1929–1931	59.1	46.0	29.2	11.8
1939–1941	62.8	47.8	30.0	12.1
1949–1951	66.3	49.5	31.2	12.8
1959–1961	67.6	50.3	31.7	13.0
1970	68.0	50.3	31.9	13.1
Sweden				
1973	72.0	53.6	34.8	14.1

Sources: National Central Bureau for Statistics, 1975; U.S. Department of Commerce, 1974; U.S. Department of Health, Education, and Welfare, 1953.

If by "well fed" we mean a diet that contributes to longevity, then the U.S. diet is average. Populations in several other developed nations, especially the Scandinavian countries, have average life expectancies greater than those in the United States. For example, a newborn male can expect to live 72 years in Sweden compared with 68 years in the United States. Life expectancies in the United States from 1900 through 1970, and in Sweden during 1973 are given in Table 5. Longevity in the United States has increased steadily during the past 70 years, although it is still not as great as that of Sweden, the developed nation with perhaps the longest life expectancy. Diet is one element in a complex of life-style factors that is capable of altering longevity.

If by "well fed" we mean a diet that minimizes the incidence of cancer, if indeed this is possible, then the American diet is obviously not improving. The major causes of death between 1900 and 1970 in the United States are presented in Table 6. It is evident that the death rate from cancer has risen steadily since the turn of the century.

It is known from animal studies that tumors are much more prevalent among older animals than younger. One would expect this to be the case for man as well. Because death from one cause or another is inevitable, those members of the population who reach maturity will eventually succumb to the diseases of aging, one of which is cancer. Thus, malignant tumor development may be inevitable if life is sufficiently prolonged. Unfortunately, our knowledge of the factors involved in tumor induction is presently so incomplete that an adequate consideration of the ultimate inevitability of tumor development is not yet possible.

Table 6.   Death rates from selected causes, per 100,000 population, 1900–1970

Cause of death	1900	1910	1920	1930	1940	1950	1960	1970
Heart disease	137.4	158.9	159.6	214.2	291.9	356.8	369.0	362.0
Malignancies	64.0	76.2	83.4	97.4	120.0	139.8	149.2	162.8
Diabetes mellitus	11.0	15.3	16.1	19.1	26.5	16.2	16.7	18.9
Pneumonia and influenza	202.2	155.9	207.3	102.5	70.1	31.3	37.3	30.9
Tuberculosis	194.4	153.8	113.1	71.1	45.8	22.5	6.1	2.6
Cirrhosis of liver	12.5	13.3	7.1	7.2	8.6	9.2	11.3	15.5
Accidental death	72.3	84.5	71.0	80.4	73.4	60.6	52.3	56.4
Certain diseases of early infancy	62.6	73.0	69.2	49.6	39.1	40.5	37.4	21.3

Source: U.S. Department of Commerce, 1950; U.S. Department of Commerce, 1974.

Population Pressures

Because the birth rates in some countries are still increasing while the death rates are declining, the world's population is growing at an increasing rate. When historians relate the dominant features of the twentieth century, population growth is likely to be a most significant characteristic. The rate of U.S. population growth has recently begun to decrease, although the absolute population size continues to increase (Table 7). This trend is emphasized by a comparison of the resident populations per square mile of land area in 1800 and today. In 1800 there were 6 people per square mile of land area, a figure that has increased over 1,000% to 61 people per square mile in 1976.

When population pressures are considered as a function of arable land, the significance of the relentless increase is thrown into clear perspective.

Table 7.   U.S. population and land area, 1800–1976

Year	U.S. population (millions)	Population increase from 1956 to 1976 (percent)	Resident population per square mile of land area (population/square mile)
1800	5.3	—	6
1820	9.6	81.1	6
1840	17.1	78.1	10
1860	31.4	83.6	11
1880	50.2	59.9	14
1900	76.2	51.8	22
1920	106.0	39.1	30
1940	132.2	24.7	37
1960	179.3	35.6	51
1976	215.2	20.0	61

Source: Urdang, 1974.

Table 8. Land available for cultivation

Year	United States		World	
	Population (in millions)	Arable land per person (in acres)	Population (in millions)	Arable land per person (in acres)
1970	205	2.1	3,500	1.00
2000 (projected)	266–321	1.6–1.3	6,267	0.56

Source: Manufacturing Chemists' Association, Inc. 1974.

Table 8 presents data on land available for cultivation in the United States and in the world as a whole for 1970 and for the year 2000, projected. If the underlying assumptions are correct, there will be about 100 million more Americans in the year 2000 than in 1970. Worldwide, population pressures are so great that the total population may nearly double during this interval. The increased concentration of people will diminish the arable land per person and thus necessitate a doubling of world food production over the 30-year time span. However, producing more food would not be enough; distribution is as critical a factor. In addition, the preservation of nutritional value of the foods during distribution will pose another serious problem.

Food preservation provided the initial rationale for the development of food additives and remains the principal reason for their use today. As population pressures increase, man must balance the advantages of food additives in averting massive death by starvation against their possible low-level health hazards to the individual user. With population pressures unrelenting at this time, there seems to be no alternative to our present course of increasing food production and stabilizing and protecting the available food supply. It is no exaggeration to suggest that our success or failure in food production and distribution is critical to the future course of mankind.

Around the world, reserves of grain stocks have shrunk dramatically since 1973 as shown by the data in Table 9. With 180,000 more mouths to feed each day (Urdang, 1974), a figure that may already have risen to 200,000, repletion and preservation of grain reserves will tax modern man's ingenuity.

Food Production and Distribution

One of the major avenues for increasing food production and distribution is through the judicious use of food additives. These chemicals, thoroughly tested, are minor constituents added to achieve specific technical effects. The United States is the world's leader in the use of food additives and

Table 9.   World food security index

Year	Reserve stocks of grain[a]	Grain equivalent of idled U.S. cropland[a]	Total reserves[a]	Reserves as days of world consumption
1961	154	68	222	95
1962	131	81	212	88
1963	125	70	195	77
1964	128	70	198	77
1965	113	71	184	69
1966	99	79	178	66
1967	100	51	151	55
1968	116	61	177	62
1969	136	73	209	69
1970	146	71	217	69
1971	120	41	161	51
1972	131	78	209	66
1973	103	20	123	37
1974 (projected)	89	0	89	27

Source: Brown, 1974.

[a] Figures given in terms of million metric tons.

processed foods. Because of this, the U.S. government has developed rather elaborate regulations for controlling the consumption of food additives and processed foods and protecting their integrity.

The Federal Food, Drug, and Cosmetic Act divides food components into two groups: generally recognized as safe (GRAS) substances, and food additives. The GRAS list that has been compiled by the Food and Drug Administration (FDA) includes some 675 substances, while the Flavor and Extract Manufacturers Association includes approximately 1,500 flavors and spices on its GRAS list. The definition of food additive by FDA regulation embodies the concept that a food additive is not GRAS, although it is safe under specified use. Additives regulated by the FDA for use in foods are listed in the Code of Federal Regulations. This list is constantly changing as new food additive petitions are reviewed by the FDA.

Every constituent of a processed food is assigned to one of the two categories, GRAS or regulated food additive. Look, for example, at the constituents of an apple pie: apples, flour, sugar, margarine, cinnamon, water, and salt. All of these ingredients are GRAS, and each is itself a food. With the exception of margarine, each has undergone minimal processing, or none at all.

In a processed food, the status of each ingredient is assessed individually. For example, the ingredients of one brand of margarine include:

partially hydrogenated vegetable oil	GRAS
water	GRAS
salt	GRAS
nonfat dry milk	GRAS
vegetable lecithin	GRAS
mono- and diglycerides	GRAS
potassium sorbate (as a preservative)	GRAS
artificial flavoring	GRAS
calcium disodium EDTA (as a preservative)	regulated food additive
vitamin A palmitate	GRAS
artificial coloring (carotene)	GRAS

Of the 11 ingredients in this brand of margarine, 10 are GRAS substances and 1 is a regulated food additive.

The GRAS list is not and never was intended to be all-inclusive. Apples are GRAS but are not found on the GRAS list. Likewise, beef, flour, and eggs are not found on any all-inclusive listing. Substances on the GRAS list, which are not as widely tested as food additives, have achieved a general recognition of safety based on their consumption by man and animals, and by analogy to tested food ingredients. Together, food additives and GRAS substances are used as preservatives, flavoring agents, emulsifiers, nutrients, antioxidants, and for some 25 other technical effects as listed in Table 10.

Flavoring agents are the most widely used food ingredients, while substances added to enhance the nutritive value of foods are the next most

Table 10. Classification of GRAS substances by technical effect

Anticaking agents, free-flow agents	Leavening agents
Antioxidants	Lubricants, release agents
Colors, coloring adjuncts	Non-nutritive sweeteners
Curing, pickling agents	Nutrient supplements
Dough conditioners	pH control agents
Drying agents	Preservatives
Emulsifiers	Processing aids
Enzymes	Propellants, aerating agents, gases
Firming agents	Sequestrants
Flavor enhancers	Solvents and vehicles
Flavoring agents	Stabilizers, thickeners
Flour-treating agents	Surface-active agents
Formulation aids	Surface-finishing agents
Fumigants	Synergists
Humectants, moisture retention agents, and antidusting agents	Texturizers

Source: Hall, 1973.

Table 11.   Adult average yearly intake of selected food ingredients

	Average yearly intake (pounds)	Percentage of diet	Percentage of total added food ingredients[a]
Sugar	102	7.2	73.1
Salt	15	1.1	10.7
32 food ingredients	9	0.6	6.4
Corn syrup	8.4	0.6	6.0
Dextrose	4.2	0.3	3.0
1,800 other ingredients	1	0.1	0.7

Source: Hall, 1973.

[a] The total diet consumed is approximately 1,420 pounds/capita/year. Added ingredients account for approximately 140 pounds of this total.

numerous isolated ingredients used in food processing. Data from the Food and Drug Administration, the National Academy of Sciences, and the Flavor and Extract Manufacturers Association indicate that approximately 2,360 isolated direct food ingredients are currently used by processors. These are comprised of the following: 1,500 GRAS flavors and spices, 407 other GRAS substances, 170 regulated flavors and spices, 250 regulated food additives, and 34 regulated color additives. Precise figures are difficult to obtain because some substances are both GRAS and regulated food additives. The status of some ingredients changes from regulated food additive to GRAS or vice versa, and some represent more than one form, for example, black pepper can be a spice, an oil, or an oleoresin.

Although the use of isolated food ingredients appears to be extensive, the percentage of the U.S. diet that consists of these substances is only 10% by weight. The average yearly intake of various isolated food ingredients for an adult is approximately 139.6 pounds in a total of 1,420 pounds of food per capita per year (Hall, 1973). The breakdown by type is approximately as follows: sugar, 102 pounds; salt, 15 pounds; corn syrup, 8.4 pounds; dextrose, 4.2 pounds; a variety of 32 different ingredients[1] including monosodium glutamate, mustard, pepper, starch, yeast, sodium carbonate, citric acid, lecithin, calcium chloride, and caramel, 9 pounds; and some 1,800 other food ingredients that account for a total of 1 pound per year.

---

[1] These 32 food ingredients are: monosodium glutamate (MSG), mustard, black pepper, hydrolyzed vegetable protein, sodium caseinate, acacia, modified starch, yeasts, monocalcium phosphate, sodium aluminum phosphate, sodium acid phosphate, sodium carbonate, calcium carbonate, dicalcium phosphate, disodium phosphate, sodium bicarbonate, hydrogen chloride, citric acid, sulfuric acid, sodium citrate, sodium hydroxide, acetic acid, phosphoric acid, calcium oxide, lecithin, mono-and diglycerides, sulfur dioxide, calcium chloride, calcium sulfate, carbon dioxide, sodium tripolyphosphate, and caramel.

The significance of these figures is most easily seen by calculating the percentages of the diet comprised of the various food ingredients and the relative frequency of each in relation to the average yearly intake of food additives (Table 11). The figures reveal that approximately 73% of the total amount of added food ingredients is sugar; 20% is made up of salt, corn syrup, and dextrose; and the remaining 7% is divided among 1,832 other ingredients (Hall, 1973).

THE DELANEY CLAUSE

The use of food additives is strictly regulated by the Food and Drug Administration. One particular section of the law, the Delaney Clause, prohibits the addition of carcinogenic additives to food. The Federal Food, Drug, and Cosmetic Act (1975) states in Section 409(c)(3)(A):

> Provided, that no additive shall be deemed to be safe if it is found to induce cancer when ingested by man or animal, or if it is found, after tests which are appropriate for the evaluation of the safety of food additives, to induce cancer in man or animal . . . .

This particular section of the Act is usually referred to as the Delaney Clause. However, there are two other similarly worded anticancer clauses pertaining to color additives and animal drugs in the Federal Food, Drug, and Cosmetic Act (Sections 706(b)(5)(B) and 512(d)(1)(H), respectively).

Oftentimes there is a great deal of misunderstanding concerning the protection provided by the Delaney Clause. The clause does not ban all carcinogens from the food supply. It does not apply to foods and other GRAS substances, which constitute more than 99% of our diets. It applies only to food additives. By definition, a food additive is "any substance the intended use of which results . . . in its becoming a component . . . of any food . . . if such substance is not generally recognized . . . to be safe under the conditions of its intended use . . ." (Federal Food, Drug, and Cosmetic Act, 1975).

The Delaney Clause requires that no food additive regulation shall be issued if a food additive "is found, after tests which are appropriate for the evaluation of the safety of food additives, to induce cancer . . ." (Federal Food, Drug, and Cosmetic Act, 1975). At most, this applies only to food additives and particularly to those situations in which tests have demonstrated the carcinogenic potential of the additive. If the testing conditions are inappropriate, the results need not be considered. However, there still remains the question of whether test conditions are appropriate when dose levels of 500- to 1,000-fold physiologic levels are administered to test animals.

Even though the Delaney Clause does not apply to foods and other GRAS substances, the American consumer is, nevertheless, protected. Section 402(a)(1) of the Federal Food, Drug, and Cosmetic Act (1975) deems a food to be adulterated "if it bears or contains any poisonous or deleterious substance which may render it injurious to health . . . ." It was under this provision that the Food and Drug Administration removed cyclamate, safrole, and coumarin.

An important difference between the Delaney Clause and Section 402(a)(1) derives from the frequent use of exaggerated doses of food additives in toxicologic studies. One can feed a man or animal 500 or 1,000 times the expected normal intake of a food additive—a situation that is impossible with foods. The fact that such high levels of compounds like cyclamate or FD&C Red No. 2 can be administered over the entire life span of an animal is taken to demonstrate the relative safety of the additive. Foods are not necessarily safer than food additives; it is only that one cannot grossly overfeed a food to test animals. If one were to feed cyclamate or FD&C Red No. 2 to laboratory animals at levels comparable to man's normal use of these substances, no untoward results would be observed. Accordingly, these differences do not represent real variations in safety, but rather different degrees of opportunity to evaluate effects under extreme or unrealistic conditions.

Although the use of carcinogenic food additives is prohibited, the law does permit the sale of foods that contain carcinogens. Section 406 of the Federal Food, Drug, and Cosmetic Act (1975) authorizes the Food and Drug Administration to set a tolerance for poisonous ingredients in food when any "such substance is required . . . or cannot be avoided . . ." This provision was invoked as the basis for setting tolerances for aflatoxin in peanuts and for selenium in animal feed.

An unintentional food additive that cannot be avoided by good manufacturing practices, such as an environmental contaminant, may be permitted in food at levels consistent with public health even though the substance is found to be carcinogenic. Examples could include:

1. *An essential nutrient that is shown, after testing, to be carcinogenic in certain animals.* That this is a real, rather than a hypothetical, example is demonstrated by the observation at Cornell University that calcium causes testicular adenomas in bulls (Krook, Lutwak, and McEntee, 1969). Does this finding mean that calcium is a carcinogen and must therefore be banned?

2. *The presence in ordinary foods of carcinogens that cannot be removed.* This is not a trivial concern but a real problem for low-level aflatoxin contamination in corn, peanuts, tree nuts, cottonseed, and other grains that are harvested in the field.

3. *Environmental contamination by:*   a) plant uptake of toxic minerals in areas of naturally high soil concentration, for example, selenium in wheat; b) intentionally added chemicals, for example, pesticides; or c) unintentionally released chemicals, for example, polynuclear aromatic hydrocarbons released in the processing and use of petrochemicals and in the burning of coal.

It is conceivable that, at some time in the future, foods will be permitted to contain known *added* carcinogens in amounts not exceeding established and safe threshold levels. On the other hand, it would be completely unrealistic to suggest that foods will ever be permitted to contain carcinogens at levels presenting a significant risk to man, even where an immediate consumer need might be perceived.

Artificial sweeteners provide an example of substances for which there is a public constituency. They are used extensively by diabetics, by patients on medical weight control programs, and by millions of people who enjoy the sweet taste while limiting their calorie intake. Removal of artificial sweeteners from the food supply has proved to be very unpopular.

We may sometimes choose to add ingredients that, at much higher dose levels, have been shown to cause cancer in laboratory animals under extreme test conditions. Three possible examples include:

1. *The use of a unique food ingredient for which there is no "safer" alternative.*   Artificial sweeteners might fall into this category.
2. *Essential nutrients that are in short supply in the diet*   and for which supplementation is necessary for optimal nutritional well-being.
3. *Foods whose production and distribution require further processing or ingredient addition.*   These may pose a risk but a *lower* one than the risk that would occur without the processing step or the ingredient addition. The processing of meat products with nitrite is a current example.

Since 1950, the Food and Drug Administration has prohibited the use of 12 compounds in foods on the basis of a finding or suspicion of carcinogenicity (Code of Federal Regulations, 1975; Food and Drug Administration, 1974). The majority of the banned compounds, listed in Table 12, are not major food ingredients, and substitutes were readily available for the food manufacturers to use. Ten of these were banned under the general safety provisions of the Federal Food, Drug, and Cosmetic Act.

The Delaney Clause has been invoked only twice to ban trivial additives used as components of articles in contact with foods. In April 1967, the Food and Drug Administration banned the use of 1,2-dihydro-2,2,4-trimethylquinoline, polymerized, and, in December 1969, 4,4'-methylenebis

Table 12.   Carcinogenic compounds delisted by the Food and Drug Administration

Date	Compound	Use of compound
1950	Dulcin	artificial sweetener
1950	P-4000	artificial sweetener
1954	Courmarin	flavoring agent
1959	Diethylstilbestrol	growth promotant for poultry
1960	Safrole, oil of sassafras, dihydro-safrole, and isosafrole	flavoring agents
1967	1,2-dihydro-2,2,4-trimethylquinoline, polymerized	component of food packaging adhesives
1968	Oil of calamus	flavoring agent
1969	4,4'-methylenebis (2-chloroaniline)	component of food packaging adhesives
1969	Cyclamic acid and its salts	artificial sweetener
1972	Diethylpyrocarbonate	preservative
1973	Mercaptoimidazoline	used in articles in contact with food
1973	FD&C Violet No. 1	food color

Sources: Code of Federal Regulations, 1975; Food and Drug Administration, 1974.

(2-chloroaniline). Recently, two other substances, diethylstilbestrol and chloroform, were proposed for banning under the Delaney Clause provision (Federal Register, 1976). Final actions are still pending on these proposed bans.

Extension of the Delaney Clause to cover other toxicologic manifestations, as has been proposed, could restrict the availability of important food ingredients. We already accept the use of food ingredients that are not universally safe for all manifestations except carcinogenesis; they are required merely to be safe under the specified conditions of use.

Should the Delaney Clause be modified to make it more scientific or to permit the application of scientific judgment on an ad hoc basis? While the suggestion is intriguing from the scientific viewpoint, any solution or suggestion for modification must represent a consensus based on the available knowledge. We need an expanded scientific base and an informed citizenry before meaningful modification is possible; neither condition is currently met.

REFERENCES

Brown, L. R. 1974. Food: Growing global insecurity. In: P. T. Piotrow (ed.), Food and Population, pp. 31–34. Report No. 19 of the Victor-Bostrom Fund for the International Planned Parenthood Federation, Washington, D.C.
Code of Federal Regulations. 1975. 21 CFR 1.17, p. 32; 21 CFR 121.106, pp. 331–333. General Services Administration, Washington, D.C.

Doll, R., Muir, C., and Waterhouse, J. (eds.). 1970. Cancer Incidence in Five Continents. Volume II, pp. 370–371. Springer-Verlag, New York.

Federal Food, Drug, and Cosmetic Act, As Amended. 1975. Sections 201(s), 402(a)(1), 406, 409(c)(3)(A). U.S. Government Printing Office, Washington, D.C.

Federal Register. 1976. Volume 41, pp. 1804–1807, 15026–15030, 19207–19210. General Services Administration, Washington, D.C.

Food and Drug Administration. 1974. Legislative history and application of the anti-cancer clauses. In: Study of the Delaney Clause and Other Anti-Cancer Clauses. Part 8 of the Hearings before the House Committee on Appropriations, "Agriculture-Environment and Consumer Protection Appropriations for 1975," pp. 180–222. U.S. Government Printing Office, Washington, D.C.

Gortner, W. A. 1975. Nutrition in the United States, 1900 to 1974. Cancer Res. 35:3246–3253.

Hall, R. L. 1973. Food additives. Nutr. Today 8:20–28.

Krook, L., Lutwak, L., and McEntee, K. 1969. Dietary calcium ultimobranchial tumors and osteopetrosis in the bull. Am. J. Clin. Nutr. 22:115–118.

Levin, D. L., Devesa, S. S., Godwin, J. D., II, and Silverman, D. T. 1974. Cancer rates and risks. U.S. Government Printing Office, Washington, D.C.

Manufacturing Chemists' Association, Inc. 1974. Food additives: What they are/how they are used. Washington, D.C.

National Central Bureau for Statistics. 1975. Statistical abstract of Sweden, Volume 62. Stockholm.

Urdang, L. (ed.). 1974. The Official Associated Press Almanac 1975. Hammond Almanac, Inc., Maplewood, N.J.

U.S. Department of Commerce, Bureau of the Census. 1950. Statistical Abstract of the United States. Washington, D.C.

U.S. Department of Commerce, Bureau of the Census. 1974. Statistical Abstract of the United States. Washington, D.C.

U.S. Department of Health, Education, and Welfare. 1953. Abridged life tables: United States, 1950. In: Vital Statistics—Special Reports: National Summaries, Volume 37. Washington, D.C.

15
Whither the Delaney Clause?

Irving I. Kessler

The regulatory principle underlying Congressman Delaney's amendment to the Food, Drug, and Cosmetic Act (1975) is one that reasonable people can readily accept. In general, food additives that may induce cancer in man should be prohibited for human consumption.

However appealing a general principle may be, the operational guidelines for carrying it out must also be acceptable. The Delaney Clause, far from resolving the cancer regulatory problem, has in some ways actually compounded it.

The assessment below of the Delaney approach to cancer control begins with a review of current federal regulations on carcinogenic substances. As a case in point, the saccharin controversy is described in the context both of existing statutes and proposed new environmental cancer regulations advocated by certain federal agencies. Arguments of important consumer-oriented public interest groups favoring Delaney are assessed and, finally, an attempt is made to answer the question posed in the title of this chapter.

CURRENT FEDERAL REGULATIONS

Many general statutory provisions for the regulation of acute and chronic toxicity in ingested substances also provide federal authorities with substantial control over carcinogenic substances as well. There are, in addition, two comprehensive statutes dealing specifically with human cancer risks, namely, the Federal Food, Drug, and Cosmetic Act and the Toxic Substances Control Act. Both contain provisions relating directly to carcinogens and both incorporate specific procedures for carcinogen control distinct from those applicable to the general problem of toxicity.

At the present time, nine federal statutes are operative in the regulation of carcinogenic substances, with the Food, Drug, and Cosmetic Act essentially taking precedence over the others. Health hazards, including cancer, that are associated with the workplace are covered by the Occupational Safety and Health Act. Potentially cancer-provoking substances used by individuals at home, at recreation, and elsewhere are regulated by the Consumer Product Safety Act and the Federal Hazardous Substances Act.

Four statutes promulgated by the Environmental Protection Agency address health hazards in the physical environment including air, water, and the use of insecticides, fungicides, and rodenticides. Certain gaps in the regulation of environmental toxins fall under the Toxic Substances Control Act, which is also administered by the Environmental Protection Agency. The types of carcinogenic substances regulated by each of the federal agencies, as well as a number of procedural details, are summarized in Table 1. It may be noted that the food provisions of the Federal Food, Drug, and Cosmetic Act are unique among the statutes in permitting no regulatory discretion. If a substance regulated by this act is determined to be a carcinogen, it *must* be banned. None of the other laws, even those dealing with health hazards of wide potential impact, mandates such action.

Policies concerning the weighing of risks versus benefits in carcinogen regulation are also diverse. This process is explicitly mandated by the Toxic Substances Control Act and permitted by most of the other statutes. On the other hand, however, risk-benefit analysis is forbidden by the Delaney Clause of the Federal Food, Drug, and Cosmetic Act.

A comprehensive treatment of federal regulations on the control of ingested substances would be beyond the scope of this chapter, although a brief digression into this rather complex subject may help to put the Delaney Amendment into a proper perspective. While the statute applies specifically to food additives, not all of them are necessarily included in the amendment's operational definition. Thus, additives that have already qualified for the Generally Recognized as Safe (GRAS) list are excluded. So, too, are pesticide chemicals used in the production, storage, or transportation of agricultural products.

Substances used as ingredients in the feed of livestock raised for food production are exempted, provided that they do not adversely affect the animals themselves and provided that no residues of the additives are found in any edible portions of the animals after slaughter or in any foods derived therefrom. Color additives, both synthetic and natural in origin, are regulated by statutes other than the Delaney Clause.

Under present law, the manufacturer of a new food additive must prove that it is both safe and effective as to the performance claimed for it, before being marketed. However, once on the market and approved, the responsibility for reconsidering evidence on safety or performance falls directly upon the Food and Drug Administration rather than the manufacturer. In discharging this responsibility, the Food and Drug Administration may proceed in one of two ways. It may apply the general safety provisions of the Food, Drug, and Cosmetic Act, in which case the evidence on harmful effects, if any, must be presented and balanced against the perceived benefits. A second option is to invoke the Delaney Clause, in which case the matter ends either with a finding that the additive is carcinogenic (leading directly to its ban) or that it is not.

The constraints under which the Food and Drug Administration must regulate food additives contrast with its policies relating to the control of drugs. In the latter instance, the agency is required to weigh the benefits of a drug against its possible risks. Thus, with respect to drugs, safety is implicitly acknowledged to be a relative concept; with respect to food additives it is absolute.

In regulating carcinogenic substances in the workplace, the Occupational Safety and Health Administration is not restricted by Delaney-type statutes. It is permitted to set limits of exposure greater than zero for substances that might cause cancer in one or more animal species. Furthermore, draft proposals of new statutes on occupational safety explicitly require a weighing of the beneficial effects of a ban against the economic consequences and associated technological problems.

An example of the "risk-benefit" type of cancer regulation is seen in the action of the Consumer Product Safety Commission to ban the chemical Tris. The Commission received evidence on the carcinogenicity of Tris, but also considered its beneficial uses, the potential economic impact of a ban, and the availability of alternative chemicals designed for the same purpose. Ultimately, a decision was made to ban Tris only for use in children's apparel. This example of regulatory discretion in carcinogen control may be contrasted with the relatively inflexible decision-making process triggered by the Delaney Clause.

THE SACCHARIN BAN

On March 9, 1977, the Food and Drug Administration proposed the removal of saccharin from the food supply, citing the Delaney Clause of the Federal Food, Drug, and Cosmetic Act. In subsequent months, the agency modified the statutory basis of its action and determined that a ban on saccharin would also be justified under the general safety provisions of the act. A congressional moratorium delaying the imposition of the ban is presently

Table 1.   Federal regulation of carcinogenic substances

	(a) Administered by	(b) Type of substances regulated	(c) Specific procedures for regulating carcinogens?
1(a) Federal Food, Drug and Cosmetic Act—food provisions	Food and Drug Administration, DHEW	Foods, food additives, other substances or residues in food	Yes, in several sections (food additives, color additives, residues of animal drugs)
1(b) Federal Food, Drug, and Cosmetic Act—drug provisions	Food and Drug Administration, DHEW	Drugs and substances in drugs	No
1(c) Federal Food, Drug and Cosmetic Act—cosmetic provisions	Food and Drug Administration, DHEW	Cosmetics and substances in cosmetics	No
2 Toxic Substances Control Act	Environmental Protection Agency	Substances such as foods, drugs, cosmetics, tobacco are not covered; all non-excluded substances are covered but if other Acts cover such substances those Acts take precedence	Carcinogenic and certain other substances are to receive priority attention; a ruling must be made on carcinogens within a specified time; but regulatory action is based on toxicity
3–6 Clean Air Act; Water Pollution Control Act; Safe Drinking Water Act; Federal Insecticide, Fungicide, and Rodenticide Act	Environmental Protection Agency	Pollutants in the respective areas of the environment	No
7 Consumer Product Safety Act	Consumer Product Safety Commission	Substances used by consumers (at home, in recreation, etc.)	No

(d) If "c" does not apply, how are carcinogens regulated?	(e) Benefit-risk analysis or consideration of factors other than safety	(f) Discretion in regulating	(g) Relationship to other federal statutes
For other sections, general safety is the criterion	Risks dominate; no such analysis permitted if color or food additives or residues from animal drugs are carcinogenic; if a naturally occurring substance in food is carcinogenic, technological feasibility of removing it may be weighed against the health risk	Carcinogenic food and color additives, and foods with carcinogenic residues of animal drugs,[a] must be banned; otherwise discretion is not prohibited	The Act takes precedence in areas of foods and related substances; for residues from pesticides there is an interagency memorandum of agreement between FDA and EPA
Carcinogenicity is considered as a risk of the drug; used in weighing safety against usefulness	Explicitly required; the benefits and the risks (safety) of a drug must be considered in regulating	Yes, FDA may permit carcinogenic drugs or substances in drugs to be marketed if the benefits outweigh the risks	Takes precedence in the area of foods
Action is taken on the basis of adulteration (unsafe or injurious)	No benefits to health are presumed; risks predominate in analysis; those "cosmetics" claiming positive health benefits are treated as drugs	Banning takes place based on the discretion allowed by the adulteration sections of the Act; public health is only criterion	Takes precedence in the area of cosmetics
Toxicity; cancer regarded as a priority class of toxicity	Explicitly required by the Act.	All regulatory actions are at the discretion of EPA	See column "b"
As environmental pollutants posing danger to public health; toxicity	Permitted	All regulatory actions are at the discretion of the Commission	At the discretion of the EPA, these acts take precedence over the Toxic Substances Control Act
As hazardous products, or imminent hazards	Explicitly required by the Act	All regulatory actions are at the discretion of the Commission	Not applicable to substances covered by Food and Drug Act; close relationship to Hazardous Substances Act

continued

Table 1.—*continued*

	(a) Administered by	(b) Type of sub-stances regulated	(c) Specific pro-cedures for regu-lating carcinogens?
8 Federal Hazardous Substances Act	Consumer Product Safety Commission	Hazardous substances (in effect, it primarily covers household products)	No
9 Occupational Safety and Health Act	Occupational Safety and Health Admin., Dept. of Labor	Hazardous substances in the workplace	No

Source: Office of Technology Assessment, U.S. Congress. 1977.

[a] There is some judicial opinion that for animal drug residues, *if regulated under general safety* some risk-benefit analysis must be made, even if carcinogenicity is indicated.

in effect. The situation provides an opportunity to consider a number of issues relating to cancer regulation in general and the Delaney Clause in particular.

The saccharin controversy stems from earlier debates on cyclamates, synthetic sweeteners marketed by Abbott Laboratories in 1950. Within 10 years following their introduction, cyclamate production had increased more than 300%, and diet drinks alone came to account for some 15% of the total soft drink market in the United States. During the same time period, a number of papers were published in which sugar consumption was associated with obesity and chronic disease.

The rising diet consciousness of Americans, as well as the increasing encroachment of non-nutritive sweeteners on sugar sales, may both have stimulated the interest of the Sugar Research Foundation to contract with the University of Wisconsin Alumni Research Foundation (WARF) for studies on the chronic toxicologic effects of cyclamates in rats. At about the same time, and perhaps in response to these efforts, Abbott Laboratories, the leading cyclamate producer, arranged for Food and Drug Research Laboratories of New York to conduct its own investigation on the safety of cyclamates.

The results of the two research efforts were ironical. The WARF studies sponsored by the sugar industry failed to demonstrate any serious adverse effects of cyclamate feeding. On the other hand, the investigation supported by the cyclamate manufacturer revealed tumors in some laboratory rats fed this substance, leading to its removal from the GRAS list in October 1969, and an outright ban a few months later.

(d) If "c" does not apply, how are carcinogens regulated?	(e) Benefit-risk analysis or consideration of factors other than safety	(f) Discretion in regulating	(g) Relationship to other federal statutes
As hazardous substances; toxicity is criterion	Not explicitly mentioned; has been interpreted as allowing it, and the Commission uses such analyses	Banning is at the discretion of the Commission; certain labeling requirements are non-discretionary	Not applicable to substances covered by Food and Drug Act
As toxic substances; there are proposed implementing regulations dealing specifically with carcinogens	Permitted by the Act; required by the implementing regulations	Yes	Takes action when other federal agencies have not, for workplace hazards

The Abbott-sponsored study upon which the cyclamate ban was largely based involved feedings of cyclamate/saccharin mixtures, rather than pure cyclamate. Thus, the hypothesized carcinogenic agent might as likely have been saccharin as cyclamate. Several years later, the shortcomings of the study were publicly acknowledged by the investigators themselves. Yet, when subsequent rat-feeding studies employing pure cyclamates yielded negative results, no reversal of the regulatory decision was forthcoming (Thomas, 1975).

Other issues relevant to carcinogen regulation come to mind with respect to the cyclamate ban. There is the question of how particular food additives are selected for the intensive scrutiny that may lead to their ultimate statutory ban. With some four million distinct chemical entities in our environment, and with perhaps more than 60,000 in common use, what rational basis is there for deciding which substances require carcinogenic testing and which do not? The Delaney Amendment triggers a decision-making process with respect to previously suspected food additives, but does not afford a mechanism for setting priorities for investigating additives according to their likelihood of being carcinogenic in man. In the generation of the evidence against cyclamates, an essential role was played by the competing commercial interests of the sugar and non-nutritive sweetener industries.

Another issue highlighted by the saccharin ban is that of the social, political, and scientific atmosphere within which the cancer regulatory process is played out. Perhaps more explicitly than ever before, the regulatory decisions on saccharin were made under the glare of klieg lights with biomedical scientists, political figures, and the press assuming essentially adversarial roles. In a recent address, President William J. McGill of Columbia University alluded to the "increasing adversary character of American public life as it affects the administration of science" and argued that scientific decisions belong largely in the domain of the scientists themselves. He suggested that:

> We are weakening America's scientific leadership by unwittingly establishing the principle that the conflicting advocacy of the Legislature or the court room is the best way to develop sound public policy in science and technology. . . . The adversary method for arriving at truth on which our legal procedures are based is, in simple language, not appropriate for arriving at sound public policy on scientific matters. Scientific questions simply cannot be settled by persuasive argument. The only effective method for resolving safety questions in nuclear or biological research is the objective analysis of experimental results by our best scientific minds. . . . What I am saying, in unvarnished simplicity, is that the use of the adversary legal process to control scientific policy is likely to lead to serious scientific errors and to badly thought-out policy (McGill, 1977).

The intrusion of political considerations and unwarranted publicity into the regulatory arena is harmful in both obvious and subtle ways. Thus, saccharin, which is one-millionth as mutagenic—and, therefore, potentially carcinogenic—as aflatoxin B on the basis of the Ames salmonella assay has been the subject of several million dollars' worth of reviews by congressional committees, the National Academy of Sciences, and other bodies, while the citizenry continues munching peanuts with aplomb.

The widely publicized and intense preoccupation of the government with saccharin almost predictably led to congressional demands for another "definitive" epidemiologic study to resolve the issue of its possible carcinogenicity. As a consequence, a $1.4 million study of 9,000 human subjects from diverse areas of the United States was commissioned for completion within 18 months. Paradoxically, the very same publicity and excessive concern wtih the potential dangers of saccharin make it unlikely that the study respondents will provide unbiased information concerning their saccharin exposures.

This is not merely an example of politics and science not mixing but, rather, of the direct interference of the one by the other. Exacerbating the situation is the fact that the commissioned saccharin study was undertaken by a federal agency of government rather than (in the more usual fashion) by university-based investigators who competed for the project and subjected themselves to traditional peer review evaluation of the quality of their proposal.

Throughout the course of the debate on cyclamate and until recently in the deliberations on saccharin, human epidemiologic investigations on the possible carcinogenicity of these substances were neither sponsored nor encouraged by the Food and Drug Administration. Notwithstanding the weaknesses imputed to epidemiologic studies by some, it is manifestly incongruous for health regulatory judgments to be made about man without a systematic effort to obtain confirmatory evidence from man. The alacrity with which rat-to-man extrapolations were made in the non-nutritive sweetener controversies may augur their eventual replacement by an even more simplistic decision-making device, namely, the short-term in vitro test. How far we seem to have strayed from Pope's dictum that "the proper study of mankind is man"!

Although the Delaney Amendment was initially cited by the Food and Drug Administration in its early pronouncements on both the cyclamate and the saccharin questions, ultimately the substances were in fact banned under the general safety provisions of the Federal Food, Drug, and Cosmetic Act. The Delaney Clause has been officially invoked to ban food additives only twice since its enactment, both times (in 1967 and 1969) with respect to food-packing adhesives. The rarity of these events in relation to the large number of putative human carcinogens suggests that the Delaney approach to carcinogen regulation may be ineffective on this basis alone.

RECENT REGULATORY PROPOSALS

Not even the most casual observer today can fail to recognize the growing importance of environmental issues in the contemporary sociopolitical arena. The origins of this, perhaps in the counterculture evolving from the Vietnam antiwar movement, need not be pursued here (Rowe, 1977). Of relevance is the vastly increasing interest of both the public and the government in environmental causes of disease, especially cancer. This is the background against which the Delaney approach to carcinogen control is being debated.

Illustrative of the government's current approach is the proposal of the Occupational Safety and Health Administration for a new general regulation concerning the "identification, classification and regulation of toxic substances posing a potential occupational carcinogenic risk" (Occupational Safety and Health Administration, 1977). An early section in the document entitled "The Increase in Cancer and Its Massive Economic, Social and Emotional Impact" emphasizes that cancer death rates "sharply exceed predictions," that the economic and social impacts of cancer are "massive and yet hard to estimate," and that "states with high rates [of cancer] are the more industrialized states." All of these statements are technically correct but seem to have been presented in a rather frightening, and perhaps distorted, context. They largely ignore the basic fact that cancer is mainly a disease of aging and that improvements in sanitation, water purity, nutrition, and working conditions, to say nothing of medical advances, have permitted ever-increasing proportions of the population to attain the ages of enhanced cancer risk.

The distortion can be illustrated with a few statistics. For example, the average loss of life expectancy at age 35 that is associated with smoking-related diseases has been estimated by the American Cancer Society to be approximately 3 years (Hammond, 1969). The total elimination of cancer as a cause of death would, in fact, not increase the average life span of a population by more than 2 years (Levin et al., 1974). These figures are not intended to minimize the seriousness of cancer as a public health menace but, rather, to put the issue into its proper biologic perspective. If human beings were potentially immortal, the elimination of cancer as a cause of death would have a far greater impact on life expectancy than has been observed. Unfortunately, we are not destined for immortality and a number of chronic diseases—particularly coronary and cerebrovascular—vie with cancer for the privilege of terminating human life at the older ages.

Thus, if the life-threatening impact of any one of these diseases were reduced through improvements in diagnosis or therapy, the apparent impact of the others would increase. This means that the secular increase in proportional mortality from cancer in advanced countries like the United States probably reflects the successful reduction in competing causes of death rather than failures in the fight against cancer. One might also suggest that the social and economic implications of cancer in the United States should have little, if any, bearing on the regulatory approaches to carcinogen control that are chosen. The frequent allusion to the growing magnitude of the cancer problem in federal proposals for cancer regulation exemplifies the degree to which the regulatory process, the political process, and science are presently confounded.

The phenomenon is also seen in such frequently repeated assertions as "some ninety percent of cancer in man is [therefore] due to chemicals" (Food and Drug Administration, 1977). Such conclusions are arrived at on the basis of deductive reasoning and statistical inference rather than through empirical scientific inquiry. They ignore two other essential elements in the epidemiologic triad of human disease etiology, namely, the host and the environment.

Most epidemiologists and many other biomedical scientists believe that chronic diseases such as cancer, as well as infectious diseases, are not simply "caused" by an agent. For example, the tubercle bacillus is not *the* cause of pulmonary tuberculosis for, if it were, most of the present adult generation would already be tuberculous as nearly all of us have ingested or inhaled mycobacteria at one time or another in our lives. To produce a clinically manifest case of tuberculosis requires an interaction between the bacterial agent and a susceptible host in an environment conducive to the interaction. Thus, the disease would be more easily acquired after exposure to the microorganism if the host's immune status were deficient, if his or her nutritional status were inadequate, or if he or she were already suffering from an intercurrent infection of another kind.

Just as the ubiquitous bacteria and viruses are not usually the necessary and sufficient causes of the diseases nominally associated with them, so should the millions of chemical agents in our macroenvironment not be considered as competent agents of disease per se. To believe otherwise would necessitate a return to the environmental purity of a Stone Age society because we do not have the resources to subject most, or even a substantial number, of the potentially harmful chemicals to the kind of scrutiny lavished upon saccharin and a tiny handful of other substances.

In the absence of a biologically rational priority system, cancer regulation may come to resemble Russian roulette, because only those substances that are selected for study stand any chance of being identified as hazardous. Who should decide which should be tested and on what basis? Applying the usual 95% confidence limits in a statistical test of significance, somewhat in excess of 200,000 of the more than four million known chemicals would yield positive (i.e., pathogenic) results *purely by chance alone*. Thus, even if governmental agencies could somehow test all four million chemicals—including the many thousands of foods and food additives—how could they then decide which of the large numbers of positive laboratory animal or bacterial system test results were spurious or biologically insignificant and which reflected genuine human cancer hazards?

Instead of dealing simplistically with viruses or chemicals in isolation as the causes of disease, the problem should be approached in terms of the agent/host/environment triad. Thus, efforts could be made toward the development of techniques to classify both the cancer risk profiles of various population subgroups as well as the chemical, biologic, and other hazards in the environment. The objective would be to minimize interactions between susceptible individuals or subgroups and specific environmental toxins that may increase their risk of cancer or other diseases.

The Occupational Safety and Health Administration now refers to environmental causes of cancer as "acting singularly or in conjunction with genetic or other susceptibles" (Occupational Safety and Health Administration, 1977). This enlightened perspective can lead to the development of a cancer regulatory system that offers a scientifically reasonable basis for deciding which of the multitude of potentially hazardous substances should be tested for carcinogenicity and which should not. The large majority of such substances will obviously never be subjected to adequate testing.

ARGUMENTS FAVORING THE DELANEY CLAUSE

A number of arguments in favor of the Delaney-type approach to carcinogen regulation have been made in recent years. These are cogently summarized in a document published by the Health Research Group (1977) and are considered in some detail here.

An early section of the document emphasizes the importance of environmental causes of cancer. The roles of asbestos, chromate, nickel, uranium, and aniline dyes in the development of cancer in man are well substantiated. On the other hand, some of the materials cited—urban residence, automobile exhausts, coke ovens, refuse, cleaning fluids, rubber, waxes, pesticides, and cosmetics—have yet to be confirmed as human carcinogens. Their inclusion tends to exaggerate the impact of individual environmental factors in human carcinogenesis and to justify such statements as "cancer has reached epidemic proportions in recent decades" (Health Research Group, 1977). Objectively, this conclusion is not well supported by the vital statistics (Lilienfeld, Levin, and Kessler, 1972). The same may be said of the Health Research Group's statement that "the good news about environmentally caused cancer is that the majority of cancers are preventable."

While conceding that food additives "are put into food products to improve their taste, appearance, texture, smell, longevity, and occasionally nutritive value," the Health Research Group document largely dismisses them as "purely cosmetic" and often as involving "outright deceit." Furthermore, "it is cheaper for the food industry to add a preservative which retards the growth of mold than to use fresh, nutritious ingredients and remove old products from the shelves." This leads to the conclusions that "should individual additives show any chance of harm to health, that risk far outweighs the limited benefits they offer" and that "in the rare case where a risky additive provides a benefit to consumers—as opposed to producers—the benefit can be provided by another additive which is safe."

As a philosophical approach to health hazard regulation, one cannot fault the first of these statements. The issue is joined, however, with respect to how one would define "any chance of harm to health." As already noted, the Delaney Amendment provides no rational mechanism for making such judgments. As for the substitution of one additive for another, this could be a reasonable basis for public policy, provided that the substitute is demonstrably safer than the additive it replaces.

Cyclamate was replaced by saccharin, which was itself later proposed for banning. In turn, aspartame, xylose, monellin, glycyrrhizin, miracle fruit, and a variety of other substances have been recommended as additive sugar ingredients. Yet none of these has been subjected to a degree of health hazard evaluation that in any way resembles that accorded saccharin (National Academy of Sciences, 1975). The Health Research Group indirectly, and others explicitly, suggest that synthetic substances are more likely to be harmful than natural foods. While the argument has considerable appeal, it ignores a substantial body of evidence on the toxic effects in man of lead, arsenic, mercury, and a large number of other natural substances.

The so-called "limitations of epidemiology" are next addressed by the Health Research Group. Their perspective is apparent from their description of the epidemiologic method, namely, "studies [which] scan hospital and other records for a correlation between a greater incidence of human cancer and exposure to a given substance" (Health Research Group, 1977). While clinical and epidemiologic studies do sometimes generate correlations, the strength of the epidemiologic method lies in its ability to generate *real data* on *real people* exposed to quantitatively determined levels of *real pathogenic agents*. A typical epidemiologic study would measure the proportion of smokers and nonsmokers who develop lung cancer and the presence or absence of a dose-response relationship between smoking and lung cancer. Correlational analyses are generated largely on the basis of data from vital statistics registries rather than in the centers of epidemiologic excellence around the country.

Presumably as an example of "good" epidemiology, the effects of diethylstilbestrol (DES) are cited: "A great rise was detected in cases of vaginal cancer, a very rare form in women" (Health Research Group, 1977). Unfortunately, the statement is inconsistent with recently published literature. Herbst and his colleagues, who made the initial observations on DES and vaginal adenosis, concede that "although most of these abnormalities were known to occur rarely in the pre-stilbestrol era, their prevalence in unexposed women examined as carefully as those who have been exposed has not been established" (Herbst et al., 1975). In other words, information sufficient to resolve the DES/vaginal cancer question is still lacking. Furthermore, animal studies involving large doses of DES have usually failed to induce vaginal neoplasia (Herbst et al., 1975, Robboy et al., 1977). To this author's knowledge, the only exception is given by Dunn who, in an editorial letter, reported the induction of vaginal cancer in mice treated with DES by injection. Significantly, however, these were squamous cell carcinomas, completely unlike the adenocarcinomas characteristically found in young women (Dunn, 1975).

A careful reading of the DES/vaginal cancer literature reveals an increasing tendency by the investigators to emphasize the association of DES in young women with adenosis, a benign condition, rather than with vaginal cancer. One may fairly conclude that the weak evidence from human epidemiologic studies and the essentially negative animal findings do not support the Health Research Group's assertion of an association between DES and vaginal cancer. In fact, the group's rather uncritical acceptance of such data as confirmatory of still another environmental cancer hazard suggests an inherent weakness in the Delaney-type approach to regulation.

As an example of the weakness of epidemiologic studies, it is stated that "if everyone smoked cigarettes, it is unlikely that lung cancer would have been traced to smoking" (Health Research Group, 1977). This is true, if only because the majority of heavy smokers—despite their carcinogenic exposure—do not develop lung cancer. That this is not a significant indictment of the epidemiologic method may be deduced by determining the likely state of our knowledge on the carcinogenic effects of cigarette smoking in man had there been no controlled epidemiologic studies in human subjects. Since, for so many years, no adequate animal models of smoking and lung cancer were developed, this question would have remained unanswered, to the enormous detriment of society. All the feeding and topical application studies of tobacco substances in rats, rabbits, mice, and other laboratory animals failed to reveal the potential carcinogenicity of tobacco for the human tracheobronchial tree. Thus, the tobacco story, rather than exemplifying a limitation of epidemiology, actually demonstrates that human epidemiologic studies can serve as an essential basis for health hazard evaluation.

It is further asserted that "epidemiologists are unlikely to spot carcinogens if they cause cancer by a single exposure, since cancer patients are unlikely to be aware of such an exposure many years back . . . [whereas] animals can get cancer from single doses of dimethylnitrosamine and aflatoxin . . ." (Health Research Group, 1977). With the possible exception of such obviously overwhelming exposures as those in Hiroshima and Nagasaki, single exposures to potentially carcinogenic substances do not usually produce cancer in man. That this occurs in some inbred laboratory animal species attests more to the inappropriateness of rat-to-man extrapolations than it does to the weaknesses of the epidemiologic method.

"Epidemiology is an after-the-fact technique," and, therefore, "human studies can only occur after there are cancer victims," according to the Health Research Group (1977). Such statements are also invalid. Retrospective, or case-control, studies are conducted after the occurrence of cancer or other diseases of interest, but prospective studies have become an important tool in the epidemiologic armamentarium.

For example, approximately 21,500 diabetic patients have been identified and followed prospectively for the development of cancer over a period in excess of 30 years (Kessler, 1971). At present, thousands of patients who underwent tonsillectomy and/or appendectomy in Baltimore between 1925 and 1936 are being prospectively studied at the University of Maryland School of Medicine. The purpose is to assess the subsequent carcinogenic risks among individuals who have lost the potential immunologic protection afforded by their lymphoid organs. In still another prospective investigation, some 17,000 patients with confirmed pulmonary tuberculosis diagnosed between 1946 and 1960 are being followed for the subsequent development of cancer, by type. The study is designed to evaluate the immunogenic potential of a prior tuberculosis infection in resisting carcinogenic pressures over the ensuing 20 to 35 years.

Accordingly, far from being an "after-the-fact" technique, epidemiology affords unique opportunities for the documentation and understanding of cancer in human beings. To be sure, not all cancer risks can be so dealt with. For example, studies involving the injection of potentially carcinogenic materials into experimental subjects would obviously have to be conducted in laboratory animals rather than in human subjects.

"Epidemiology," it is averred, "usually cannot spot the less potent carcinogens. . . . Yet, it is assuredly the less potent carcinogens that seem to be more important in human cancer" (Health Research Group, 1977). To the best of this author's knowledge, there is no evidence to support the latter statement. Perhaps the assertion is made in tacit recognition of the fact that the etiology of so few human neoplasms has yet been elucidated, despite many thousands of experiments in animal models. It is likely that the enigma of human carcinogenesis remains unresolved largely because of a biologically myopic emphasis on cancer agents in isolation, rather than on the development of pathogenic models that take into account the agent, the host, and the interactive environment.

In supporting the Delaney Clause, the Health Research Group argues that "because the collection of human data has so many limitations, scientists have traditionally relied on the results of animal tests to determine whether substances entail a risk of cancer for humans." The assertion is supported by the subsequent claim that "with the possible exception of arsenic . . . all chemicals and other agents found to be carcinogenic in man have also caused animal cancer." The latter statement, taken from the address of a federal official, is not based upon comprehensive studies of human and animal carcinogens. Rather, it derives from uncontrolled clinical observations, a variety of assumptions and inferences, as well as a very flexible definition of the term *cancer*.

Thus, the occurrence of any kind of neoplasm in an animal is regarded as a positive finding. It may be reported, for example, that the administration of chemical X in 50 laboratory animals produced a significant excess of cancers when compared with 50 untreated animals. When the results are examined in detail, it is seen that the test animals did not develop one characteristic tumor type in response to the chemical but, rather, a wide variety of neoplasms, both benign and malignant, in many topographic sites.

To some investigators, cancer is cancer is cancer. However, to the oncologist treating cancer patients every day, and to the clinical epidemiologist studying the natural history of cancer in man, this notion is invalid. Neoplasms of even the same topographic site may differ in histopathology, prodroma, clinical course, case fatality, and known or suspected etiologic factors. To lump such a diversity of diseases together is to ignore much of what has already been learned about the neoplastic process from the observations and experiments of thousands of clinicians and bioscientists around the world over the past century. This practice may make it easier to draw conclusions about the significance of animal study findings, but in no way does it help to resolve the fundamental, and as yet insoluble, dilemma of extrapolating the results of such studies to man.

A minor caveat is then introduced, namely, "cancer scientists believe that while the fact that a substance causes cancer in animals does not make it certain that it has the same effect in humans, with a well-designed experiment, it is highly probable that a similar effect would occur in humans." However, it is quickly added that "it is almost incredible that our species could be exempt from such causes of cancer when other species are susceptible" (Health Research Group, 1977).

In this fashion, the Health Research Group would appear, in effect, to have turned one of their previous arguments on its head. For even if, as they assert, all chemicals found to be carcinogenic in man also cause cancer in animals, it does not follow that all—or most, or even some—animal carcinogens behave similarly in humans. Much evidence to the contrary may be found in the voluminous literature on animal carcinogenesis. The Special Virus Cancer Program of the National Cancer Institute invested millions of dollars over more than a decade attempting to link RNA viruses that cause tumors in animals to cancers in humans—without success. In fact, when Nobel Prizes were awarded for viral carcinogenesis to two distinguished investigators in 1975, both were careful to de-emphasize the relevance of their work to human cancer. Thus, the Delaney Amendment's emphasis on the pertinence of animal findings to man may be attractive to federal regulators seeking to simplify the decision-making process, but there is as yet little objective evidence to support the feasibility of such a "push-button" approach.

"Animal tests yield knowledge about weak carcinogens when human evidence is unlikely ever to be obtained." This essentially valid statement by the Health Research Group (1977) serves as part of the rationale for the use of nonphysiologic doses of test drugs in laboratory animal studies. Three other reasons are offered by the Health Research Group (1977): "(1) to compensate for the short life span of animals as compared to humans; (2) to compensate for the very fast metabolism and excretion of chemicals by animals as compared to humans; and (3) to compensate for the small number of test animals compared to the number of humans exposed to the chemicals."

While each of these explanations is acceptable, none addresses the basic inferential problem. One would like to determine, for example, whether the amount of saccharin that is usually ingested by people in the course of their daily lives poses any carcinogenic risks to them. On the other hand, only the experimental biologist, but certainly not the health regulator, would be interested in such theoretical questions as the risk of cancer following ingestion by artificial means of enormous quantities of saccharin that no human could, in fact, possibly tolerate.

Miniscule or demographically insignificant cancer risks can certainly elude statistical detection, but the essential issue concerns the risk level at which governmental regulation should be invoked. For example, if the risk of bladder cancer from saccharin were limited to immunodeficient patients, should society as a whole be deprived of this substance's perceived benefits, or should the endangered class of individuals alone be protected by specific legislation?

Assessments of low level carcinogenic hazards can be mischievous if one simply multiplies the risk factor (1% or 0.1% or 0.01%, etc.) by the U.S. population of 215 million. Thus, instead of describing a potential risk attributable to saccharin as 0.01%, one may define it in terms of a risk that potentially affects 21,500 people. Such statistical manipulations tend to be demagogic because the scientific community presently lacks the means to detect such low risks—if they do indeed exist—against the variety of background noises involved.

It can also be asserted that human epidemiologic studies are not necessarily ineffective in detecting weak carcinogenic effects. While each individual investigation on the saccharin question, for example, may have been inadequate because of sample size to rule out very small carcinogenic effects, the statistical power of *all* the epidemiologic studies combined may be considerable. Since each of the studies was conducted under somewhat different circumstances and among different population groups, one might expect that a small but consistent carcinogenic risk attributable to saccharin would not easily remain undetected for long. This point has not yet been given the attention it deserves.

The weaknesses ascribed to epidemiologic studies should be weighed against the weaknesses of laboratory studies conducted on inbred animal strains under highly contrived conditions. Those cancers that arise naturally in human society are probably a response to a complex of interactions between environmental agents and host factors such as genotype, constitution, hormone balance, and immunologic status. From this perspective, epidemiologic studies conducted in the natural milieu of cancer are eminently appropriate and realistic. They contrast favorably with what might be regarded as the rather abstract setting of the typical laboratory experiment.

"Even at high doses, only a tiny fraction of chemicals tested cause cancer" (Health Research Group, 1977). The Health Research Group supports this statement by noting that "since the Delaney Clause was enacted in 1958, out of over 3,000 food additives in use, only about ten have been banned for causing cancer" (1977). By no means should this imply that 10 of the additives are carcinogenic and that 2,990 are not because only a small minority of the 3,000 were systematically tested in any fashion, let alone with the intensity characterizing the saccharin studies, for example.

"Because of the complexity of the many factors influencing the cause of cancer in humans, including the wide variety of other chemicals to which humans are exposed, a 'no-effect' dose in animal studies cannot predict a safe dose for humans." Furthermore, "the principle of a zero tolerance for carcinogenic exposures should be retained in all areas of legislation covered by it and should be extended to cover other exposures as well" (Health Research Group, 1977). This, in essence, is the "bend over backward to play it safe" regulatory argument. In fact, the suggested process would merely confer an illusion of safety upon those tested substances that yielded negative laboratory animal results, while setting off an alarm concerning those which did not.

In view of the numerous arbitrary elements—which substances are being tested, with what degree of intensity, which laboratory animal species are to be selected for testing, which doses and other experimental conditions are to apply, etc., etc.—the effect of a zero tolerance criterion would be to increase the number of suspect carcinogens without in any way increasing the precision of our knowledge concerning them. This would scarcely qualify as increasing the public's margin of protection against cancer.

"Advances in detection methodology provide a greater awareness of the hazards and a better means to determine total environmental exposures to known dangers. . . . For example, in 1954, FDA permitted DES to be added to cattle feed to stimulate growth, in the belief that none of the cancer causing chemical ended up in table meat. Chemical analytical methods have improved over the years, and DES residues can now be detected in meat, with the result that FDA has proposed to ban DES in feed." These statements of the Health Research Group (1977) suggest that there are no means presently at hand to determine safe doses of carcinogens and, therefore, support the notion of zero tolerance.

While this premise is correct, the conclusion is faulted. Consider the example of DDT, which by preventing crop contamination has probably saved millions of children and others from starvation around the world until it was banned. The ban did not follow the compilation of new evidence concerning its pathogenicity in man but, rather, the development of more refined technologies capable of measuring parts per billion residues of DDT.

One might suppose that our air, water, and food all contain parts per billion of theoretically hazardous substances of all kinds that cannot be eliminated without a drastic restructuring of Western civilization. Thus, we are not dealing here with simplistic alternatives, good versus evil, or the public versus industry.

> Instead, the true conflict is between competing good values, all of which we as a democratic nation support and value. The true confrontation in these cases is between such lofty and valued societal objectives as protecting the public against exploitation and protecting personal freedom (Crout, 1978).

The Health Research Group (1977) denies that the Delaney Clause rules out the valid exercise of scientific reason and interpretation: "The Delaney Clause gives FDA the scientific discretion to decide whether the food additive has in fact been shown to cause cancer. FDA can examine the test design, the way the additive was administered, the purity of the additive used, the reliability of the diagnosis of cancer, etc., to determine if the tests are methodologically acceptable to the scientific community." While all this is true, the fact remains that the Delaney Clause must be triggered if an appropriately designed laboratory test yields tumors in animals that are fed a suspect additive. In other words, the Delaney Clause takes for granted that animal results may properly be extrapolated to human beings despite the fact that people may not even be able to metabolize the additive and irrespective of the doses that may far exceed the capacity of anyone to absorb them over an entire lifetime.

It is noted that "the judgment that Congress has made [relating to the Delaney Clause] is a social one. No additive is worth the risk of cancer" (Health Research Group, 1977). It would be difficult to challenge this statement. On the other hand, one can support the statement while remaining less than enthusiastic about the protections afforded against cancer by the Delaney Clause.

An important statement of the Health Research Group (1977) concerns pressures against consumer protection at the Food and Drug Administration. It is posited that "the FDA is over-influenced by the industries it is supposed to regulate" and that "FDA is subject to high level political pressures against safety." While these accusations may very well be true, the fair-minded reader should also recognize that thousands of people now owe their livelihoods to the existence of regulatory agencies and research laboratories concerned with the human cancer problem. These individuals constitute what may be termed a *cancer constituency*, because they benefit personally from governmental decisions, for example, that saccharin causes human bladder cancer. Were saccharin and a number of other suspect substances deemed safe for human consumption, this would contract the activities of the regulatory agencies and research laboratories, thereby reducing employment or promotion possibilities for the many individuals therein. Clearly, therefore, political pressures of many hues are operative in the cancer regulatory arena.

THE REGULATORY DILEMMA

One wonders what has happened to the classic triad of agent, host, and environment. In the highly contrived setting of the animal laboratory, tumor induction may sometimes be produced by straightforward exposure of test animals to known carcinogens. In the real and complex world of human beings, however, the situation is far different.

Although heavy cigarette smokers incur an eight- or tenfold greater risk of lung cancer than nonsmokers, most heavy smokers will never develop lung cancer at all. The same is probably true for all the known human carcinogens. The enormous variability of tumor inductibility in man is related in part to the genetic, immunologic, hormonal, and other constitutional differences among individuals; in part to the degree and duration of carcinogenic exposure; and in part to other factors as yet unknown.

The multifactorial nature of human cancer etiology presents serious problems to the investigator, to the regulator, and to the general public. The investigator is obliged to conduct experiments in such fashion as to take account of as many of the host and environmental factors that might affect the agent's potency as possible. For all its shortcomings, the epidemiologic method of studying the development of cancer in human subjects in their natural habitat under controlled conditions is a rational and effective approach to this challenge. For all its evident simplicity, the classic toxicologic testing situation—although it may contribute greatly to our knowledge of carcinogenic mechanisms—is in fact quite artificial, particularly if one wishes to extrapolate findings from animals to man.

To the health regulator, the epidemiologic triad poses an especially vexing problem because the government, having undertaken to protect the citizenry against cancer, must make good its promise. Unfortunately, governments tend to be impatient with complex situations and, in the present instance, with our rather enormous ignorance concerning cancer.

Therefore, bureaucratically simple mechanisms for decision-making on the carcinogenicity of suspected substances tend to earn high priority.

While those in academia may be content to advance knowledge at a deliberate and careful pace, government regulators are under enormous public pressure to make decisions and to make them rapidly. This explains their frequently expressed disenchantment with epidemiologic studies that usually require 3 or 4 years for completion and that are basically unsuited for randomized testing of suspected carcinogens to which human populations have not been spontaneously exposed. This also explains their reliance upon laboratory animal studies in which potential confounding factors such as species specificity, strain specificity, experimental conditions, and extrapolation problems remain unresolved. In good measure, this also explains the enthusiasm with which the short-term in vitro tests for mutagenicity are supported, despite their obvious limitations.

The regulatory dilemma today is due, in part, to the very real fact that the prevalence of cancer is increasing. This in turn stems from our increasing longevity and possibly from the increasing number and variety of chemical substances in the environment. Because of the relatively sudden appearance of these agents, our normal evolutionary adaptive mechanisms may be inadequate. The regulatory dilemma also stems from the increasingly consumer-oriented society in which we live. Disease is no longer regarded as an act of God but rather as a challenge to the government, which is held responsible for protecting us therefrom, regardless of whether or not the means are at hand.

One gains the impression that the regulatory agencies are more interested in positive (i.e., cancer-associated) results than in negative findings among studies that are equally well designed. In fact, a number of high-level regulatory officials have publicly supported the notion that positive epidemiologic findings should be taken seriously by the government, but that negative findings may be ignored because of the inherent weaknesses of the epidemiologic method. This approach is logically and scientifically untenable.

A crucial factor in the regulatory situation is introduced by the Delaney Amendment itself. This tends to make the regulatory process more perfunctory, automatic, and bureaucratic, and to influence it by statistical rather than biologic considerations. Should the question of saccharin's safety, for example, be resolved on the basis of the statistical significance of differences between case and control groups or in terms of the power of the statistical test at given α and β levels?

In fact, regulatory issues like those posed by saccharin should be regarded as biologic questions to be resolved primarily by the application of scientific reasoning to the data at hand. Thus, instead of focusing upon the statistical significance of the findings, one should assess the biologic significance. The fact that man does not metabolize saccharin is, for example, a biologic reality that cannot simply be dismissed on statistical grounds or otherwise ignored. Coherence of observations with previously established facts is another essential element in the process of imputing cancer to saccharin or to other suspected agents.

Epidemiologic evidence on saccharin and other putative carcinogens should be taken seriously. The purported weakness of epidemiologic studies is, in a sense, contradicted by the argument that they are not based upon large enough samples of individuals to permit definitive tests of the hypotheses. The argument is specious because it is made by the same critics who defend the use of 40 or 50 animals per experiment in the toxicologic setting as representing a reasonable approach. This limitation necessitates the feeding of nonphysiologic doses of test substances, with all the inferential consequences this entails.

We should not have it both ways. If epidemiologic studies are defective because of inadequate sample size—generally 500 to 1,000 subjects per series—this would also apply to the classic rat-feeding study. If it is difficult and expensive to investigate 1,000 people, it would certainly be less difficult and less expensive to investigate 1,000 rats. Yet, with very few exceptions, this is not being done. If the saccharin issue is sufficiently important to justify Congressional hearings, National Academy of Sciences evaluations and other activities, the use of 10,000 or even 100,000 rats exposed to varying doses of saccharin down to physiologic levels is also justified. At the least, studies of this type would help to answer the question of whether thresholds exist for cancer induction by such substances.

The threshold question is a crucial one if only because it evokes the question of absolute safety. Some have argued that the food and drug laws should be applied so as to ensure the public of the absolute safety, that is, the total absence of carcinogenic risk, of all foods and food additives. Absolute safety could be ensured for substances in which there is a dose threshold. Without it, the only other option would be a total ban of the suspected substance.

In light of the complexity of the human carcinogenic process, however, the concept of absolute safety is difficult to defend. For example, how should one regulate a substance if it is proved to be weakly carcinogenic only in babies or pregnant women? Would it be more rational to banish the substance from the general marketplace or to make special provision for protecting the susceptibles?

Regrettably, little or no consideration is being given these days to host factors in human cancer. Government regulators appear to be taking a simplistic course in which they seek to characterize saccharin as a carcinogen without in any way determining the conditions under which it may or may not be carcinogenic. Elucidation of host factors that protect most of us but predispose some of us to cancer would represent an eminently rational approach to cancer control at the public level.

The Delaney-based orientation of our current regulatory system is well intentioned but unduly susceptible to bureaucratic whim. It singles out cancer to the exclusion of cardiovascular and other chronic diseases that kill and disable most of us. It calls for judgments on the basis of *appropriate tests* without providing any definition of the term. Does one positive test override three negatives? Should seven well-designed negative studies refute one positive study? Will the controversial "quick" tests in tissue culture eventually replace even the laboratory animal experiments (Kolata, 1976; Sivak, 1976)?

The Delaney approach permits no balancing of the presumed risks of saccharin against the benefits to the obese, the carious, or the diabetic. It does not represent a bending over backward to protect the public against carcinogenic risk because these risks are generally species specific. Under the Delaney Clause, a negative saccharin-feeding study might be regarded as implying the safety of the substance, when in fact other species, including man, might actually test positive. Thus, the injudicious application of the Delaney Clause could confer a false sense of security with respect to many substances to which we are exposed and that happen to prove negative in the particular animal species tested.

THE PRESENT REGULATORY SYSTEM

The present regulatory system, while based upon explicit law and giving the appearance of providing a straightforward method for decision making, is based in part upon some rather dubious scientific assumptions:

1. *That all species of animals and man react similarly to the same environmental agents.* In fact, the various species respond quite differently, depending upon their metabolic systems, etc. For example, the chemical β-naphthylamine causes bladder cancer quite readily in dogs, less frequently in mice, and only rarely in rats and rabbits.
2. *That strains or types of animals of a given species react similarly to environmental agents.* In fact, inbred strains of laboratory animals may respond quite differently to the same agent. For example, while breast cancer is a major cause of death in some strains of mice, it is rare in others (MacKenzie and Garner, 1973; Smith, Walford, and Mickey, 1973).

3. *That the experimental conditions of study are relatively unimportant.* In fact, doses of drugs used, the duration of their use, the age of the animals tested, as well as the routes of administration of the test materials, are all critically important in determining whether or not the disease becomes manifest.

4. *That when a drug or chemical fails to produce cancer in rats or other laboratory animals, it may be presumed safe for man as well.* If test findings are negative in the rat, will they necessarily be so in the mouse, in the monkey, or in man? That this assumption tends to confer upon us a false sense of security should be evident from the species differences in responses to toxic challenges noted previously. This particular shortcoming of the present regulatory system is often ignored by those who regard the Delaney Amendment as erring, if at all, "on the safe side."

5. *That the findings of scientific investigations tend to be highly consistent.* In fact, the reverse is often true. For example, earlier studies on the possible adverse effects of artificial sweeteners yielded highly diverse results, with a few experiments suggesting carcinogenic effects, some revealing none, and others yielding equivocal or uninterpretable results. What should be the regulatory decision when, for example, the results of one rat study (say, on saccharin and bladder cancer) are positive while the results of other studies in rat or monkey or man are negative? Should one positive study outweigh the negatives, irrespective of quality? Should two (or 5 or 10) negative studies outweigh one positive? Present law tends to ignore such subtleties and to invoke regulatory action whenever *any* studies are positive, irrespective of the number or quality of negative studies. Statistically, one can expect a proportion of studies to be spuriously "positive" on the basis of chance alone.

The Delaney-type approach to cancer regulation may also be characterized as permitting undue attention to extremely weak carcinogens such as saccharin and distracting attention and scientific resources from other cancer problems far more urgently in need of study. For example, although cervical cancer is one of the most common malignancies, some 30%–40% of American women at high risk of this disease are not receiving the benefits of Papanicolaou testing on a regular basis. It appears that no serious attempts are under way to deal with this important subgroup of the population. Similarly, although 90% of lung cancer is attributable to cigarette smoking, no congressional hearings are contemplated to demand more effective action against this principal cancer killer of United States males.

The point is that, in a sense, the Delaney Amendment sits waiting to be invoked by positive findings in whatever study happens to be undertaken for whatever reason. One wonders about the myriad of substances that are *not* being tested simply because researchers are not interested in them. Naturally, since no studies are being done, no positive findings are being reported and, under the law, the substances are construed as safe.

ALTERNATIVES TO THE DELANEY APPROACH

We should be striving for a regulatory system that: 1) recognizes our present fallibility and the incompleteness of our knowledge about cancer, 2) is not based upon simplistic "black-and-white" criteria, 3) permits a reasoned assessment of the benefits and risks of each regulatory decision, 4) reduces public anxiety and the polarization of public opinion, 5) encourages the cooperation of industry in testing food and drug safety, rather than alienating it, and 6) relieves government of political pressures to make hasty regulatory decisions.

The decision-making process on health questions should not be locked in a rigid box that permits only two modes of operation, wide open or tightly shut. If the crucial decisions are made on an ad hoc basis by panels of scientists expert on the particular regulatory question at issue, a system flexible enough to take into account all the relevant factors can be developed. Our regulatory system could benefit from substitution of expert opinion for the rigid legal box of the Delaney Amendment. Such an arrangement could readily be accommodated by the existing general safety provisions of the Food Additives Amendment of 1958, which requires that food additives be safe for human consumption.

Ad hoc panels on particular regulatory questions could be established by the Food and Drug Administration and legislation enacted to grant their decisions the same legal authority as that previously vested in the Delaney Amendment process. A given panel, consisting of researchers in the scientific area of inquiry, as well as representatives of government, industry, and the general public could: 1) periodically review existing knowledge and recommend action in their mandated area of interest, 2) identify related problems requiring research, 3) recommend the provision of funds for studies, in both man and animals, of such questions, and 4) assist the Food and Drug Administration in establishing a more systematic monitoring of the impact of foods and drugs on the health of the public. There is, of course, no logical reason to restrict their mandate to questions relating to cancer. Birth defects, cardiovascular disease, and all other important killers and maimers of society could be regulated in this fashion.

The expert panels would make ad hoc decisions on the basis of the best available data, with special emphasis on implications for human disease. A wide variety of decisions would be possible, including: 1) immediate ban, 2) delayed ban, 3) warning labels, 4) prescription-restricted sales, and 5) incentives to industry for developing potentially safer substitute products.

A more flexible and scientific (as opposed to legalistic) regulatory system for foods and drugs would be appreciated by the public and supported by industry, prove administratively effective for government, and be conducive to the advancement of our knowledge on human health and disease.

REFERENCES

Crout, J. R. 1978. The Nature of Regulatory Choices. Center for the Study of Drug Development, PS 7812. University of Rochester, Rochester, N.Y.

Dunn, T. B. 1975. Carcinogenic action of estrogens (letter to the editor). N. Engl. J. Med. 285:1147.

Food and Drug Administration, Department of Health, Education, and Welfare. 1977. Saccharin and its salts: Proposed rule and hearing. Federal Register 42:19996–20010.

Hammond, E. C. 1969. Life expectancy of American men in relation to their smoking habits. J. Natl. Can. Inst. 43:951–962.

Health Research Group. 1977. Cancer Prevention and the Delaney Clause. Rev. Ed. 2000 P Street, N.W., Washington, D.C.

Herbst, A. 1976. Summary of changes in the human female genital tract as a consequence of maternal diethylstilbestrol therapy. J. Toxicol. Environ. Health 1(suppl):13–20.

Herbst, A. L., Poskanzer, D. C., Robboy, S. J., Friedlander, L., and Scully, R. E. 1975. Prenatal exposure to stilbestrol: A prospective comparison of exposed female offspring with unexposed controls. N. Engl. J. Med. 292:334–339.

Kessler, I. I. 1971. Mortality experience of diabetic patients: A 26-year follow-up study. Am. J. Med. 51:718–724.

Kolata, G. B. 1976. Chemical carcinogens: Industry adopts controversial "quick" tests. Science 192:1215–1217.

Levin, D. L. Devesa, S. S., Godwin, J. D., and Silverman, D. T. 1974. Cancer rates and risks. 2nd Ed. U.S. Department of Health, Education, and Welfare, Publication No. (NIH) 75-691, Washington, D.C.

Lilienfeld, A. M., Levin, M. L., and Kessler, I. I. 1972. Cancer in the United States. Vital and Health Statistics Monograph Series, American Public Health Association, Harvard University Press, Cambridge, Mass.

McGill, W. J. 1977. Quoted in unsigned article, Point of View. Science 198:275.

MacKenzie, W. F., and Garner, F. M. 1973. Comparison of neoplasms in six sources of rats. J. Natl. Cancer Inst. 50:1243–1257.

National Academy of Sciences. 1975. Sweeteners: Issues and uncertainties. Academy Forum, Washington, D.C.

Occupational Safety and Health Administration, Department of Labor. 1977. Identification, classification and regulation of toxic substances posing a potential occupational carcinogenic risk. Federal Register 42:54148–54247.

Office of Technology Assessment, U.S. Congress. 1977. Cancer testing technology and saccharin. Library of Congress catalog card No. 77-600051, Washington, D.C.

Robboy, S. J., Scully, R. E., Welch, W. R., and Herbst, A. L. 1977. Intrauterine diethylstilbestrol exposure and its consequences. Arch. Pathol. Lab. Med. 101:1–5.

Rowe, W. D. 1977. Governmental regulation of societal risks. George Washington Law Rev. 45:944–968.

Sivak, A. 1976. The Ames assay (letter to the editor). Science 193:272–273.

Smith, G. S., Walford, R. L., and Mickey, M. R. 1973. Lifespan and incidence of cancer and other diseases in selected long-lived inbred mice and their F_1 hybrids. J. Natl. Cancer Inst. 50:1195–1213.

Thomas, D. L. 1975. Bitter and the sweet: The ban on cyclamate was a triumph of pseudo-science. Barron's pp. 3–12.

Index

Additives in food, *see* Food additives
Advice rules, in CANSCREEN, 86–87
Aflatoxin
 carcinogenicity of, 238, 250, 256
 in foodstuffs, 220, 238
AFP, *see* Alpha-fetoprotein
Agamma-globulinemic state, sex-linked,
  immune response in, 40
Age groups
 breast fluid analysis in, 166–167, 177,
  179
 mortality rates in, 8–9, 184–185, 189
 and risk for cancer, 4, 62, 67, 74, 89,
  90, 92, 252
  animal studies of, 231
  in breast cancer, 46, 47, 62, 67,
   183, 184–185, 186, 187–188,
   190, 191
 site-specific screening in, 62, 64, 67,
  74, 183, 184–185, 186,
  187–188, 190, 191
AG-e screening, in cervical cancer
  detection, 22–23, 39
AG-4, associated with uterine cervical
  cancer, 22, 39, 42, 48
Air monitoring, for carcinogenic
  agents, 24
Alcohol use
 counseling affecting, 97, 98
 as risk factor, 90, 92
Alkylating agents, in chemotherapy,
  156
Alpha-fetoprotein (AFP) in immunodiagnosis, 128–129, 131, 132
 false-positive results with, 129
 used with other monkeys, 131
American Cancer Society, establishment of, 3
American Society for Control of
  Cancer, establishment of, 3
Amino acid deficiency, cancer risk in,
  40
Aminopterin, in chemotherapy, 156
Anemia, pernicious, assessing cancer
  risk in, 42, 90
Angiography
 in brain cancer, 201, 202, 203
 compared to computerized tomography, 201, 202

in pancreatic cancer, 200
Aniline dyes, occupational exposure to,
  6, 20–21
Animal feeds, carcinogenic material in,
  209, 217, 219, 237, 238, 244,
  260
Animal studies
 on aflatoxin, 220, 256
 on age and risk for cancer, 231
 applicability to humans, 23–25,
  217–218, 238, 251, 256,
  257–266
 of breast cancer, 265
 of chemotherapy, 158, 159, 160
 of cyclamates and saccharin,
  248–249, 250–251
 of DDT, 220
 in Delaney Clause, 209, 212,
  215–216, 217, 238, 259, 260,
  264
 of diethylstilbestrol, 255–256
 dose levels in, 217, 238, 259–260,
  264, 266
Antibiotics, in chemotherapy, 156
Antibody production
 antitumor, and cancer progression,
  27
 BCG vaccination affecting, 26
 in cancer patients, 132, 133–134, 137
Antigens, tumor-associated
 AG-e, 22–23, 39
 AG-4, 22, 39, 42, 48
 carcinoembryonic, 23, 65, 113–116,
  123, 126–128, 131, 132
 detection of antibodies to, 137
 in immunodiagnosis of cancer,
  122–123, 126–132, 134–138
 in production of vaccines against
  cancer, 26
 tissue, 123
 virus-induced, 22–23, 24–25, 26, 39,
  42, 48, 123, 137–138
Antimetabolites, in chemotherapy, 156
Appendectomy, cancer incidence after,
  257
Arsenic
 in leukemia, 155
 occupational exposure to, 6, 15
 toxic effects of, 255

Aryl hydrocarbon hydroxylase inducibility in lymphocytes, for screening cigarette smokers, 65
Asbestos exposure, cancer related to, 15, 21, 93
Assigned marketing system for consumer protection (AMSCOP), 25
Australia, cancer mortality rate in, 16
Austria, cancer mortality rate in, 16

BCG vaccine, 26–29
Belgium, cancer mortality rate in, 16
Benefit-risk considerations, 63–65, 68, 69, 74–76
  bias inherent in, 45, 97
  in brain cancer screening, 201, 202
  in breast cancer screening, 43–48, 63–64, 69, 74, 92, 98, 105, 113, 183, 188–192
  in consumer protection, 215, 218–220, 239–240, 244, 259, 263–264, 265
  cost factors in, 47–48, 65, 69, 70, 81, 105–106, 112–113, 116–117, 190, 191, 201
  decision-making process in, 44–48, 79–101, 105–106
  in immunodiagnosis, 124, 135
  in ROC analysis, 105, 112–113, 116–117
Benzol, occupational exposure to, 6, 15
3,4-Benzpyrene, as carcinogenic agent, 21
Beta emitters, in elimination of neoplastic microfoci, 42
Biases in screening program assessment, 45, 97
  in immunodiagnosis, 122
  lead time, 45, 97, 125, 186, 187, 190
  length, 45, 97
  selection, 97
Biochemical analysis of breast fluid, 165, 166, 170–177
Biochemical markers, in assessing cancer risk, 42
Biopsies, after breast cancer screening, 73, 74, 191

Birth control pills, as risk factor, 91
Bladder
  cancer of, 151–152
    age to begin screening for, 62
    animal studies on, 265
    CANSCREEN approach to, 81
    cytologic examination in, 151
    early detection of, 41
    external carcinogenic agents in, 6, 15, 20–21, 151
    incidence of, 4, 9, 10, 12, 13, 63, 224, 227
    in occupational groups, 6, 14, 20–21
    stages of, 151–152, 153
    surgical treatment of, 17
    survival rate in, 9, 12–13, 18
  papillomas of, cancer risk in, 42
Blood pressure, and hypertension as cancer risk factor, 91
Bone cancer
  carcinogenic agents related to, 15, 21
  mortality rate in, 13
Bowel cancer, see Gastrointestinal cancer
Brain cancer, 193, 200–202
  mortality rate in, 12
  screening for
    benefit-risk considerations in, 201, 202
    computerized tomography in, 200–202, 203
    costs of, 201
  survival rate in, 18
Breast aspiration pump, procedure for using, 166
Breast cancer, 65, 66, 183–192
  age-related risk for, 46, 47, 62, 67, 183, 184–185, 186, 187–188, 190, 191
  animal studies on, 265
  benefit-risk considerations in screening for, 43–48, 63–64, 69, 74, 92, 98, 105, 113, 183, 188–192
  biopsy recommended in, 73, 74, 191
  breast fluid analysis in, 165–180
  CANSCREEN approach to, 81, 82, 83
  carcinoembryonic antigen in, 126, 127

chemotherapy in, 157, 158, 159, 161
costs of screening for, 113, 190, 191
demonstration program for detection
    of, 43–44, 45, 46, 69, 70, 72,
    73–74
duration of stages in, 58
environmental carcinogenic agents in,
    177, 179
false-negative diagnosis of, 70
false-positive diagnosis of, 69,
    111–112, 191
follow-up after screening for, 188,
    190
HIP study on, 43, 44, 45, 46, 47,
    63–64, 74, 112, 113, 185, 187,
    188, 189–191
hormonal dependency of, 156
immunodiagnosis of, 135, 136, 137
incidence of, 4, 6, 9, 10, 12, 13, 62,
    63, 224
in situ, detection of, 165
lead time in, 186, 187, 190
mammography in, 43–48, 69, 73, 74,
    83, 98, 105, 110–112, 113,
    188, 189, 190–191
metastases at time of diagnosis of, 61
mortality rate in, 184–188, 189
paramedical personnel in screening
    for, 68–69
periodicity of screening for, 189–190
physical examination in, 65, 71, 73
pregnancy affecting risk for, 179
self-examination for, 83, 98
surgical treatment of, 17, 156, 158,
    170, 172, 175, 176
survival rate in, 18
thermography in, 65, 69, 72, 73
and transmission of carcinogenic
    influences, 24
viruses associated with, 123, 137
Breast Cancer Detection Demonstration
    Program (BCDDP), 43–44,
    45, 46, 69, 70, 72–74
Breast disease
  breast fluid cytology in, 168, 169
  as risk factor, 91
Breast fluid analysis, 163–180
  age variations in, 166–167, 177, 179
  biochemical, 165, 166, 170–176
  cytologic, 165, 166, 167–170
  and earwax type, 166–167, 168
  extrinsically derived substances in,
      176–177, 179
  histologic, 168–169
  immunologic, 170–176
  and procedure for obtaining fluid,
      166
  racial variations in, 166–167, 177
Bronchoscopy, in lung cancer, 72, 195,
    202–203
Buccal cavity cancer, 6, 12, 14
Burkitt's lymphoma
  chemotherapy in, 156, 157
  Epstein-Barr virus associated with,
      123, 137
  vaccination against, 26

Calamus oil, FDA regulation of, 216,
    240
Canada, cancer in, 16, 31, 225
Cancer basic protein, and lymphocyte
    stimulation in immunodiagno-
    sis, 136–137
CANSCREEN program, 80–88
  advice rules in, 86–87
  control population compared to,
      98–101
  decision logic in, 83–86, 94, 95–96
  evaluation of outcomes in, 96–101
  false-negative results in, 95–96
  follow-up in, 87
  health counseling in, 82, 86–87,
      97–98
  health history questionnaire in, 83,
      91–92, 94–95
  multisite screening in, 81–82
  nurse examiner in, 83, 95
  objective of, 81
  primary prevention in, 97–98
  risk factors in, 90–92, 93–94
    self-reporting of, 83, 91–92, 94–95
  secondary prevention in, 96–97
  validity and reliability of, 94–101
Carcinoembryonic antigen (CEA), 23,
    65, 123
  in breast cancer, 126, 127
  and CEA-S test, 128
  false-positive results with, 126, 128,
      131

Carcinoembryonic antigen (CEA)—
  continued
  in gastrointestinal cancer, 113–116,
    126–128, 131, 132
  in lung cancer, 126, 127
  sensitivity of testing with, 65
  used with other markers, 131
Carcinogenesis
  external agents in, *see* External
    carcinogenic agents
  stages of, *see* Stages of cancer
Carcinoma in situ, definition of, 147
Cell-mediated immunity, 27, 40
  cytotoxicity assays of, 134, 135–136
  delayed hypersensitivity tests in, 27,
    134, 135
  leukocyte adherence inhibition assay
    of, 134, 136
  leukocyte migration inhibition assay
    of, 134, 136
  lymphocyte proliferation in, 134,
    136–137
  macrophage electrophoretic mobility
    test of, 134, 136
  in melanoma, 27, 135, 136
  to tumor antigens, 25, 26, 123, 133,
    134–136
Cellular alterations in cancer
  nucleus in, 144, 147, 148
  prevention of, 11, 18, 20, 40–42
Cervix uteri cancer
  accuracy of screening for, 36, 150
  age at time of screening for, 62
  antigens associated with, 22–23, 26,
    39, 42, 48, 123, 137
  CANSCREEN approach to, 81, 83
  colposcopic examination in, 34, 151
  disappearance of precancerous
    lesions, 148–149
  duration of stages in, 59, 96, 148,
    149–150, 153
  dyskaryosis in, 148
  dysplasia as precursor of, 48, 148,
    149, 151
  early detection of, 41
  effectiveness of screening for, 32–36,
    39, 49, 64
  fitter cell theory of, 144, 147–148
  histologic examination in, 150–151
  incidence of, 13, 34, 35, 36, 63, 224,
    226

interpretation of screening for,
    150–151
  intraepithelial lesions of, 149–150
  metastases at time of diagnosis of, 61
  mortality rate in, 32–34, 35, 49
  origins of, 144, 145–151
  Pap test in, 3–4, 30–39, 48–49, 64,
    65, 74, 83, 147, 150
  precancerous lesions of, 148–150
  risk for, 42, 92, 93
  self-screening for, 37–39, 49, 65
  squamocolumnar junction in, 147
  surgical treatment of, 17
  survival rate in, 18, 34
  transformation zone in, 147
Chemical structure of substances,
    related to carcinogenic activ-
    ity, 21–22
Chemical tests in screening programs,
    65, 71, 72
Chemotherapy for cancer control, 41,
    43, 155–161
  adjuvant, 158–159
  after irradiation, 158, 159
  after surgery, 158, 160
  animal models of, 158, 159, 160
  antitumor compounds in, 156
  combinations of drugs in, 156, 158
  growth rate of tumor affecting,
    157–158, 159, 160
  historical aspects of, 155–157
  proliferative rebound in, 159
  remission with, 60, 156, 157
  tumors responsive to, 157–158
Childhood neoplasms
  chemotherapy in, 158
  genetic mechanisms in, 24, 39
Chile, cancer mortality rate in, 16
Chimney sweeps, cancer in, 21
Chloroform, proposed banning of, 240
Choriocarcinoma
  chemotherapy in, 156, 157
  screening programs for, 72
Cigarette smoking
  counseling affecting, 82, 97
  and immunodiagnosis, 124
  and lung cancer, 194, 195, 255, 256,
    262, 266
  and pancreatic cancer, 198
  as risk factor, 25, 39, 42, 62, 65,
    67–68, 90, 92

interaction of other factors with, 93
Coal miners, cancer in, 15, 21
Coal tar derivatives
  need for proper study of, 219
  occupational exposure to, 6, 15
Colombia, cancer incidence in, 225
Colon cancer, see Gastrointestinal cancer
Colonoscopy, in colon cancer screening, 69, 72
Color additives in food, regulation of, 209, 237, 244
Colposcopy, in cervical cancer detection, 34, 151
Computerized tomography
  in brain cancer, 200–202, 203
  in pancreatic cancer, 200
Conditional probability
  false-negative, 109–110
  false-positive, 109–110
  true-negative, 109–110
  true-positive, 109–110
Confidence threshold, concept of, 107–108
Consumer Product Safety Act, 244, 246–247
Consumer protection from carcinogenic agents, 24, 25
  assigned marketing system for, 25
  benefit-risk considerations in, 215, 218–220, 239–240, 244, 245, 254, 259, 263–264, 265
  Delaney Clause in, see Delaney Clause
Contamination effect, in mammographic screening program, 46–47
Contraceptives, oral, as risk factor, 91
Costs of screening procedures
  benefits compared to, 47–48, 65, 69, 70, 81, 105–106, 112–113, 116–117
  in brain cancer, 201
  in breast cancer, 113, 190, 191
  ROC analysis of, 112–113
Coumarin, FDA regulation of, 240
Counseling, health, in CANSCREEN, 82, 86–87, 97–98
Cyclamates
  banning of, 216, 238, 248–249

FDA regulation of, 240
  testing of, 216, 238, 248–249, 250–251, 254–255
Cyclophosphamide, in metastatic Burkitt's lymphoma, 156
Cytologic examination, 40–41, 144–145, 147
  applications of, 65
  in bladder cancer, 151
  of breast fluid, 165, 166, 167–170
    in dysplasia, 168, 169
    in hyperplasia, 168, 169
  circulating, 71
  epidemiologic significance of data in, 143–153
  exfoliative, 70, 71
    false diagnosis in, 36, 48
    irrigation method, 37–39
    Pap procedure for, 3–4, 30–39, 48–49, 64, 65, 74, 83, 147, 150
    sensitivity of, 64
  in precancerous states, 152
  self-administered, 37–39, 49, 65
  of sputum, in lung cancer, 59, 65, 69, 194–198, 203
Cytotoxicity
  assays in immunodiagnosis of cancer, 134, 135–136
  cell-mediated, 134, 135–136
  humoral factors in, 134, 136

DDT, in foodstuffs, 220, 261
Death rate in cancer, see Mortality rate
Decision-making process
  in CANSCREEN, 83–86, 94, 95–96
  negative decisions in, 107, 108
  positive decisions in, 107, 108
  risk-factor analysis in, 44–48, 79–101, 105–106
  ROC analysis in, 105–117
  and true states, actually positive or negative, 107
Delaney Clause, 207–268
  alternatives to, 267–268
  animal studies in, 209, 212, 215–216, 217, 238, 259, 260, 264
  arguments favoring, 254–262
  basis of, 265–267
  evolution of, 209–213
  need for, 218–220

Delaney Clause—*continued*
political factors affecting, 249–250
requirements in, 209
zero tolerance principle in, 216–218,
        220, 260
Delayed hypersensitivity tests, 136
in cell-mediated immunity, 27, 134,
        135
primary sensitization in, 132, 133
with recall antigens, 132, 133
tumor extracts in, 134, 135
Denmark, cancer in, 16, 225
Diabetes, and cancer incidence, 40, 256
Diagnostic procedures, 67–76, 80
age factors in, 62, 64, 67, 74, 183,
        184–185, 186, 187–188, 190,
        191
benefit-risk considerations in, *see*
        Benefit-risk considerations
benign disease and cancer distin-
        guished in, 121–122, 124–125
biases in, 45, 97, 122, 125, 187, 190
in brain cancer, 200–202, 203
in breast cancer, *see* Breast cancer
and cancer control, 18, 19, 30–40,
        42, 43–48, 49, 57–66, 79
in CANSCREEN method, 80–101
in cervical cancer, *see* Cervix uteri
        cancer; Pap test
chemical tests in, 65, 71, 72
combination of approaches in, 72–73
confidence threshold in, 107–108
costs of, *see* Costs of screening
        procedures
cytologic, *see* Cytologic examination
decision criteria in, *see* Decision-
        making process
endoscopy in, 71, 72, 200
extent of disease determined in, 62,
        68, 121, 127
false-negative results in, 36, 68, 70,
        95–96, 107–110, 116
false-positive results in, *see* False-
        positive diagnosis
and follow-up phase, 87, 188, 190
in gastrointestinal cancer, *see* Gastro-
        intestinal cancer
hard-to-reach groups in, 90
high-risk population identified in,
        62–65, 66, 67–76, 121, 124,
        126

history-taking in, 70, 71, 83, 91–92,
        94–95
imaging in, *see* Imaging in screening
        programs
immunodiagnosis in, *see* Immuno-
        diagnosis
interpretation of variations in,
        152–153
in lung cancer, *see* Lung cancer
multisite, 81–82
nonacceptance of, 68, 69, 74, 75
nonavailability of, 74, 75
in pancreatic cancer, 71, 72, 131,
        132, 198–200
paramedical personnel in, 68–69, 83,
        86–87, 95, 188
physical examination in, 65, 70, 71,
        73, 83, 95
presence or absence of cancer deter-
        mined in, 62, 107–117, 121
requirements in, 68–70
ROC analysis of, 105–117
self-screening in, *see* Self-screening
        procedures
signal detection theory in, 105–117
and stage of cancer, 59–62, 66, 68,
        125
traditional approach to, 80
true negative and positive results in,
        107–110
Dibenzanthracene variations, carcino-
        genicity of, 22
Diet
and cancer, 40, 42, 225, 227
Delaney Clause regulating carcino-
        genic agents in, 207–268
GRAS substances in, 234–236, 244
and life expectancy, 231
trends in changes of, 227–231
and yearly intake of selected items,
        236–237
Diethylprocarbonate (DEPC), FDA
        regulation of, 216, 240
Diethylstilbestrol (DES)
in animal feeds, 209, 219, 260
animal studies on, 255–256
FDA regulation of, 216, 217, 240,
        255–256, 260
and vaginal cancer, 255–256
and vertical transmission of carcino-
        genic influences, 24

1,2-Dihydro-2,2,4-trimethylquinoline, polymerized, FDA regulation of, 239, 240
7,12-Dimethylbenzanthracene, carcinogenicity of, 22
Dimethylnitrosamine, carcinogenicity of, 256
Dinitrochlorobenzene (DNCB), in delayed hypersensitivity tests, 132, 133
DNA synthesis, and tumor susceptibility to drugs, 157
N-Dodecane, animal studies on, 218
Dose levels
    of chemicals in animal studies, 217, 238, 259–260, 264, 266
    of radiation exposure, and cancer risk, 45, 74, 190
Down's syndrome, cancer risk in, 42
Drugs in cancer control, see Chemotherapy
Dulcin, FDA regulation of, 240
Dyskaryosis, and uterine cervix carcinogenesis, 148
Dysplasia
    of breast, cytologic examination in, 168, 169
    of uterine cervix, 48, 148, 149, 151

Earwax type, and breast secretions, 166, 167, 168
Education
    in CANSCREEN approach, 83, 86–87, 97–98
    in prevention of cancer, 80
Electrostatic x-ray imaging, 71
Endocrine abnormalities, cancer risk in, 42
Endoscopy, in screening programs, 71, 72, 200
    in pancreatic cancer, 72, 200
England, cancer in, 16, 225, 227
Environmental agents in cancer, see External carcinogenic agents
Environmental Protection Agency, 244, 246–247
Enzymes
    in cancer screening, 71, 72
    in chemotherapy, 156

Epidemiologic studies
    of breast cancer and breast secretory activity, 176–180
    cytologic and histologic data in, 143–153
    of environmental agents as carcinogens, 256–258, 262, 263, 264
    of pancreatic cancer, 198
    of risk for cancer, 89–90
    triad in, 25, 252–253, 257, 260, 262
    variables affecting, 152
Epstein-Barr virus (EBV)
    tumors associated with, 24, 123, 137
    vaccination against, 26
Esophageal cancer
    incidence of, 5, 6, 10, 12
    mortality rate in, 12, 13
    in occupational groups, 6, 14
Estrogen therapy, see also Diethylstilbestrol
    in prostate cancer, 156
    as risk factor, 91
Ewing's sarcoma, chemotherapy in, 157, 158
External carcinogenic agents, 6, 14–15, 19–25, 151
    agent/host triad in, modifying effects of, 11, 18, 20, 25–30, 252–253, 257, 260, 262, 264–265
    animal studies of, 23–25, 209, 212, 215–218, 220, 238, 248–251, 255–266
    benefit-risk considerations of, 215, 218–220, 239–240, 244, 245, 254, 259, 263–264, 265
    in bladder cancer, 151
    breast epithelium exposure to, 177, 179
    chemical structure of, 21–22
    clinical studies of, 20–21
    combination of effects of, 218
    dose effects of, 217–218, 238, 256, 259–260, 261, 266
    environmental monitoring of, 24
    epidemiologic studies of, 256–258, 262, 263, 264
    experimental techniques in identification of, 21–23
    and genetic transmission of carcinogenic influences, 24, 39–40
    immunologic studies of, 25

External carcinogenic agents—*continued*
  immunopotentiation reducing effects
      of, 26–29
  incidence of cancer caused by, 80,
      223, 252–253, 254, 255
  in vitro test systems for, 23
  macromolecular indicators of, 22–23
  National Cancer Program Plan for,
      11, 18, 19–25
  occupation-related, *see* Occupational
      carcinogenic agents
  regulation of
    alternatives to, 267–268
    current statutes for, 244, 245,
        246–249, 265–267
    Delaney Clause for, *see* Delaney
        Clause
    dilemma in, 262–265
    recent proposals for, 251–253
  viral, 22–23, 24–25, 26, 39, 42, 48,
      123, 137–138
  and zero tolerance principle,
      216–218, 220, 260, 265

False-negative diagnosis, 68, 70, 107
  in breast cancer, 70
  in CANSCREEN, 95–96
  in colon cancer, 116
  frequency of, 107–110
    conditional probability of, 109–110
  in Pap test, 36
False-positive diagnosis, 68, 69, 107
  in alpha-fetoprotein testing, 129
  in breast cancer, 69, 111–112, 191
  in CANSCREEN, 96
  in carcinoembryonic antigen assay,
      126, 128, 131
  in colon cancer, 115
  frequency of, 107–110
    acceptable levels of, 125–126
    conditional probability of, 109–110
  in Pap test, 48
  problems associated with, 125
  in tuberculosis, 109, 110
Farmers, cancer risk in, 6, 14
Federal Cancer Control Program, 4
Federal Hazardous Substances Act,
    244, 248–249

Females
  mortality rate in cancer, 7–8, 8–9,
      12–13, 16
  risk for cancer, 4–5, 6, 10, 62,
      223–226
Fetal cells, tumor antigens associated
    with, 123
Fetoprotein, *see* Alpha-fetoprotein
Fiberoptic bronchoscopy
  in lung cancer, 195, 202–203
  in neoplasm localization, 195
Finland, cancer in, 7, 16, 225
Fitter cell theory of carcinogenesis,
    144, 145, 146
  immortal and mortal cells in, 144,
      145, 146
  in uterine cervix cancer, 144, 147–148
Fluoroscopy, in artificial pneumo-
    thorax, 44, 45
Follow-up studies
  after breast cancer screening, 188,
      190
  in CANSCREEN, 87
Food, intake of, *see* Diet
Food additives
  benefit-risk analysis of, 218–220,
      239–240, 244, 254, 261, 265
  definition of, 237
  population pressures affecting use of,
      232–233
  regulation of
    current laws for, 243–244, 246–247
    Delaney Clause in, *see* Delaney
        Clause
  testing procedures for, 215, 237–238,
      244–245, 248–251, 254–262
  tolerance levels for, 238–239
Food and Drug Administration (FDA),
    regulation by, 237–240
  of artificial sweeteners, 216, 238,
      239, 240, 243, 245–251,
      254–255
  Delaney Clause in, *see* Delaney
      Clause
  of diethylstilbestrol, 216, 217, 240,
      255–256, 260
  drugs and food additives compared
      in, 245, 246–247
  GRAS lists in, 234–236, 244

political pressure affecting, 249–250, 261–262

Food, Drug and Cosmetic Act, 243–244, 245, 246–247

and Delaney Clause Amendment, *see* Delaney Clause

Food packaging procedures, 250, 251

France, cancer mortality rate in, 16

Gamma emitters, in neoplastic micro-foci detection, 42

Gastrointestinal cancer, 65
  age to begin screening for, 62
  CANSCREEN approach to, 81, 83
  carcinogenic agents related to, 15
  colonoscopy in, 69, 72
  drug susceptibility of, 157
  immunodiagnosis of, 121, 122, 126–128, 131, 132, 135
    carcinoembryonic antigen in, 113–116, 126–128, 131, 132
    fetal sulfoglycoprotein antigen in, 130–131
    multiple markers in, 131, 132
  incidence of, 4, 5–6, 10, 13, 62, 63, 224, 225, 227
  metastases at time of diagnosis of, 61
  mortality rate in, 12, 13
  in occupational groups, 14
  surgical treatment of, 17
  survival rate in, 18

Genetic mechanisms
  and carcinogenicity of external agents, 24, 30, 39–40
  in childhood neoplasms, 24, 39
  in fitter cell theory, 144, 146
  in risk factor approach, 90, 91, 92, 93
  in secretory activity of breast, 167
  in thyroid cancer, 129

Germany, cancer in, 16, 225

Gonadotropin, chorionic, in immuno-diagnosis, 131

GRAS (generally recognized as safe) food substances, 234–236, 244

Growth rate of tumors
  assessment of, 59
    tritiated thymidine in, 157, 159

and drug susceptibility, 157–158, 159, 160

and lead time, 125

Hazardous Substances Act, 244, 248–249

Head and neck cancer, viruses asso-ciated with, 123, 137

Health counselor, in CANSCREEN approach, 86–87, 97

Health Insurance Plan (HIP) of Greater New York, breast cancer screening study by
  benefit-risk considerations in, 43, 44, 47, 63, 74, 113, 185–192
  on costs of screening procedures, 113
  as definitive study, 45–46, 63–64
  dose exposures in, 45, 190–191
  incidence data from, 112

Hemochromatosis, and cancer risk, 42

Hepatoma, alpha-fetoprotein in screen-ing for, 128–129

Herpesvirus antigens
  AG-e, 22–23, 39
  AG-4, 22, 39, 42, 48
  HSV-2, 22, 24, 25, 26
    carcinogenic effects of, 24, 25
    humoral and cell-mediated immun-ity to, 25, 26
    uterine cervix cancer associated with, 22, 26
    vaccines against, 26
    uterine cervical cancer associated with, 22–23, 26, 39, 42, 48, 123, 137

Herpesvirus infections
  genital
    incidence of, 34
    Pap testing in, 48
  vaccination against, 26

Histologic examination
  of breast fluid, 168–169
  epidemiologic significance of data from, 143–153
  in uterine cervical cancer, 150–151

History-taking in screening program, 70, 71
  in CANSCREEN, 83, 91–92, 94–95

280   Index

Hodgkin's disease
  BCG vaccination in, 28–29
  chemotherapy in, 156, 157
  incidence of, 224
  mortality rate in, 12, 13, 18, 159
  survival rate in, 9, 12, 18
Hormones
  in chemotherapy, 156
  in screening for cancer, 71, 72
Humoral immune responses, 25, 26,
      40, 123, 134, 136
Hungary, cancer in, 225, 227
Hydatidiform mole, screening programs
      in, 72
Hyperplasia of breast, cytologic exami-
      nation in, 168, 169
Hypersensitivity, delayed, see Delayed
      hypersensitivity tests
Hypertension, as cancer risk factor, 91

Imaging in screening programs, 71–72
  confidence threshold in, 107–108
  frequency of incorrect interpretations
      in, 108–109
  isotopic, 42, 71, 201, 202
  mammography in breast cancer,
      43–48, 69, 73, 74, 83, 98, 105,
      110–112, 113, 188–191
  ROC analysis of, 107–108, 109,
      110–112
  thermography, 65, 69, 71, 72, 73
  ultrasound, 65, 71, 200
  x-ray, 65, 71, 194–198, 202, 203
Immortal cells, in fitter cell theory,
      144, 145, 146
Immune competence, diminished
  antibody production in, 132, 133–134
  and cancer risk assessment, 42, 123,
      132–134
  delayed hypersensitivity tests in,
      132, 133
  lymphocyte function in, 132, 133
  lymphocyte proliferation in, 132, 133
  macrophage function in, 132, 133
Immune response
  cell-mediated, 25, 26, 27, 40, 123,
      133, 134–137
  humoral, 25, 26, 40, 123, 134, 136
  immunopotentiation enhancing,
      26–29

  serum factor blocking, 123, 134, 136
  to tumor or virus-associated antigens,
      25, 26, 123, 133, 134–138
Immune response genes, 40
Immunodiagnosis, 121–138
  accuracy of, 121–122, 123–126
  alpha-fetoprotein in, 128–129, 131,
      132
  benefit-risk analysis of, 124, 135
  benign disease and cancer distin-
      guished in, 121–122
  bias in evaluation of, 122
  of breast cancer, 135, 136, 137
  cancer basic protein in, 136–137
  carcinoembryonic antigen in, 23, 65,
      113–116, 123, 126–128, 131,
      132
  clinical applications of, 121, 126–127,
      134
  current status of, 126–132
  cytotoxicity assays in, 134, 135–136
  delayed hypersensitivity tests in,
      27, 132, 133, 134, 136
  diminished immune competence in,
      42, 123, 132–134
  fetal sulfoglycoprotein antigen in,
      130–131
  leukocyte adherence inhibition assay
      in, 134, 136
  leukocyte migration inhibition assay
      in, 134, 136, 137
  lymphocyte function in, 132, 133
  lymphocyte proliferation in, 132,
      133, 134, 136–137
  macrophage electrophoretic mobility
      test in, 134, 136
  in monitoring of known cancer, 121,
      127
  multiple markers in, 131
  as screening procedure, 121, 126, 129
  thyrocalcitonin radioimmunoassay
      in, 129–130
  tumor antigens in, 122–123, 126–132,
      134–138
    soluble extracts prepared with 3 M
      KCl, 136
Immunoglobulins, in breast fluid,
      175–176
  in normal and cancer patients,
      170–176
Immunologic studies
  of breast fluid, 170–176

of cancer risk, 40, 71, 72, 257
of carcinogenic agents, 25
Immunopotentiation, and immune
    response to carcinogenic chal-
    lenge, 26–29
Immunotherapy, 26–29, 43
India, cancer incidence in, 225
International variations in cancer inci-
    dence, 16, 225, 227
Intestinal cancer, 12, 13, 14, 135
    see also Gastrointestinal cancer
Iodine-131, in thyroid cancer, 42
Ireland, cancer mortality rate in, 16
Irrigation pipette technique, in self-
    screening for cervical cancer,
    37
Isotopic imaging in screening programs,
    42, 71, 201, 202
Israel, cancer in, 16, 225
Italy, cancer mortality rate in, 16

Jamaica, cancer incidence in, 225, 227
Japan, cancer in, 16, 225

Kidney cancer
    CANSCREEN approach to, 81
    incidence of, 224
    mortality rate in, 12

Laparotomy, in pancreatic cancer diag-
    nosis, 199–200
Laryngoscopy, in screening programs,
    72
Larynx cancer
    CANSCREEN approach to, 81
    incidence of, 12, 13, 224
    survival rate in, 9, 12, 13, 18
Lead time bias in assessment, 45, 97,
    125, 186, 187, 190
Length bias in assessment, 45, 97
Leukemia
    BCG vaccination in, 27, 28
    carcinogenic agents related to, 6, 15
    chemotherapy in, 155, 156, 157
    immunodiagnosis in, 135, 136
    immunologic response in, control of,
    40
    incidence of, 6, 12, 224, 225
    mortality rate in, 12, 18, 28

in occupational groups, 6, 14
survival rate in, 9, 12, 18
and transmission of carcinogenic
    influences, 24
Leukocytes
    adherence inhibition assay, 134, 136
    migration inhibition assay, 134, 136,
    137
Life expectancy in cancer, 252
    Sweden and US compared, 231
    see also Survival rate
Liver cancer
    alpha-fetoprotein in screening for,
    128–129
    incidence of, 227
Lung cancer, 65, 193, 194–198, 202–203
    accuracy of screening for, 69
    age to begin screening for, 62, 67
    bronchoscopy in screening for, 72,
    95, 202–203
    calcitonin levels in, 130
    CANSCREEN approach to, 81, 82
    carcinogenic agents related to, 6, 15
    CEA assay in, 126, 127
    chemotherapy in, 158
    and cigarette smoking, 194, 195, 255,
    256, 262, 266
    duration of stages in, 59
    early detection of, 41
    incidence of, 4, 5, 6, 10, 12, 62, 63,
    194, 223, 224, 225, 227
    metastases at time of diagnosis of, 61
    occupational factors in, 6, 14–15, 21
    risk factor approach to, 93
    sputum cytology in, 59, 65, 69,
    194–198, 203
    survival rate in, 18, 194, 203
    x-ray screening for, 194–198, 203
Lymphocyte enumeration
    cancer basic protein in, 136–137
    in cell-mediated immunity, 134,
    136–137
    in diminished immune competence,
    132, 133
    rosette assay for, 132, 133
    tumor extracts treated with 3 M KCl
    in, 136
Lymphoma
    Burkitt, see Burkitt's lymphoma
    frequency of, 63, 224
    histiocytic, chemotherapy in, 157
    Hodgkin's, see Hodgkin's disease

Macromolecular indicators of carcinogenic agents, 22–23
Macrophage functions in cancer, 132,
133
electrophoretic mobility test of, 134,
136
Males
mortality rate in cancer, 7–8, 8–9,
12–13, 16
risk for cancer in, 4–5, 6, 10, 62,
223–226
Mammography in breast cancer screening, 43–48, 69, 73, 74, 105,
110–112, 188, 189, 190–191
in CANSCREEN, 83, 98
contamination effect in, 46–47
costs of, 113, 192
effectiveness of, 188, 189
false-positive diagnosis in, 111–112
risk-benefit analysis of, 43–48, 69,
74, 98, 105, 190–191
Massachusetts, statewide cancer control
programs of, 3
Mastectomy in breast cancer
breast fluid analysis after, 170, 172,
175, 176
chemotherapy after, 158
Mastitis, cystic, and cancer risk, 42, 46
Melanoma
BCG vaccination in, 27
cell-mediated immunity in, 27, 135,
136
incidence of, 227
surgical treatment of, 17
survival rate in, 18
Menarche, age of, as risk factor, 91
Mercaptoimidazoline, FDA regulation
of, 240
Metabolic considerations in cancer risk,
29–30, 39–40
Metastatic disease
chemotherapy in, 155–161
at time of diagnosis, 59, 60–62, 66,
68, 125
Methotrexate, in choriocarcinoma, 156
4,4'-Methylenebis, FDA regulation of,
239–240
Mitotic inhibitors, in chemotherapy,
156
Mortal cells, in fitter cell theory, 144,
145

Mortality rate in cancer, 4–11, 16, 225,
226, 231, 252
by age groups, 8–9, 184–185,
187–188, 189
chemotherapy affecting, 159–160,
161
compared to other diseases, 7, 8–9,
232, 252
and Delaney Clause, 212–213
international variations, 6–7, 16
male/female ratio of, 7–8, 8–9,
12–13, 16
occupation-related, 14
site-related, 12–13, 18
Mutagenicity assays, for prediction of
carcinogenicity, 23
Mycobacterium tuberculosis, immunization against, and cancer
resistance, 26–29
Mycosis fungoides, chemotherapy in,
157
Myeloma, multiple, survival rate in,
9, 18

β-Naphthylamine, animal and human
studies of, 218, 265
Nasal cavity cancer, carcinogenic agents
related to, 15
Nasopharyngeal cancer, Epstein-Barr
virus associated with, 123, 137
National Cancer Institute, 3, 4
National Cancer Program Plan, 4,
11–51
control components of, 11, 18, 19,
20, 43
diagnostic procedures in, 11, 18, 19,
20
objectives of, 11, 18, 19
Operational Plan of, 11
Overall Strategic Plan in, 11
prevention in, 11, 18, 20, 41–42
rehabilitation in, 18, 19, 20, 43
research components of, 11, 18, 19
risk assessment in, 11, 18, 19–40, 42
treatment assessment in, 18, 19, 20,
43–48, 49–51
Negative diagnosis
false, *see* False-negative diagnosis
true, 107–110

Netherlands, cancer mortality rate in, 16

New York, statewide cancer control programs of, 3

New Zealand, cancer in, 16, 225, 227

Nigeria, cancer incidence in, 225

Nitrates in food products, safety of, 239

Nitrogen mustard, in chemotherapy, 156

Norway
  cancer incidence in, 225
  cancer mortality rate in, 7, 16

Nurse examiner, in CANSCREEN approach in, 83, 95

Nutrition, see Diet

Obesity, as risk factor, 91

Occupational carcinogenic agents, 6, 15, 20–21, 24, 25
  regulation of, 244, 245, 248, 249, 253
    recent proposals for, 251–252
  as risk factors, 6, 14, 20–21, 42, 62, 90, 91–92, 93
  sites affected by, 6, 14, 15, 20–21, 151

Occupational Safety and Health Act, 244, 245, 248–249

Orchiectomy, in prostate cancer, 156

Ovariectomy, in breast cancer, 156

Ovary cancer
  incidence of, 4, 6, 10, 12, 63, 224
  surgical treatment of, 17
  survival rate in, 18

P-4000, FDA regulation of, 240

Pancreatic cancer, 193, 198–200, 203
  and cigarette smoking, 198
  clinical indications of, 203
  endoscopy in screening for, 72, 200
  immunodiagnosis of, 131, 132
  incidence of, 5, 6, 9, 10, 12, 63, 198, 224, 225
  laparotomy in diagnosis of, 199–200
  metastases at time of diagnosis of, 61, 62
  mortality rate in, 198
  surgical treatment of, 17

survival rate in, 9, 11, 12, 18, 198, 200

ultrasound in screening for, 71

Pap test for cervical cancer, 3–4, 30–39, 65, 147, 150
  accuracy of, 36, 48
  in CANSCREEN approach, 83
  effectiveness of, 31, 32–36, 48–49, 64
  nonacceptance of, 38, 49, 74
  self-screening compared to, 37–39

Para-aminodiphenyl, and bladder cancer risk, 151

Paraffin exposure, and cancer, 21

Paramedical personnel in screening programs, 68–69, 83, 86–87, 95, 188

Pharynx cancer
  early detection of, 41
  incidence of, 6, 12
  in occupational groups, 6, 14

L-Phenylalanine mustard, in breast cancer therapy, 158

Physical examination in screening programs, 65, 70, 71
  in breast cancer, 65, 71, 73
  in CANSCREEN, 83, 95

Pneumoencephalography, compared to computerized tomography, 201, 202

Pneumothorax, artificial, fluoroscopy in treatment of, 44, 45

Poland, cancer incidence in, 225

Polyposis
  intestinal, 40
    and cancer risk, 90
  multiple, and cancer risk, 42, 93

Population growth, and food additive use, 232–233

Portugal, cancer mortality rate in, 7, 16

Positive diagnosis
  false, see False-positive diagnosis
  true, 107–110

Precancerous lesions
  in bladder cancer, 151
  cytology in detection of, 152
  in uterine cervix caner, 148–150

Pregnancy, and breast cancer risk, 179

Prevention of cancer
  education in, 80
  in National Cancer Program Plan, 11, 18, 19, 20, 41–42

Prevention of cancer—*continued*
  primary, 43, 97–98
  secondary, 43, 96–97
  tertiary, 18, 19, 20, 43
Proctoscopy, in CANSCREEN, 83
Proctosigmoidoscopy, in screening
    programs, 69, 72
Prognosis in cancer, *see* Mortality rate;
    Survival rate
β-Propiolactone, carcinogenicity of, 22
Prostate cancer, 65
  age to begin screening for, 62
  CANSCREEN approach to, 81, 83
  incidence of, 4, 6, 9, 10, 12, 13, 63,
    224, 225
  metastases at time of diagnosis, 61
  risk in prostate infections, 90
  surgical treatment of, 17, 156
  survival rate in, 9, 12, 18
Psychological problems
  in false-positive diagnosis, 135
  and prognosis in cancer, 42
  in rehabilitation of cancer patient, 43
Puerto Rico, cancer incidence in, 225

Racial groups
  breast fluid in, 166–167, 177
  cancer risks in, 4, 5–6, 10
  cervical cancer in, 32, 33, 35, 36
Radiation exposure
  diagnostic, 65, 71
    in computerized tomography, 202
    dose-related risk of, 45, 73, 190
    electrostatic imaging method in, 71
    in lung cancer, 194–198, 203
    in mammography, 43–48, 69, 73,
      74, 83, 98, 105, 110–112, 113,
      188–191
    in pancreatic cancer, 200
    risk-benefit analysis of, 43–48, 69,
      90, 98, 105, 190–191
    silver halide method in, 71
  occupational, 6, 15, 21
  to sun, and effects of counseling,
    97, 98
  therapeutic, 43
    chemotherapy after, 158, 159
Radioactive dust, as carcinogenic agent,
    15, 21

Receiver Operating Characteristic
    (ROC) analysis, 105–117
  average cost and net benefit in,
    112–113
  in breast cancer diagnosis, 110–112
  in colon cancer screening, 113–116
  confidence threshold concept in,
    107–108
  conventional curve in, 108–110
  negative and positive diagnosis in,
    107–110
Rectal cancer, 14, 17, 18
Red Dye No. 2, carcinogenicity of,
    216, 238
Rehabilitation of cancer patient, 18, 19,
    20, 43
Remission, in chemotherapy, 60, 156,
    157
Research
  funding priorities in, 50–51, 198–199,
    203
  and National Cancer Program Plan,
    11, 18, 19
Reticuloendothelial system, BCG vacci-
    nation affecting, 26, 28
Retinoblastoma
  chemotherapy in, 157, 158
  and transmission of carcinogenic in-
    fluences, 24, 39
Rhabdomyosarcoma, chemotherapy in,
    157, 158
Rhodesia, cancer incidence in, 225
Risk-benefit considerations, *see*
    Benefit-risk considerations
Risks of developing cancer, 4–6, 81
  in age groups, 4, 62, 67, 74, 89, 90,
    92, 231, 252
  biochemical markers in assessment
    of, 42
  in breast cancer, 46, 47, 62, 67, 183,
    184–185, 186, 187–188, 190,
    191
  CANSCREEN approach to, 80–88,
    90–92, 93–95
  in cervical cancer, 42, 92, 93
  and decision-making in screening,
    44–48, 79–101, 105–106
  early detection in reduction of, 30–36
  environmental factors in, 6, 14–15,
    19–25

epidemiologic considerations in,
89–90
genetic considerations in, 24, 30,
39–40, 90, 91, 92, 93, 129,
144, 146
identification of high-risk population, 62, 66, 67, 75, 124, 126
immunodiagnosis in assessment of,
121, 124, 126, 129
immunopotentiation in reduction of,
26–29
interaction of factors in, 93–94
metabolic considerations in, 29–30,
39–40
modifying individuals to minimize
risk, 11, 18, 20, 25–40
and National Cancer Program Plan,
11, 18, 19–40, 42
occupational, 6, 14, 20–21, 42, 62,
90, 91–92, 93
in racial groups, 4, 5–6, 10, 32, 33,
35, 36
self-reporting of, 83, 91–92, 94–95
in sex groups, 4–5, 6, 10, 62, 223–226
site-related, 62–63
ROC, see Receiver Operating Characteristic analysis
Romania, cancer incidence in, 225
Rosette assay, in lymphocyte enumeration, 132, 133
Rubber gaskets in contact with food,
FDA regulation of, 216

Saccharin
assessing risk of, 23, 24, 259,
263–264, 265
controversy in regulation of, 216,
239, 243, 245–251, 254–255
Safrole, FDA regulation of, 216, 238,
240
Salmonella/Ames test, 23, 250
Sarcoma
BCG vaccination in, 27
and transmission of carcinogenic
influences, 24, 39
Sassafras oil, FDA regulation of, 216,
238, 240
Scotland, cancer mortality rate in, 16

Screening procedures, see Diagnostic
procedures
Scrotal cancer, carcinogenic agents in,
21
Selection bias, in screening program
assessment, 97
Selenium, tolerance level for, 238, 239
Self-screening procedures
for breast cancer, 83, 98
for cervical cancer, 37–39, 49, 65
Sex hormones in animal feeds, regulation of, 217
Sexual behavior, in risk factor approach, 90, 91, 92, 93
Signal detection theory, in early diagnosis of cancer, 105–117
Silver halide x-ray imaging, 71
Site of cancer
carcinogenic agents related to, 6, 15,
20–21
and mortality rate, 8–11, 12–13, 18
Skin cancer
CANSCREEN approach to, 81,
83–85
carcinogenic agents related to, 6, 15
melanoma, see Melanoma
occupational factors in, 6, 14–15, 21
Skin tests, see Delayed hypersensitivity
tests
Smoking, see Cigarette smoking
Socioeconomic groups, risk factors in,
90, 93
Soot exposure, and cancer, 21
South Africa, cancer in, 16, 225
Sputum cytology, in lung cancer screening, 59, 65, 69, 194–198, 203
Stages of cancer, 57–60, 143–144, 145
in bladder cancer, 151–152, 153
in breast cancer, 58, 61, 165
and carcinoma in situ, 146–147,
148–150, 151, 152, 153
in cervical cancer, 56, 96, 144,
145–151, 153
and drug susceptibility, 157–158
duration of, 56, 58–59, 65, 96,
149–150, 152, 153
fitter cell theory of, 144, 145, 147
squamocolumnar junction in, 147
at time of diagnosis, 59–62, 66, 68,
125, 129, 130, 165

Stages of cancer—*continued*
  transformation zone in, 147
Stomach cancer, *see* Gastrointestinal
  cancer
Strang Clinic, 3
Sugar consumption, yearly, 236–237,
  248
Surgery in cancer, 43
  in breast cancer, 156, 158, 170, 172,
    175, 176
  chemotherapy after, 158, 160
  in localized disease, 8–9, 17
  in prostate cancer, 156
Survival rate in cancer, 9–11, 12, 13, 18
  chemotherapy affecting, 157
  lead time bias in, 45, 97
  normal population compared to, 60,
    61
  screening programs affecting, 66, 79,
    129, 130
Sweden
  cancer in, 16, 225, 227
  life expectancy in, 231
Sweeteners, artificial
  benefit-risk analysis of, 239, 259,
    263–264, 265
  FDA regulation of, 216, 238, 240,
    243, 245–251, 254–255
  testing of, 23, 24, 248–249, 250–251,
    254–255, 259, 266
Switzerland, cancer mortality rate in,
  7, 16

T-globulin test, for immunodiagnosis
  of cancer, 122
Tar exposure, and cancer, 21
Teratomas, alpha-fetoprotein in screening for, 128
Testicles
  cancer of
    CANSCREEN approach to, 81, 83
    chemotherapy in, 157
  orchiectomy in prostate cancer, 156
  undescended, and cancer risk, 90
Thalidomide, congenital malformations from, 25
Thermography in screening programs,
  65, 69, 71, 72, 73
Thymidine, tritiated, in tumor growth
  assessment, 157, 159

Thyrocalcitonin radioimmunoassay, in
  thyroid cancer screening,
  129–130
Thyroid cancer
  CANSCREEN approach to, 81
  genetic predisposition to, 129
  iodine-131 in, 42
  mortality rate in, 13, 18
  survival rate in, 9, 13, 18
  thyrocalcitonin radioimmunoassay
    in, 129–130
Thyroiditis
  Hashimoto's, as risk factor, 91
  subacute, calcitonin levels in, 130
Tissue antigens, tumor-associated, 123
Tobacco chewing, as risk factor, 91
Tobacco smoking, *see* Cigarette
  smoking
Tomography, *see* Computerized tomography
Tongue cancer, incidence of, 13
Tonsillectomy, cancer incidence after,
  257
Toxic Substances Control Act,
  243–244, 246–247
Transformation zone, and carcinogene-
  sis in uterine cervix, 147
Tris, benefit-risk considerations for,
  245
True-negative diagnosis, 107
  frequency of, 107–110
True-positive diagnosis, 107
  frequency of, 107–110
Tuberculosis
  cancer antagonism with, 26–29
  false-positive diagnosis of, 109, 110

Ulcer, gastric, cancer risk in, 42, 90, 93
Ultrasound techniques in cancer diagnosis, 65, 71
  in pancreatic cancer, 71, 200
Uranium mining, as risk factor, 93
Urethane, in leukemia, 155
Urinary bladder, *see* Bladder
Uterine cancer, 17, 18, 60, 61, 62, 224
  age to begin screening for, 62
  cervical, *see* Cervix uteri cancer
  incidence of, 5, 6, 10, 62, 63, 224
  metastases at time of diagnosis, 60,
    61

surgical treatment of, 17
survival rate in, 18

Vaccines in cancer, 26–29, 43
Vaginal cancer
  and DES exposure, 255–256
  and transmission of carcinogenic
      influences, 24
Vaginal irrigation technique, 37
Venereal diseases, and cancer risk, 90
Violet No. 1, FDA regulation of, 216
Viruses, 22–23, 24–25
  antigens associated with, 22–23,
      24–25, 26, 39, 42, 48, 123,
      137–138
  as carcinogenic agents in animals and
      humans, 24–25
  Epstein-Barr, 24, 26, 123, 137
  herpes, 22–23, 24, 25, 26, 34, 39,
      42, 48, 123, 137
  tumors associated with, 123, 137–138
    breast cancer, 123, 137
    Burkitt's lymphoma, 123, 137
    cervical carcinoma, 22–23, 26, 39,
        42, 48, 123, 137
    head and neck cancer, 123, 137

nasopharyngeal carcinoma, 123,
    137
  vaccines against, 26
Von Recklinghausen's neurofibroma-
    tosis, and cancer risk, 42

Water monitoring, for carcinogenic
    agents, 24
Wilms' tumor
  chemotherapy in, 157, 158
  and transmission of carcinogenic
      influences, 24, 39

Xenylamine exposure, and bladder
    cancer risk, 151
Xeroderma pigmentosum, 40, 42
X-rays, see Radiation exposure

Yugoslavia, cancer incidence in, 225

Zero tolerance principle, for carcino-
    gens in food, 216–218, 220,
    260